Bioinformatics Tools for Pharmaceutical Drug Product Development

Scrivener Publishing
100 Cummings Center, Suite 541J
Beverly, MA 01915-6106

Publishers at Scrivener
Martin Scrivener (martin@scrivenerpublishing.com)
Phillip Carmical (pcarmical@scrivenerpublishing.com)

Bioinformatics Tools for Pharmaceutical Drug Product Development

Edited by

Vivek Chavda

Department of Pharmaceutics and Pharmaceutical Technology, L. M. College of Pharmacy, Ahmedabad, India

Krishnan Anand

Department of Chemical Pathology, School of Pathology, University of the Free State, Bloemfontein, South Africa

and

Vasso Apostolopoulos

Institute for Health and Sport, Immunology and Translational Research Group, Victoria University, Melbourne, Australia

Scrivener Publishing

WILEY

This edition first published 2023 by John Wiley & Sons, Inc., 111 River Street, Hoboken, NJ 07030, USA and Scrivener Publishing LLC, 100 Cummings Center, Suite 541J, Beverly, MA 01915, USA

For more information about Scrivener publications please visit www.scrivenerpublishing.com.

Wiley Global Headquarters
111 River Street, Hoboken, NJ 07030, USA

For details of our global editorial offices, customer services, and more information about Wiley products visit us at www.wiley.com.

Library of Congress Cataloging-in-Publication Data

ISBN 978-1-119-86511-7

Cover image: Pixabay.Com
Cover design by Russell Richardson

Set in size of 11pt and Minion Pro by Manila Typesetting Company, Makati, Philippines

Printed in the USA

Contents

Preface

For a new drug to be developed and brought to market, approximately US$1.8 billion and a minimum of 15 years in development are required. In most instances, only a few drugs make it to market because the process of creating a new drug can fail at different steps along the way, with most of them failing in the final stages of development. Some reasons for this can be attributed to the lack of extensive clinical data, unexpected toxicities and long-term side effects; as well as the highly competitive market, which puts a strain on the development of new drugs. A way to reduce some of the costs and increase the likelihood of success is to maximize the information gained via basic science and the design of better translational approaches and clinical trials. As such, bioinformatics approaches are becoming more essential in drug discovery and vaccine design, not only in academia, but also in the pharmaceutical industry. Bioinformatics involves the use of software tools and computer programming to understand biological data, particularly when the data is large and complex. The development of large data warehouses and algorithms to analyze large data, the identification of biomarkers and novel drug targets, computational biochemistry, genomics, drug discovery and design have all been at the forefront of translational drug discovery in recent years. Bioinformatics has revolutionized disease-based and drug-based approaches as well as improved knowledge of biological targets. It has ushered in a new era of research with the aim to accelerate the design and development of drug and vaccine targets, improve validation approaches as well as facilitate in identifying side effects and predict drug resistance. As such, this will aid in more successful drug candidates from discovery to clinical trials to the market and, most importantly, make it a more cost-effective process overall.

Since there has been much emphasis placed on developing bioinformatics tools for pharmaceutical drug development, this book is a timely and important addition to the evolving field. The 17 chapters are categorized into three sections. The first section presents the latest information on bioinformatics tools, artificial intelligence, machine learning, computational methods, protein interactions, peptide-based drug design and omics technologies. The following two sections include bioinformatics tools for the pharmaceutical and healthcare sectors.

In this book, experts from around the world provide comprehensive overviews of the many important steps involved in—and the critical insights needed for—the successful development of therapeutic drug products with the help of bioinformatics, artificial intelligence and machine learning. The amount of work put into these 17 chapters required significant collaboration and input, and there are many people who are worthy of our thanks. We thank the support of over 20 thought leaders in AI/ML from across the globe who contributed to the chapters. Without their contributions, the book would not have been possible. We offer our sincere gratitude to the Department of Pharmaceutics and Pharmaceutical Technology, L.M. College of Pharmacy, Ahmedabad-Gujarat, India; the Department of Chemical Pathology, School of Pathology, University of the Free State, Bloemfontein campus, Free State, South Africa; and Victoria University, Institute for Health and Sport for their ongoing support in publishing this volume. We also thank Scrivener Publishing and their staff for their editorial support throughout the publication process.

The Editors
Vivek Chavda
K. Anand
Vasso Apostolopoulos
December 2022

Part I

BIOINFORMATICS TOOLS

1

Introduction to Bioinformatics, AI, and ML for Pharmaceuticals

Vivek P. Chavda[1*], Disha Vihol[2], Aayushi Patel[3], Elrashdy M. Redwan[4,5] and Vladimir N. Uversky[6†]

[1]*Department of Pharmaceutics and Pharmaceutical Technology, L. M. College of Pharmacy, Ahmedabad, Gujarat, India*
[2]*Department of Phytopharmacy and Phytomedicine, School of Pharmacy, Gujarat Technological University, Ahmedabad, Gujarat, India*
[3]*Pharmacy Section, L. M. College of Pharmacy, Ahmedabad, Gujarat, India*
[4]*Department of Biological Sciences, Faculty of Sciences, King Abdulaziz University, Jeddah, Saudi Arabia*
[5]*Therapeutic and Protective Proteins Laboratory, Protein Research Department, Genetic Engineering and Biotechnology Research Institute, City of Scientific Research and Technological Applications, New Borg EL-Arab, Alexandria, Egypt*
[6]*Department of Molecular Medicine and Byrd Alzheimer's Research Institute, Morsani College of Medicine, University of South Florida, Tampa, FL, USA*

Abstract
Bioinformatics is a growing field that has emerged in recent years. The use of computational applications for protein sequence analysis in the early 1960s created the groundwork for bioinformatics. Alongside, developments in molecular biology techs evolved DNA analysis, leading to simpler manipulation of DNA, its sequencing, and computer science, suggesting the development of compatible and more powerful computers with innovative software for performing bioinformatics tasks. Biological Big Data collection when analyzed with bioinformatics tools leads to powerful predictive results with repeatability. Due to advancements in the merging of computer science and biology, even subdisciplines like synthetic biology, systems biology, and whole-cell modeling are emerging rapidly.

**Corresponding author*: vivek7chavda@gmail.com
†*Corresponding author*: vuversky@usf.edu: ORCID: https://orcid.org/0000-0002-4037-5857

Vivek Chavda, Krishnan Anand and Vasso Apostolopoulos (eds.) Bioinformatics Tools for Pharmaceutical Drug Product Development, (3–18) © 2023 Scrivener Publishing LLC

Keywords: Bioinformatics, artificial intelligence, machine learning, AI/ML, pharmaceuticals, drug product development

1.1 Introduction

In the context of Artificial Intelligence (AI), Machine Learning (ML), and Big Data, the healthcare industry explores the medication research process, evaluating how emerging technologies can enhance efficacy [1]. Artificial intelligence and machine learning are seen as the way of the future in a variety of fields and sectors, including pharmaceuticals. In a world, where a single authorized medicine costs millions of dollars and requires years of rigorous testing before being licensed, saving money and time is a priority.

Producing new pharmacological compounds to combat any disease is an expensive and time-consuming procedure, yet it goes unchecked. The most important aspect of drug design is to take advantage of the collected data and seek fresh and unique leads. Once the medication target has been determined, numerous multidisciplinary domains collaborate to develop enhanced pharmaceuticals using AI and ML technologies [2]. These technologies are utilized at every phase of the computer-aided drug discovery process, and combining them results in a proven track record of success in finding hit molecules. Furthermore, the fusion of AI and ML with high-dimension data enhanced the capabilities of computer-aided drug discovery and design [3]. Clinical trial output prediction using AI/ML integrated models might decrease the costs of the clinical trial, while simultaneously increasing their success rates. In this study, we will be covering the potential of AI and ML technologies in enabling computer-aided drug creation, along with challenges and opportunities for the pharmaceutical sector.

1.2 Bioinformatics

When biological data along with genetic information is analyzed using computer technology for calculating and obtaining mathematically and statistically approved results, is called Bioinformatics. The computational means are utilized for addressing data-intensive, large-scale biological challenges [4]. It includes the development and application of databases, algorithms, computational and statistical tools, and theory to tackle formal and practical issues emerging from biological data administration and analysis [5, 6].

Bioinformatics allows rapid molecular modeling of biological processes from the collected big data for obtaining meaningful conclusions through various stages such as compilation of the statistical information from biological data, creation of a computational model, the resolution of computational modeling issues, and the assessment of the resulting computational algorithm [7]. Genomics and proteomics are the branches of bioinformatics that aim at understanding the organizing principles encoded inside the nucleic acid and protein sequences, respectively. Image and signal processing enables usable conclusions to be extracted from vast volumes of raw data [5]. It helps in decoding genetics by facilitating text mining of biological literature, comparing, analyzing, and interpreting genetic, genomic, and proteomic data, assessing gene and protein expression, detecting mutations, sequencing and annotating genomes, and interpreting evolutionary aspects with disease pathways [8, 9]. Moreover, it helps to simulate and model DNA, RNA, proteins, and biomolecular interactions in structural biology. All of these can be achieved by correlating the biological data for understanding the effect of the diseased condition on the body's normal cellular functions [10]. Hence, bioinformatics has progressed now to the point, where analysis and interpretation of diverse forms of data is the most important challenge.

Omics technologies offer a chance to investigate changes in DNA, RNA, proteins, and other biological components across intraspecies and interspecies. The analysis of these components is interesting from a toxicity assessment view as they can alter in response to chemical or drug exposure in cells or tissues. Genomic research, which generates enormous amounts of data, is one area, where bioinformatics is very valuable. Bioinformatics aids in the interpretation of data, which may then be used to provide a diagnosis for a patient suffering from a rare ailment, track and monitor infectious organisms as they spread across a community, or determine the best therapy for a cancer patient [11]. Genomics sequences assemble and analyze the structure and function of genomes using recombinant DNA, DNA sequencing technologies, and bioinformatics. Various software used in bioinformatics includes accessibility of protein surface and secondary structure predictions using NetSurfP, prediction of beta-turn sites in protein sequences using NetTurnP, and AutoDock for Automated Docking Tool Suite [4].

Rapid advances in genomics and other molecular research tools, along with advances in information technology, have resulted in a massive volume of molecular biology knowledge during the last few decades [12]. Bioinformatics will continue to advance as a result of the integration of many technologies and techniques that bring together professionals from

Table 1.1 Various bioinformatics and AI-driven tools applied in the pharmacy department and industry.

Computational tools	Application	Reference
BLAST	The Basic Local Alignment Search Tool (BLAST) is used for searching local similarity regions between sequences and compares to the available database for calculating the statistical significance of matches. The matching infers functional and evolutionary relationships between sequences and identifies genetically related families.	[15]
ChEMBL	ChEMBL is designed manually to maintain a database of bioactive molecules. It correlates genomic data with chemical structure and bioactivity for the development of new drugs.	[16]
geWorkbench	The genomics Workbench (geWorkbench) comprises the tools for performing management, analysis, visualization, and annotation of biomedical data. It supports data for microarray gene expression, DNA and Protein Sequences, pathways, Molecular structure – prediction, Sequence Patterns, Gene Ontology, and Regulatory Networks	[11]
GROMACS	It is software for high-performance molecular dynamics and output analysis, especially for proteins and lipids.	[7]
IGV	Integrative Genomics Viewer (IGV) is a high-performance, user-friendly, interactive tool for the visualization and exploration of genomic data.	[17]
MODELLER	A protein three-dimensional structural homology or comparative modeling tool.	[18]
SwissDrugDesign	SwissDrugDesign provides a collection of tools required for Computer-Aided Drug Design (CADD).	[19]

(*Continued*)

Table 1.1 Various bioinformatics and AI-driven tools applied in the pharmacy department and industry. (*Continued*)

Computational tools	Application	Reference
UCSF Chimera	UCSF Chimera is an interactive tool for the visualization and analysis of molecular structures.	[20]
AlphaFold	It is an AI system developed to computationally predict protein structures with unprecedented accuracy and speed.	[21]
Cyclica	The ML tool address challenges faced across the drug discovery life cycle by correlating biophysics, medicinal chemistry, and systems biology.	[21]
DeepChem	It is a deep learning framework for drug discovery.	[18]
DeltaVina	Gives docking scores for protein-ligand binding affinity	[17]
Exscientia	The AI engineers precision medicines more rapidly and efficiently by accelerating pre-clinical drug discovery phases through monitoring and analysis of drug design and experiments.	[13]
Hit Dexter	It estimates how likely a small molecule is to trigger a positive response in biochemical and biological assays.	[4]
ORGANIC	Objective-Reinforced Generative Adversarial Network for Inverse-design Chemistry (ORGANIC) is a tool for creating molecules with desired properties.	[8]
Somatix	It is a real-time gesture detection technology that enables passive data collection of indoor and outdoor patients for enhancing medication adherence rates, data reliability, and cost-effectiveness.	[22]

other domains to build cutting-edge computational and informational tools tailored to the biomedical research business [4, 9]. Table 1.1. represents various bioinformatics and AI-driven tools, which can be applied in the pharmacy department and industry.

1.2.1 Limitations of Bioinformatics

In the case of drug discovery by applying *in silico* approaches, prediction of ligand affinity and inhibitory activity, where adequate training data are available is possible at certain levels but search for the mechanism-based inhibitors remains a highly challenging task. In structure-based approaches to various binding affinities, free energy calculations without extensive data collection at times leads to adequate results but high chances of false-positive rates remain a limiting factor. While chemical structure mining, the bioinformatics tools are efficiently able to produce a large number of metabolites but it is by no means possible to find ways of ranking metabolites accurately. Prediction of metabolic rates is generally not possible with bioinformatics tools. The *in vivo* predictions by applying bioinformatics for assessing biological activity and toxicological effects detect most toxicophores but the prediction of time-dependent inhibitors remains a difficult task [13].

Furthermore, it requires a sophisticated laboratory for the in-depth study and collection of biomolecules, and the establishment of such laboratories requires significant funds. The system operation is a complex mechanism so specially trained individuals are required for handling computer-based biological data. Uninterrupted electricity supply for biological investigations using computational applications is the basic requirement, abrupt interruption can lose huge data from the system memory. The system must also be virus-protected, which, if not controlled, can lead to the deletion of data and corruption of the programs [14].

1.2.2 Artificial Intelligence (AI)

Artificial intelligence (AI) is a branch of computer science that unlike natural intelligence is demonstrated by machines or computers and is defined as a system that analyzes its environment and performs a series of actions to achieve goals similar to a human-being process. The objectives of AI include gathering information, establishing rules on usage of the information, reasoning, data representation, organizing, planning, learning, problem-solving, processing, and the ability to manipulate data or self-correction [9, 21].

In the pharmaceutical industry, AI plays role in providing technologies for drug discovery, such as drug target identification, optimization, designing, formulation development, manufacturing, break-down R&D costs, analyzing biomedicine information for recruiting suitable patients for clinical trials, drug repurposing, diagnostic tools and assistance, and optimizing medical treatment processes [23]. Moreover, AI optimizes innovation, enhances the efficiency of research by data management, and creates computational tools for researchers, physicians, and regulators with minimizing human intervention and errors [24]. Generally, two main classes of AI technology developments are incorporated in the case of drug discovery. The first component comprises computing methodologies including systems simulating human experiences along with outputs. The second one consists of models mimicking Artificial Neural Networks (ANNs) for real-time data correlation with the management of AI technology evolution [25].

Various *in silico* models predict pharmacokinetics and simulate molecular docking of the drugs to ease down drug discovery phases along with predictions of *in vitro* and *in vivo* responses [26, 27]. AI in drug development includes predictions of probable synthetic pathways for drug-like molecules, pharmacokinetic and dynamic properties, protein identification and characterization, bioactivity, drug-target, and drug-drug interactions [18, 28, 29]. Moreover, AI incorporates various omics for identifying new disease pathways with targets using novel biomarkers and therapeutic targets [30]. In the case of clinical trials, AI improves candidate selection criteria by identifying the best patients with human-relevant biomarkers of disease and gene targets for the study and ensuring the most suitable trial results. It also helps in removing the trail hindering elements and reduces the time for conducting large database analysis [24]. An example of such an AI platform is AiCure, a mobile application subjected to phase 2 clinical trial patients with schizophrenia for assessing improvement in patient medication adherence [31]. The AI-driven PAT (Process analytical technology) proves to be a necessary tool in terms of quality control and assurance while manufacturing. Improvements can be observed in product yield, utilization, and cost-saving with less waste generation [32]. To assess real-time manufacturing aspects, the Manufacturing Execution System (MES) is utilized. It complies with regulatory guidelines and ensures high-quality product development through risk management, shortened production cycles, optimized resource use, and controlled batch release [33]. Then the Automatic Process Control System (APCS) is used for ensuring a safe and profitable process by monitoring and optimizing process variables like concentration, flow, pressure, temperature, and vacuum [34].

Furthermore, AI can be utilized in drug repurposing, where a drug gets qualified to enter Phase II trials for different use without going through Phase I clinical trials and toxicology testing which reduces costing and time of the trials [35]. Not only AI can be used for drug discovery, but it can also be used in polypharmacology, the 'one-disease–multiple targets theory. Databases such as BindingDB, ChEMBL, DrugBank, Ligand Expo, PubChem, PDB, and ZINC are available for information on binding affinities, biological activities, chemical properties, crystal structures, drug targets, and pathways [36].

The digitalization of health and medicine has created an opportunity for AI in hospital pharmacies for performing tasks, such as maintaining electronic medical records and patients' medication history, designing treatment approaches and dosage forms, medication safety, drug interactions, ADME consultations, and providing healthcare aid to patients. This way AI agrees with share-risk agreements and decision-making in Pharmacy and Therapeutics Committees [37, 38]. Electronic health records (EHR) are collected routinely and can be classified into structured and unstructured data. Structured data refers to the collection of data in an organized manner with standard units and ranges (e.g., vital signs), unlike unstructured data with unclear management (e.g., imaging results) [39]. This data is collected by AI in real-time for analyzing clinical data management and practice which can give insights into novel drug discovery, pharmacovigilance, drug-associated adverse events, patient medication adherence, and prescription errors [40]. With the information of EHR, various patient-omics data (i.e., genomics, microbiomics, proteomics) can be integrated for the creation of the Electronic Medical Records and Genomics (eMERGE) network which helps in identifying unknown diseases with associations to the gene bank obtained [41]. AI can also predict an epidemic outbreak. Even predictions of shipment times of therapeutics can be carried out efficiently by incorporating AI tools in the case of e-pharmacy. Moreover, AI can be used as a diagnostic tool for disease analysis and status by grading system with reproducibility. It improves the accuracy of the treatment decisions and predicts prognosis. Even data can be collected from uncooperative patients [42].

Advantages of AI include providing real-time data management, error minimization and producing efficient output, multitasking, patient data management, adverse effects or side effects data collection, medication designing with disease correlation, streamlining tasks, inventory management, and assisting research in the development of drug delivery formulations. Nevertheless, disadvantages are also a part of the AI and they are the need for human surveillance, expensive building and launching of AI tools, chances of false report generation, lack of data collection and method standardization, may overlook social variables, raises unemployment, no creativity, the risk of data leakage and mass-scale destruction, and acceptance within the healthcare sector [37, 43].

1.3 Machine Learning (ML)

Machine learning (ML) is a subclass of AI, where algorithms process big data to detect patterns, learn from them, and solve problems statistically and autonomously. ML is categorized into supervised, unsupervised, and reinforcement learning. Supervised learning includes the application of regression and classification methods which forms a predictive model upon data insertion from input and output sources. The predictive models can be disease diagnosis or drug efficacy and ADMET predictions [44]. In unsupervised mode, solely input data are utilized and interpreted using clustering and feature-finding methods. The output comprises discovering a disease with its probable targets [45, 46]. Lastly, reinforcement learning depends majorly on decision-making in the applied or specific environment with maximum performance ability. By applying modeling and quantum chemistry, outputs such as de novo drug design can be executed with this learning mode [47].

ML includes a subdivision consisting of Deep Learning (DL), which engages Artificial Neural Networks (ANNs) for adapting and learning the experimental data. These networks are similar to human biological neurons responsible for electrical impulses transmission in the brain, which allows real-time data collection and interpretation [48]. This big data in association with algorithm application can help in discovering new drugs with more potency and can improve the personalized medicine sector based on genetic markers [47].

Machine learning in healthcare performs multiple tasks, such as classification, recommendations, clustering and correlation of cases, prediction, anomaly detection, automation, and ranking of information [49]. The disease progression and development mechanism within a body is a complex system that cannot be understood by simple data collection. Usually, real-time data collection and compilation are carried out by high throughput approaches such as the usage of the pre-defined set of machine learning applications. This software not only provides diagnostic approaches but also helps in identifying hypothetical therapeutics for drug development. The benefits of incorporating machine learning are infinite availability of data storage and high flexibility in its management. Various data sets include assay information, biometrics, images, omics data, textual information, and data collected from wearables [50, 51]. Various ML applications such as Python, Spark, MLLib, and Jupyter notebooks have been utilized by pharma industries for data mining and predictive intelligence for solving daily tasks along with moderately tedious challenges [52].

1.3.1 Applications of ML

a) Research and development of new drug:

ML utilizes a feedback-driven drug development process by interpreting existing results from sources, such as computational modeling data, literature surveys, and high-throughput screening. This process helps in identifying lead compounds with efficiency and reduced randomness, errors, and time-lapse. In the approach such as de novo design, inputs require a compound library gained through *in silico* methods and virtual screening applications which mimic bioactivity and toxicity models [53]. The drug discovery can be carried out by following a series of steps starting from the identification of novel bioactive compounds through docking studies and molecular dynamics. A hit compound can be found while screening chemical libraries, computer simulation, or screening naturally isolated materials, such as plants, bacteria, and fungi. Then the recognized hits are screened in cell-based assays consisting of animal models of disease to assess efficacy and safety. Once the activity of the lead molecule is confirmed, chemical modifications can be carried out in search of a novel compound consisting of maximal therapeutic benefits with minimal harm [54, 55]. Hence, incorporating algorithm datasets in conjugation with chemical structures and targets is utilized for the optimization of new leads and is preferable to the laborious target-specific lead identification for the R&D sector of a pharma company.

b) Claims Databases for finding patients:

The Claims Database includes the use of applications such as APLD (Anonymized Patient-Level Data) and Truven Marketscan for identifying patients exhibiting characteristic symptoms correlating to the diagnosis code available in the software, with this, an undiagnosed case can also be identified. This approach can be utilized for finding orphan diseases, which are often left undiagnosed. By applying ML, early disease progression can be identified, and pharma companies can utilize this information for creating orphan drugs which are usually very expensive per patient revenue compared to the cost allotted for drug discovery. Some examples of ML-based approaches for identifying rare diseases are CART (Classification and Regression Tree) models such as C5, standard decision trees, and random forests.

c) Patient medical history and treatment pathways:

A patient medical history reveals the journey through various treatment and therapy approaches which can be further utilized to identify disease

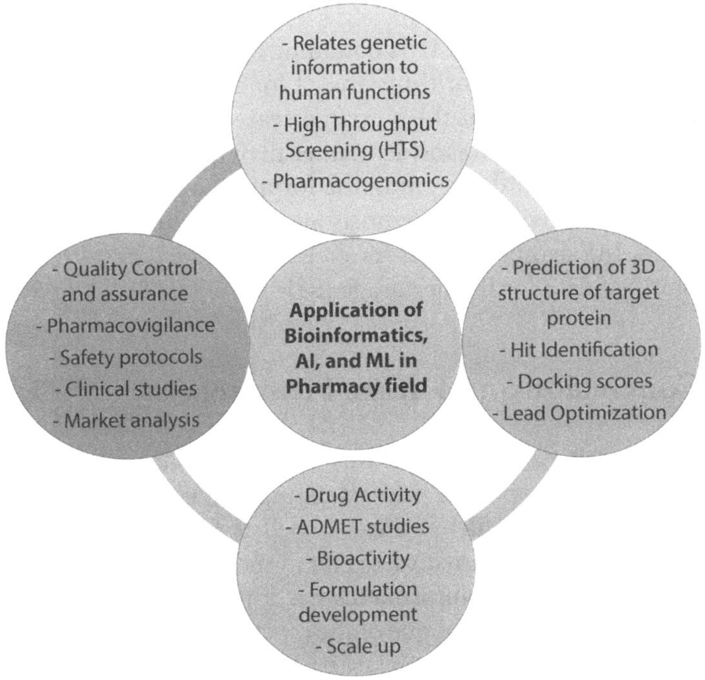

Figure 1.1 Applications of bioinformatics, AI, and ML in the pharmacy sector.

pathways and dosage regimens [52]. In this sector, machine learning is utilized as means of avoiding data clustering from scoring models by creating a time series data correlated with treatment pathways for faster processing and improved efficiency, by incorporating database tools like kdb+, and Tensorflow.

d) Enhancing Commercial market survey:
Physical methods as means of surveying physicians' drug prescribing patterns is often a tedious task for marketing individuals in the pharma sector. These surveys are usually conducted for identifying dosage trends that can be further utilized for new drug developments [52]. ML models, such as Associative Rules Mining or "apriori", make the laborious task easier by providing quantitative variables related to Rx records, which can then be applied for large data assessment. Figure 1.1 summarizes some of the applications of bioinformatics, AI, and ML in the pharmacy sector.

1.3.2 Limitations of ML

The major issue while using ML is obtaining accurate diagnostic values. In ML, a predefined set of algorithms are set for a particular disease but it is not generally quantitative as the human diseased state is due to innumerable complex pathways going inside. Rather than quantitative assessment in identifying a disease and designing the formulation for them, experience and expertise are needed for diagnosis and dose requirement calculation. Nevertheless, ML can be utilized for creating a huge dataset that can give fairly quantified data for further usage [52].

1.4 Conclusion and Future Prospects

It is determined that a summary of this interdisciplinary subject is formed by producing a unique precise understanding that is provided by the reaction of biology and computer science, as well as certain evaluation aspects such as statistics and mathematics, to end in the recently hatched field after this powerful reaction. Bioinformatics has a promising outlook in many biological and living fields, but one of the most critical difficulties that must be addressed is the integration of a large and diverse set of data sources and databases for the improvement of life and a massive biological change.

References

1. Quazi, S., *Role of Artificial Intelligence and Machine Learning in Bioinformatics: Drug Discovery and Drug Repurposing*, 2021. https://www.preprints.org/manuscript/202105.0346/v1
2. Selvaraj, C., Chandra, I., Singh, S.K., Artificial intelligence and machine learning approaches for drug design: Challenges and opportunities for the pharmaceutical industries. *Mol. Divers.*, 3, 1893–1913, 2021.
3. Henstock, P.V., Artificial intelligence for pharma: Time for internal investment. *Trends Pharmacol. Sci.*, 40, 8, 543–546, 2019.
4. Chen, C., Hou, J., Tanner, J.J., Cheng, J., Bioinformatics methods for mass spectrometry-based proteomics data analysis. *Int. J. Mol. Sci.*, 21, 8, 2873, 2020.
5. Can, T., Introduction to bioinformatics. *Methods Mol. Biol.*, 1107, 51–71, 2014.
6. Najarian, K., Deriche, R., Kon, M.A., Hirata, N.S.T., Bioinformatics and biomedical informatics. *Sci. World J.*, 2013, 591976, 2013.
7. Chakraborty, C., Doss, C.G.P., Zhu, H., Agoramoorthy, G., Rising strengths Hong Kong SAR in bioinformatics. *Interdiscip. Sci.*, 9, 2, 224–236, 2017.
8. Pallen, M.J., Microbial bioinformatics 2020. *Microb. Biotechnol.*, 9, 5, 681–686, 2016.
9. Wooller, S.K., Benstead-Hume, G., Chen, X., Ali, Y., Pearl, F.M.G., Bioinformatics in translational drug discovery. *Biosci. Rep.*, 37, 4, BSR20160180, 2017.
10. Pop, M. and Salzberg, S.L., Bioinformatics challenges of new sequencing technology. *Trends Genet.*, 24, 3, 142–149, 2008.
11. Tillett, R.L., Sevinsky, J.R., Hartley, P.D. *et al.*, Genomic evidence for reinfection with SARS-CoV-2: A case study. *Lancet Infect. Dis.*, 21, 1, 52–58, 2021.
12. Rothberg, J., Merriman, B., Higgs, G., Bioinformatics. Introduction. *Yale J. Biol. Med.*, 85, 3, 305–308, 2012.
13. Mbah, C.J. and Okorie, N.H., Pharmaceutical bioinformatics: Its relevance to drug metabolism. *Madridge J. Bioinform. Syst. Biol.*, 1, 1, 19–26, 2019. [Internet] Available from: https://madridge.org/journal-of-bioinformatics-and-systems-biology/mjbsb-1000104.php.
14. Bayat, A., Science, medicine, and the future: Bioinformatics. *BMJ*, 324, 7344, 1018–1022, 2002.
15. Altschul, S.F., Gish, W., Miller, W., Myers, E.W., Lipman, D.J., Basic local alignment search tool. *J. Mol. Biol.*, 215, 3, 403-410, 1990.
16. Davies, M., Nowotka, M., Papadatos, G. *et al.*, ChEMBL web services: Streamlining access to drug discovery data and utilities. *Nucleic Acids Res.*, 43, W1, W612–W620, 2015. [Internet] Available from: https://www.ebi.ac.uk/chembl/.

17. Thorvaldsdottir, H., Robinson, J.T., Mesirov, J.P., Integrative genomics viewer (IGV): High-performance genomics data visualization and exploration. *Brief. Bioinform.*, 14, 2, 178–192, 2013. [Internet] Available from: https://academic.oup.com/bib/article-lookup/doi/10.1093/bib/bbs017.
18. Nascimento, A.C.A., Prudêncio, R.B.C., Costa, I.G., A multiple kernel learning algorithm for drug-target interaction prediction. *BMC Bioinf.*, 17, 1, 46, 2016. [Internet] Available from: http://www.biomedcentral.com/1471-2105/17/46.
19. Daina, A. and Zoete, V., Application of the SwissDrugDesign online resources in virtual screening. *Int. J. Mol. Sci.*, 20, 18, 4612, 2019.
20. UCSF Chimera. [Internet] Available from: https://www.rbvi.ucsf.edu/chimera/.
21. Jumper, J., Evans, R., Pritzel, A. *et al.*, Highly accurate protein structure prediction with AlphaFold. *Nature*, 596, 7873, 583–589, 2021. [Internet] Available from: https://www.nature.com/articles/s41586-021-03819-2.
22. Snijder, E.J., Decroly, E., Ziebuhr, J., The nonstructural proteins directing coronavirus RNA synthesis and processing. *Adv. Virus Res.*, 96, 59–126, 2016.
23. Mamoshina, P., Vieira, A., Putin, E., Zhavoronkov, A., Applications of deep learning in biomedicine. *Mol. Pharm.*, 13, 5, 1445–1454, 2016. [Internet] Available from: https://pubs.acs.org/doi/10.1021/acs.molpharmaceut.5b00982.
24. Schneider, P., Walters, W.P., Plowright, A.T., Sieroka, N., Listgarten, J., Goodnow, R.A. Jr, Fisher, J., Jansen, J.M., Duca, J.S., Rush, T.S., Zentgraf, M., Hill, J.E., Krutoholow, E., Kohler, M., Blaney, J., Funatsu, K., Luebkemann, C., Schneider, G., Rethinking drug design in the artificial intelligence era. *Nat. Rev. Drug Discov.*, 19, 5, 353–364, 2020.
25. Agatonovic-Kustrin, S. and Beresford, R., Basic concepts of artificial neural network (ANN) modeling and its application in pharmaceutical research. *J. Pharm. Biomed. Anal.*, 22, 5, 717–727, 2000.
26. Sakiyama, Y., The use of machine learning and nonlinear statistical tools for ADME prediction. *Expert Opin. Drug Metab. Toxicol.*, 5, 2, 149–169, 2009.
27. Gobburu, J.V.S. and Chen, E.P., Artificial neural networks as a novel approach to integrated pharmacokinetic—Pharmacodynamic analysis. *J. Pharm. Sci.*, 85, 5, 505–510, 1996.
28. Merk, D., Friedrich, L., Grisoni, F., Schneider, G., De novo design of bioactive small molecules by artificial intelligence. *Mol. Inform.*, 37, 1–2, 1700153, 2018. [Internet] Available from: https://onlinelibrary.wiley.com/doi/10.1002/minf.201700153.
29. Klopman, G., Chakravarti, S.K., Zhu, H., Ivanov, J.M., Saiakhov, R.D., ESP: A method to predict toxicity and pharmacological properties of chemicals using multiple MCASE databases. *J. Chem. Inf. Comput. Sci.*, 44, 2, 704–715, 2004. [Internet] Available from: https://pubs.acs.org/doi/10.1021/ci030298n.

30. Hamet, P. and Tremblay, J., Artificial intelligence in medicine. *Metabolism*, 69, S36–S40, 2017. [Internet] Available from: https://linkinghub.elsevier.com/retrieve/pii/S002604951730015X.
31. Bain, E.E., Shafner, L., Walling, D.P. *et al.*, Use of a novel artificial intelligence platform on mobile devices to assess dosing compliance in a phase 2 clinical trial in subjects with schizophrenia. *JMIR mHealth uHealth*, 5, 2, e18, 2017. [Internet] Available from: http://mhealth.jmir.org/2017/2/e18/.
32. Sharma, T., Mankoo, A., Sood, V., Artificial intelligence in advanced pharmacy. *Int. J. Sci. Res. Arch.*, 2, 1, 047–054, 2021. [Internet] Available from: https://ijsra.net/content/artificial-intelligence-advanced-pharmacy.
33. Mundy, L., Trowman, R., Kearney, B., Improving access to high-cost technologies in the Asia region. *Int. J. Technol. Assess. Health Care*, 35, 3, 168–175, 2019.
34. Technologies, O., Automatic process control control (APCS). Access date 03/05/2022; https://rivs.ru/en/asu_tp#:~:text=Automated%20process%20control%20system%20(APCS,mathematical%20support%20and%20operational%20personnel.
35. Corsello, S.M., Bittker, J.A., Liu, Z. *et al.*, The drug repurposing hub: A next-generation drug library and information resource. *Nat. Med.*, 23, 4, 405–408, 2017. [Internet] Available from: http://www.nature.com/articles/nm.4306.
36. Mak, K.-K. and Pichika, M.R., Artificial intelligence in drug development: Present status and future prospects. *Drug Discovery Today*, 24, 3, 773–780, 2019. [Internet] Available from: https://linkinghub.elsevier.com/retrieve/pii/S1359644618300916.
37. Das, S., Dey, R., Nayak, A.K., Artificial intelligence in pharmacy. *Indian J. Pharm. Educ. Res.*, 55, 2, 304–318, 2021.
38. Del Rio-Bermudez, C., Medrano, I.H., Yebes, L., Poveda, J.L., Towards a symbiotic relationship between big data, artificial intelligence, and hospital pharmacy. *J. Pharm. Policy Pract.*, 13, 1, 75, 2020.
39. Weber, G.M., Mandl, K.D., Kohane, I.S., Finding the missing link for big biomedical data. *JAMA*, 24, 2479–2480, 2014.
40. Luo, Y., Thompson, W.K., Herr, T.M. *et al.*, Natural language processing for EHR-based pharmacovigilance: A structured review. *Drug Saf.*, 40, 11, 1075–1089, 2017.
41. Gottesman, O., Kuivaniemi, H., Tromp, G. *et al.*, The electronic medical records and genomics (eMERGE) network: Past, present, and future. *Genet. Med.*, 15, 10, 761–771, 2013.
42. Abdullah, Y.I., Schuman, J.S., Shabsigh, R., Caplan, A., Al-Aswad, L.A., Ethics of artificial intelligence in medicine and ophthalmology. *Asia-Pac. J. Ophthalmol.*, 10, 3, 289–298, 2021.
43. Trenfield, S.J., Awad, A., McCoubrey, L.E. *et al.*, Advancing pharmacy and healthcare with virtual digital technologies. *Adv. Drug Deliv. Rev.*, 182, 114098, 2022.

44. Gunčar, G., Kukar, M., Notar, M. *et al.*, An application of machine learning to haematological diagnosis. *Sci. Rep.*, 8, 1, 411, 2018. [Internet] Available from: http://www.nature.com/articles/s41598-017-18564-8.
45. Koohy, H., The rise and fall of machine learning methods in biomedical research. *F1000Res.*, 6, 2012, 2018. [Internet] Available from: https://f1000research.com/articles/6-2012/v2.
46. Young, J.D., Cai, C., Lu, X., Unsupervised deep learning reveals prognostically relevant subtypes of glioblastoma. *BMC Bioinf.*, 18, S11, 381, 2017. [Internet] Available from: http://bmcbioinformatics.biomedcentral.com/articles/10.1186/s12859-017-1798-2.
47. Chen, H., Engkvist, O., Wang, Y., Olivecrona, M., Blaschke, T., The rise of deep learning in drug discovery. *Drug Discovery Today*, 23, 6, 1241–1250, 2018. [Internet] Available from: https://linkinghub.elsevier.com/retrieve/pii/S1359644617303598.
48. Beneke, F. and Mackenrodt, M.-O., Artificial intelligence and collusion. *IIC-Int. Rev. Intellect. Prop. Compet. Law*, 50, 1, 109–134, 2019. [Internet] Available from: http://link.springer.com/10.1007/s40319-018-00773-x.
49. Tkachenko, N., Machine learning in healthcare: 12 real-world use cases to know, in *IEEE Access*, 2021. [Internet] Available from: https://nix-united.com/blog/machine-learning-in-healthcare-12-real-world-use-cases-to-know/; Bharadwaj, H.K. *et al.*, A review on the role of machine learning in enabling IoT based healthcare applications. *IEEE Access*, 9, 38859–38890, 2021.
50. Vamathevan, J., Clark, D., Czodrowski, P. *et al.*, Applications of machine learning in drug discovery and development. *Nat. Rev. Drug Discovery*, 18, 6, 463–477, 2019.
51. Mamoshina, P., Volosnikova, M., Ozerov, I.V. *et al.*, Machine learning on human muscle transcriptomic data for biomarker discovery and tissue-specific drug target identification. *Front. Genet.*, 242, 9, 2018.
52. Dasgupta, N., Real-world use cases for AI & ML in pharma. Access date 03/05/2022; https://www.rxdatascience.com/blog/top-use-cases-for-machine-learning-in-pharma
53. Yuan, Y., Pei, J., Lai, L., Ligbuilder 2: A practical *de novo* drug design approach. *J. Chem. Inf. Model.*, 51, 5, 1083–1091, 2011. [Internet] Available from: https://pubs.acs.org/doi/10.1021/ci100350u.
54. Zhu, T., Cao, S., Su, P.-C. *et al.*, Hit identification and optimization in virtual screening: Practical recommendations based on a critical literature analysis. *J. Med. Chem.*, 56, 17, 6560–6572, 2013. [Internet] Available from: https://pubs.acs.org/doi/10.1021/jm301916b.
55. Anderson, A.C., Structure-based functional design of drugs: From target to lead compound. *Methods Mol. Biol.*, 2012, 359–366, 2012. [Internet] Available from: http://link.springer.com/10.1007/978-1-60327-216-2_23.

2

Artificial Intelligence and Machine Learning-Based New Drug Discovery Process with Molecular Modelling

Isha Rani[1], Kavita Munjal[2], Rajeev K. Singla[3,4] and Rupesh K. Gautam[5]*

[1]Spurthy College of Pharmacy, Marasur Gate, Bengaluru, Karnataka, India
[2]MM College of Pharmacy, MM (Deemed to be) University-Mullana, Ambala, Haryana, India
[3]Institutes for Systems Genetics, Frontiers Science Center for Disease-Related Molecular Network, West China Hospital, Sichuan University, Chengdu, China
[4]iGlobal Research and Publishing Foundation, New Delhi, India
[5]Department of Pharmacology, Indore Institute of Pharmacy, IIST Campus, Rau, Indore (M.P.), India

Abstract

Drug development is a time-consuming, expensive and extremely risky procedure. Up to 90% of drug concepts are discarded due to challenges such as safety, efficacy and toxicity resulting in significant losses for the investor. The use of artificial intelligence (AI), namely machine learning and deep learning algorithms, to improve the drug discovery process is one technique that has arisen in recent years. AI has been effectively used in drug discovery and design. This chapter includes these machine learning approaches in depth, as well as their applications in medicinal chemistry. The current state-of-the-art of AI supported pharmaceutical discovery is discussed, including applications in structure and ligand-based virtual screening, *de novo* drug design, drug repurposing, and factors related, after introducing the basic principles, along with some application notes, of the various machine learning algorithms. Finally, obstacles and limits are outlined, with an eye towards possible future avenues for AI-supported drug discovery and design.

Keywords: Artificial intelligence, drug development, drug discovery, lead optimization, molecular modelling, virtual screening, *de novo* drug design, drug repurposing

**Corresponding author*: drrupeshgautam@gmail.com

Vivek Chavda, Krishnan Anand and Vasso Apostolopoulos (eds.) Bioinformatics Tools for Pharmaceutical Drug Product Development, (19–36) © 2023 Scrivener Publishing LLC

Abbreviations

AI	Artificial intelligence
RNA	Ribonucleic acid
R & D	Research and develoment
ML	Machine Learning
SBVS	Structure-based virtual screening
VS	Virtual screening
CADD	Computer aided drug design
PDB	Protein data bank
SAS	Synthetic accessibility score

2.1 Introduction

The development of pharmaceutical drugs is a time-consuming and costly process. Pharmaceutical and biotechnology companies often spend over $1 billion to develop a drug to the market, and can take anywhere from 10 to 20 years. This process is extremely risky with up to 90% of new drug concepts are discarded due to difficulties such as safety and efficacy, resulting in significant loss for the investor [1, 2]. Traditional drug discovery methods are target-driven, in which a known target is used to screen for small molecules that either interact with it or affect its function in cells. These approaches work well for easily druggable targets with well-defined structures and well-understood cellular interactions. However, due to the complex nature of cellular interactions and limited knowledge of intricacies, these methods are severely limited [1, 3].

The term "artificial intelligence" (AI) refers to intelligence displayed by computers. When a computer exhibits cognitive behavior similar to that of humans, such as learning or problem solving, this term is employed [4]. AI makes use of systems and software that can read and learn from data in order to make independent judgments in order to achieve certain goals. Machine learning, for example, is a well-established technology for learning and predicting novel features [5]. By finding novel relationships and inferring the functional importance of distinct components of a biological pathway, AI can overcome these obstacles. Complex algorithms and machine learning are employed by AI to extract useful information from enormous datasets. As such, a dataset of RNA sequencing can be used to discover genes whose expression correlates with a specific biological situation. AI can also be used to discover compounds that could bind to 'undruggable targets,' or proteins with unknown structures. A predicted collection of compounds may be easily identified in a relatively short length of time by iterative simulations of different compounds' interactions with tiny portions of a protein [6]. Companies that are commercializing AI drug discovery platforms and AI-discovered pharmaceuticals have demonstrated that using algorithms can reduce the multi-year process down to a few months [7]. This large reduction in development time, as well as the quantity of compounds that must be manufactured for laboratory testing provides for significant cost savings, addressing two key challenges in pharmaceutical R&D. The drug development process covers mainly virtual screening, *de novo* drug design, lead optimization (predicting and optimizing compound properties), planning chemical synthesis, pre-clinical testing, translation to human clinical trials, as well as manufacturing processes, scale up etc. All of these procedures add to the difficulty of identifying effective drugs to treat an illness. As a result, the most important concern facing pharmaceutical businesses is how to manage the process's cost and pace [8–10].

All of these issues need to be answered in a simple and scientific manner, reducing the time and expense of the procedure. Furthermore, the rise in data digitization in the pharmaceutical and healthcare industries stimulates the use of AI to solve the issues of analyzing complicated data [11, 12]. This chapter will comprise the role of AI in drug discovery with respect to virtual screening (VS), *de novo* design, synthesis planning, quality control and quality assurance etc. Various AI applications in drug design and discovery, including primary and secondary screening, drug toxicity, drug pharmacokinetics, medication dose efficacy, drug repositioning, polypharmacology, and drug-target interactions etc. all of which are presented herein.

2.2 Artificial Intelligence in Drug Discovery

The drug industry has seen a significant surge in knowledge digitization in recent years. Using an AI algorithm in drug development is a step-by-step procedure that begins with an identification of the problem [13]. This method includes processes such as problem recognition, AI architecture design, analysis of data, model assessment and evaluation, and understanding and presenting the data. To be more particular, prior to making any specific design decisions, one must have a thorough understanding of the problem (step 1). With the goal of AI programming in sight, the next stage is to create a model architecture that is suitable for this project (step 2). This stage entails selecting an appropriate algorithm and determining appropriate set of parameters initial values. Once settling on a tentative design, data is collected (step 3 in Figure 2.1). The quality, amount, and generalizability

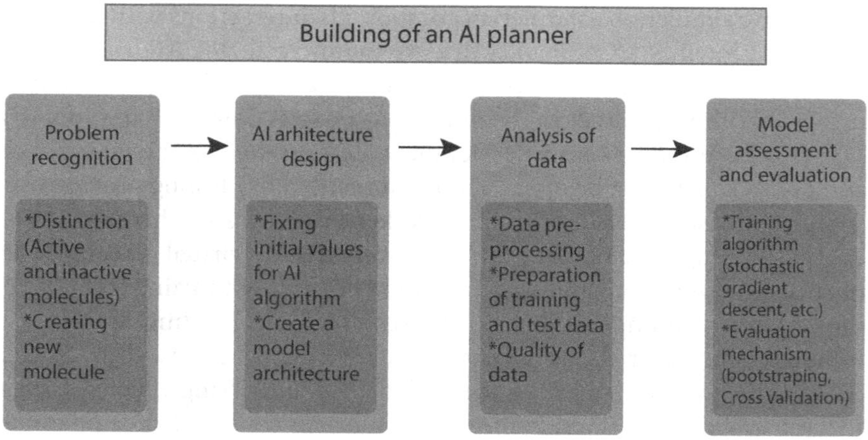

Figure 2.1 The process of constructing an AI planner in general.

of initial data have a significant effect on the performance of an AI system. After the basic architecture and data repositories have been developed, learning algorithm and validation begins (step 4). The goal of the training process is to determine a set of conditions that will limit the forecast error. The completed AI model is expected to articulate the underlying relationship among both molecular descriptions and professional goals [14].

2.2.1 Training Dataset Used in Medicinal Chemistry

A constant input string is the most commonly utilized input data format in drug development (e.g. bitstrings, real-valued digits vector) [15]. Many AI-assisted drug development tools produce numerical values as output

Table 2.1 Input and output data patterns for the development of AI algorithms in drug discovery.

Data format	
Input X	• Subsequent data (e.g. SMILES String, data from time period) • Structure of macromolecules structures, crystal structure of molecules, retrieving receptor-ligand interaction vector with a predefined size (bitstrings, real-valued digits vector)
Output Y	• Binary numbers for binary classification tasks • Numeric values for cluster analysis, • Legitimate numbers for regression issues • Subsequent data (e.g. SMILES String, Series of amino acids) • Solitary learning relates to a single input column; multitasking process with respect to the many data columns

data, such as binary numbers for binary classification tasks, numeric values for cluster analysis, and legitimate numbers for regression issues, which typically incorporate genuine biological outcomes [16]. Table 2.1 represents various data patterns used as input and output for the development of AI algorithms in drug discovery.

2.2.2 Availability and Quality of Initial Data

It is necessary to give extra attention to the original data's predictive value and attribute values. To commence, evaluate if the efficiency of the training set is acceptable or not (Figure 2.2). If it is satisfactory on training set then the performance of test set need to be checked. If the training set's result are not up to par, alterations to the AI architecture is required [17]. Collecting more data will be one of the most effective methods if the difference between training and test-set effectiveness is unacceptable. To acquire an understanding of the model's representativeness and stability, functionality the input data and retrain the model with varying proportions of every stratum selected evenly, as well as arbitrarily. Almost usually, it is desirable to obtain good-quality raw data at a lower cost. A more common

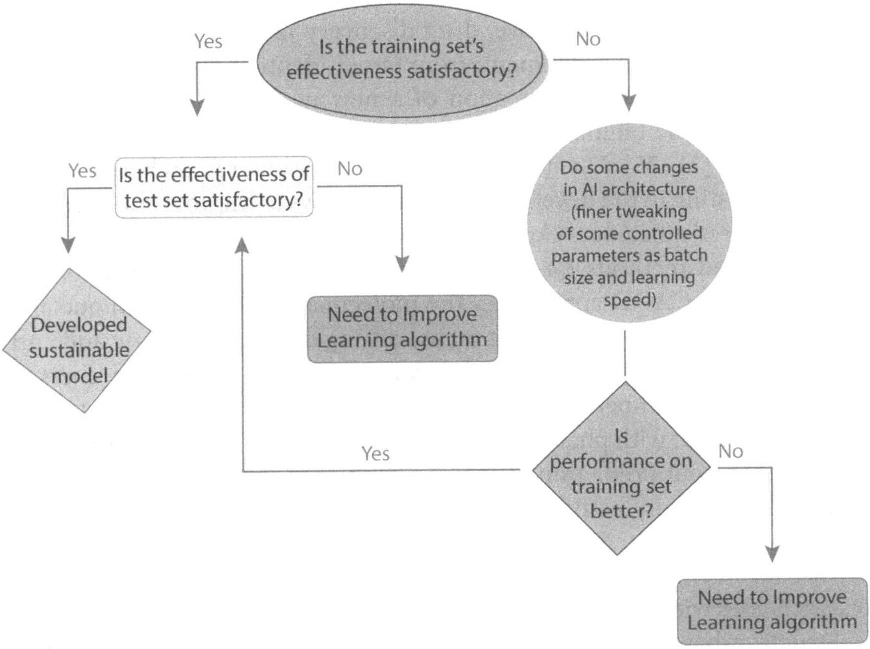

Figure 2.2 General flowchart to describe model optimization techniques.

case is that such procedures are prohibitively expensive or impossible to implement, as is frequently the case in medication development using biological information [18, 19]. To enhance the model with knowledge about related data, the training set can be supplemented by creating multitasking or transferable learning processes [20]. Based on the problem at mind, the simulation can be enhanced by hyper-parameter tuning, regularization or the use of additional specialized neural net topologies. If the test dataset efficiency is still significantly lower than the training sample after tweaking the regularization hyperparameters, and collecting additional training data is impractical, the simplest solution to reduce the generalization error may be to enhance the deep learning model itself. The GAN method, for example, may be used to efficiently construct artificial molecule structures with desired attributes from both restricted labelled and unlabeled input.

2.3 AI in Virtual Screening

The main goal of the drug development process is to find bioactive molecules that can help in disease therapy. The process begins with the discovery of molecular targets for a specific drug (natural or synthetic) and ends with the confirmation of those targets. The drug development procedure is lengthy and very costly. As stated above, drug discovery journey goes through all phases of new drug development, from target identification through drug registration. Moreover, the creation of a new medicines/drugs can costs between $1 and $2 billion USD on average and can take 10–20 years for its development [21–23]. Due to such problematic issues, researchers are continually investing in the development of novel ways to improve the drug discovery process' efficiency. Computer-aided drug design is one of the most widely utilized methods for reducing medication development costs and time (CADD). CADD approaches the molecular modeling technique and enables for improved experiment focus, cutting down on the time and cost of medication development [24]. Molecular modeling allows researchers to examine a large number of molecules in a short amount of time, illustrating how they interact with pharmacological targets even before they are synthesized. It starts out prediction of various important characteristics of molecules such as toxicity, activity, bioavailability, and efficacy etc. and then after validation and proper interpretation of above stated parameters, it moves further for *in vitro* and *in vivo* testing. Thus, by following such techniques, research goes with proper planning and direction [25–27].

Structure-based virtual screening (SBVS), one of the most promising *in silico* tools for drug research, is resilient and useful in this context. Virtual screening (VS) can help with hit discovery (finding active drug candidates) and lead optimization (transforming biologically active compounds into appropriate pharmaceuticals by increasing their physicochemical qualities). Finally, these improved leads go through preclinical and clinical testing before being approved by regulatory agencies [28]. For VS, large databases of known 3D structures are analyzed automatically utilizing computational approaches. Initially, thousands of possible active ligands are screened for a target. The probable ligands are selected using VS with AutoDock Vina. DOCK 6 is then used for carrying out molecular dynamics simulations. By this way, active compounds with promising results are selected for further experimental testing. This leads to the most promising synthesized molecules. VS techniques do even wonders by identifying if any compound is toxic. It gives proper ADMET (absorption, distribution, metabolism, excretion and toxicity) analysis of tested molecule. At the binding site, search algorithms are utilized to systematically evaluate ligand orientations and conformations. In rigid docking, the search algorithms make use of translational and rotational degrees of freedom to explore alternative positions of ligands at the active binding site, whereas in flexible docking, conformational degrees of freedom are added to the translations and rotations of the ligands. Search algorithms use a variety of strategies to anticipate the correct conformation of ligands, including checking the chemistry and geometry of the atoms involved (DOCK 6, FLEXX and genetic algorithm) [29–31]. Further, SBVS uses scoring functions to evaluate the force of non-covalent contacts between a ligand and a molecular target, and it tries to anticipate the optimum interaction mode between two molecules to form a stable complex [32].

The availability of a 3D structure of the target protein and the ligands to be docked is a need for executing VS [33, 34]. Some databases have been built to store 3D molecular structures, such as, Protein Data Bank (PDB), PubChem, ChemSpider, Brazilian Malaria Molecular Targets (BraMMT), Drugbank [35].

2.4 AI for *De Novo* Design

The purpose of *de novo* design is to find new bioactive molecules that can meet a variety of important performance parameters, including as activities, selection, physiochemical characteristics, and ADMET qualities, all at the same time [36]. Numerous approaches and software solutions have been introduced [37]. But *de novo* design has not seen a widespread use in drug discovery. This is at least partially related to the generation of compounds, which are synthetically difficult to access. The field has seen some revival recently due to developments in the field of artificial intelligence. An interesting approach is the variational autoencoder, which consists of two neural networks, an encoder network and a decoder network [38]. The encoder network converts the chemical constituents described by the SMILES description into a legitimate constant vector. The decoding section can convert variables from the latent space into active compounds. An *in-silico* model employed this feature to search for best solution in subspace, and the decoder networks used this feature to reverse translate such matrices into actual molecules. For the majority of reverse translates, one molecule predominate, while minor structural changes occur with a lower likelihood. The researchers trained a framework on the QED drug-likeness rating [39] and the synthetic accessibility score SAS [40] using the latent feature model. It might be possible to create a track of compounds with specific targeted qualities. A generating model generates unique chemical structures in the antagonistic learning algorithm. While the predictive model tries to mislead the discriminative model, a second discriminative adversarial model is trained to distinguish genuine molecules from produced ones. In generating mode, the antagonistic algorithm created considerably more acceptable architectures than the variational learning algorithm. Novel structures anticipated to be effective in opposition to the dopamine receptor type 2 might be produced using an *in-silico* approach. A generative adversarial network (GAN) was utilized by Kadurin *et al.* to suggest chemicals with suspected anticancer characteristics [41]. Numerous distinct architectures have just been constructed, each of which is possible to produce complete and effective new structures one of them is, Recursive neural networks (RNN) [42]. These approaches can be used to explore a novel chemical space, with the created molecules' property distributions being similar to the training space. The methodology's initial potential application was successful, with four out of five molecules exhibiting the anticipated activity. However, further expertise with the vastness of the chemical space examined and chemical validity of the defined compounds is required.

2.5 AI for Synthesis Planning

Molecule synthesis is one of the most difficult problems in organic chemistry, and a chemist's conventional method to solving a problem is based on experience and is a repeated, time-consuming operation that frequently results in non-optimized solutions [43, 44]. Artificial intelligence and machine learning have shown their potential usefulness in small molecule predictive chemistry and synthetic planning; at least a few businesses have reported using *in silico* synthetic planning into their overall approach to obtaining target molecules. Despite the fact that chemistry has a reputation for being a conservative science that is hesitant to adopt new ideas, AI is rapidly being researched across chemical disciplines [43]. Computational approaches have long been used in medicinal chemistry, supplemented by computer-aided drug design and cheminformatics, to aid in the search for and optimization of active molecules [45]. The synthesis planning is a key element in the drug discovery process. New computational approaches such as, prediction of outcomes of a reaction based on given set of inputs, prediction of yield of chemical reactions, and, involvement of retrosynthetic planning are utilized. Knowledge-based systems based on expert-derived rules or rules directly derived from reaction datasets dominate retrosynthetic planning. According to a recent study, a variety of computer strategies were utilized to forecast forward synthesis. They rate routes based on the retro synthesis technique. In one technique, chemical descriptors from quantum mechanics are merged with manually programmed rules and machine learning to anticipate the reaction and its products at the conclusion. This approach or process is used to forecast the outcome of a multi-step analytical response [46].

2.6 AI in Quality Control and Quality Assurance

The balancing of numerous factors is required to manufacture the required product from raw materials [47]. Manual intervention is required for product quality control tests and also batch-to-batch uniformity. This highlights the necessity for AI implementation at this level [48]. The Food and drug administration changed the Current Good Manufacturing Practices (cGMP) by proposing a "Quality by Design" plan to better understand the important operations and specifications that determine the final quality of pharmaceutical products [49]. Gams *et al.* employed a mix of human and AI efforts to examine early data from manufacturing batches and create regression trees. Those were then turned into principles, which the personnel assessed in order to lead the manufacturing cycle [47]. With the use of ANN, Goh *et al.* investigated the dissolution rate, a measure of batch-to-batch uniformity of some drugs [50]. AI could be used to regulate in-line production processes in order to reach the target product standard [49]. The freeze-drying process is monitored using an ANN that employs a mixture of self-adaptive progression, local search, and backpropagation methods. This could be utilized to estimate temperature and desiccated-cake thickness at a later time point (t + Dt) for a wide range of operating circumstances, thereby assisting in the quality checks of the finished product [51]. The quality control of the product can be ensured using an automated information input platform, such as an Electronic Lab Notebook, in conjunction with advanced, intelligent procedures [52]. In the Total Quality Management inference engine, data gathering and various knowledge discovery techniques can also be used as helpful approaches in making complicated judgments and developing new technologies for intelligent quality control [53].

2.7 AI-Based Advanced Applications

The use of AI in drug development has the potential to transform the existing time and scope of drug research. For drug discovery, AI does not rely on predetermined targets. As a result, there is no subjective bias or prior information in this medication development process. AI makes use of the most recent developments in biology and computation to create cutting-edge drug discovery algorithms. AI has the potential to level the playing field in drug research, with to rapid increases in computing capacity and lower processing costs. When it comes to defining relevant interactions in a drug screen, AI has a greater predictive power. As a result, by carefully setting the parameters of the test in question, the risk of false positives can be decreased. Most crucially, AI has the ability to shift drug screening from the bench to a virtual lab, where findings can be produced more quickly and intriguing targets can be prioritized without requiring extensive experimental input or personnel hours [6, 54]. So, some of the advanced applications of AI in drug development process have been mentioned below.

2.7.1 Micro/Nanorobot Targeted Drug Delivery System

Micro/nanorobots have gained popularity as a research field in recent years. It has a lot of potential in medical therapy because it may be used for targeted medicine delivery, surgery, illness diagnostics, and so on. Unlike traditional medication distribution, which relies on blood circulation to reach the target, the proposed micro/nanorobots may move independently, allowing pharmaceuticals to be delivered to difficult-to-reach locations [55, 56]. Nanotechnology can be used to improve medication solubility, modify drug distribution in diverse tissues and organs, adjust release rates to provide sustained and controlled release patterns, and induce drug aggregation in its target [57]. Nanorobots are primarily made up of integrated circuits, sensors, power supplies, and secure data backup, all of which are maintained using computational technologies such as artificial intelligence. They are programmed to avoid collisions, identify targets, detect and attach to them, and then excrete from the body. Nano/microrobot advancements enable them to go to the desired region based on physiological parameters like pH, boosting efficacy and lowering systemic side effects. Microchip implants are utilized for both programmed release and detecting the implant's position in the body [3].

2.7.2 AI in Nanomedicine

Nanomedicines combine nanotechnology and medicine to diagnose, treat, and monitor diseases such as infectious diseases, cancer, malaria, asthma, and a variety of inflammatory diseases. Because of their improved efficacy and therapy, nanoparticle-modified drug delivery has been increasingly relevant in the field of therapeutics and diagnostics in recent years. As the nanomedicine field has progressed, multifunctional techniques to concurrently combine therapeutic and diagnostic chemicals onto a single particle or deliver numerous nanomedicine-functionalized therapies in tandem have been explored. These techniques may improve treatment outcomes by targeting multi-agent distribution while preserving medication synergy, similar to the goals of traditional combination therapy [58]. Nanomedicine-based drug delivery is also frequently investigated at fixed doses, similar to conventional/unmodified combination therapy. Many formulation development difficulties could be solved with a mix of nanotechnology and artificial intelligence. For example, the creation of silicasomes, which are made up of iRGD, a tumor-penetrating peptide, and irinotecan-loaded multifunctional mesoporous silica nanoparticles, was aided by artificial intelligence. Because iRGD improves silicasome transcytosis, this resulted in a three- to fourfold increase in silicasome uptake, with improved treatment outcomes and overall survival [3].

2.7.3 Role of AI in Market Prediction

The ongoing expansion and growth of a company's business is the key to its success. Despite having access to large cash, the pharmaceutical industry's R&D production is declining due to companies' failure to adopt new marketing technologies. The 'Fourth Industrial Revolution' in digital technologies is assisting innovative digitalized marketing through a multicriteria decision-making approach that collects and analyses statistical and mathematical data and implements human inferences to make AI-based decision-making models explore new marketing methodology [59]. Under the influence of AI, small pharma businesses dramatically alter their research and development, master data management, analysis and reporting, and human resource business operations. AI is being used by big pharma to transform their production, sales, marketing, and analysis operations. Medium-sized businesses, on the other hand, are in the center and, based on their specialization, modify their business operations separately [60].

Furthermore, AI aids in a comprehensive examination of a product's core requirements from the customer's perspective, as well as evaluating the market's need, which aids in decision-making using prediction tools. It can also forecast sales and conduct market research. By displaying adverts that drive people to the product site with only a click, AI-based software engages customers and raises awareness among physicians [3]. Several business-to-business (B2B) organizations have introduced self-service solutions that allow free browsing of health items, which can be easily located by providing specifications, as well as placing orders and tracking their delivery. To meet the unmet requirements of patients, pharmaceutical companies are launching online programs such as 1 mg, Medline, Netmeds and, Ask Apollo [61].

2.8 Discussion and Future Perspectives

Artificial intelligence has recently garnered a lot of consideration, and it has also been successful in the realm of medication discovery. In the drug discovery process, many machine learning algorithms, such as QSAR methods and Random Forests, are well-known. As can be seen in multiple benchmarking studies comparing deep learning to traditional machine learning, innovative algorithms based on deep neural networks, such as deep learning models, provide even more benefits for property projections. The usefulness of these unique methods has been established for a variety of applications, including physicochemical qualities, bioactivities, toxic effects, and so on. Free software versions of machine learning for drug discovery benefit greatly from access to software libraries that allow for the building of complicated neural nets. As a result, open source frameworks such as Tensorflow [62] and Keras [63] are extensively utilized in drug discovery to create various neural network topologies. In addition, the Deepchem collection includes a Tensorflow wrapper that makes it easier to process chemical structures [64]. Artificial intelligence algorithms' implementations have broadened significantly in recent years, currently including new genetic design and retrosynthetic assessment, indicating that we will find many more uses in domains where vast datasets are accessible.

With advancements in these domains, we can anticipate a trend toward more and more computer-assisted drug discovery. Large advancements in robots, in particular, will hasten this process. Artificial intelligence, on the other hand, is far from flawless. Many techniques with a strong theoretical foundation will continue to be relevant, in part because they benefit from increased compute power, allowing larger systems to be simulated with more precise approaches. Moreover, there still are gaps in the data, such as innovative ideas, making a mix of human and machine intellect a viable option a great point of view. In spite of current recent constraints, collaboration between pharmaceutical industries and organizations focused on developing machine learning algorithms strategies could aid in the discovery of novel chemical compounds, the development of new treatment methods, and the tracking of enormous health data through the use of appropriate technologies. Given the high expense of developing new and innovative treatments in terms of time, resources, and effort, as well as lower approval numbers, it is acceptable to depend on computational models aimed at improving drug research efficiency while lowering error rates. These breakthroughs will aid in the advancement of medical services, targeted therapy, and therapeutic efficacy [65].

2.9 Conclusion

In this chapter we presented a variety of machine learning methods that may be utilized for *in silico* drug screening, as well as providing instances of alternate techniques. These algorithms, which provide a broad range of exploratory capabilities, enable the identification of biomolecules whose inhibition or augmentation could increase the efficacy of therapeutic treatments. Furthermore, relevant geneto-drug response connections can be captured when data-mining algorithms are employed. We also present an overview of useful machine learning algorithms used in drug repurposing, which is a different approach to traditional drug development. To summarize, the current analysis demonstrates that the discipline of AI, which includes machine learning as well as methodologies such as deep learning, may be used in clinical settings.

References

1. Patel, V. and Shah, M., A comprehensive study on artificial intelligence and machine learning in drug discovery and drug development. *Intell. Med.*, 2021 (*in press*).

2. Taylor, D., The pharmaceutical industry and the future of drug development, in: *Pharmaceuticals in the Environment*, pp. 1–33, Royal Society of Chemistry (RSC) Publishing, Cambridge, United Kingdom, 2016.
3. Paul, D. *et al.*, Artificial intelligence in drug discovery and development. *Drug Discov. Today*, 26, 1, 80–93, 2021.
4. Hessler, G. and Baringhaus, K.H., Artificial intelligence in drug design. *Molecules*, 23, 10, 2520, 2018.
5. Kersting, K., Machine learning and artificial intelligence: Two fellow travelers on the quest for intelligent behavior in machines. *Front. Big Data*, 1, 6, 1, 6, 2018.
6. Jiménez-Luna, J. *et al.*, Artificial intelligence in drug discovery: Recent advances and future perspectives. *Expert Opin. Drug Discov.*, 16, 9, 949–959, 2021.
7. Verma, S. *et al.*, Artificial intelligence in marketing: Systematic review and future research direction. *Int. J. Inf. Manag. Data Insights*, 1, 1, 100002, 2021.
8. Yang, X. *et al.*, Concepts of artificial intelligence for computer-assisted drug discovery. *Chem. Rev.*, 119, 18, 10520–10594, 2019.
9. Bhisetti, G. and Fang, C., Artificial intelligence-enabled de novo design of novel compounds that are synthesizable. *Methods Mol. Biol.*, 2390, 409–419, 2022.
10. Grebner, C., Matter, H., Hessler, G., Artificial intelligence in compound design. *Methods Mol. Biol.*, 2390, 349–382, 2022.
11. Soto, R. *et al.*, Data science and AI-based optimization in scientific programming. *Sci. Program.*, 2019, 7154765, 2019.
12. Tripathi, M.K. *et al.*, Evolving scenario of big data and artificial intelligence (AI) in drug discovery. *Mol. Divers.*, 25, 3, 1439–1460, 2021.
13. Schneider, G., Mind and machine in drug design. *Nat. Mach. Intell.*, 1, 128–130, 2019.
14. Lo, Y.-C., Rensi, S.E., Torng, W., Altman, R.B., Machine learning in chemoinformatics and drug discovery. *Drug Discov. Today*, 23, 1538–1546, 2018.
15. Todeschini, R. and Consonni, V., *Molecular Descriptors for Chemoinformatics: Vol. I: Alphabetical Listing/Vol. II: Appendices, References*, John Wiley & Sons, Weinheim, Germany, 2009.
16. Blaschke, T., Olivecrona, M., Engkvist, O., Bajorath, J., Chen, H., Application of generative autoencoder in *de novo* molecular design. *Mol. Inf.*, 37, 1700123, 1–2, 2018.
17. Srivastava, N., Hinton, G., Krizhevsky, A., Sutskever, I., Salakhutdinov, R., Dropout: A simple way to prevent neural networks from overfitting. *J. Mach. Learn. Res.*, 15, 1929–1958, 2014.
18. Chawla, N.V., Bowyer, K.W., Hall, L.O., Kegelmeyer, W.P., SMOTE: Synthetic minority over-sampling technique. *J. Artif. Intell. Res.*, 16, 321–357, 2002.
19. Maciejewski, T. and Stefanowski, J., Local neighbourhood extension of SMOTE for mining imbalanced data. *2011 IEEE Symposium on*

Computational Intelligence and Data Mining, Paris, France, Nov. 16, 2010, CIDM, pp. 104–111, 2011.
20. Altae-Tran, H., Ramsundar, B., Pappu, A.S., Pande, V., Low data drug discovery with one-shot learning. *ACS Cent. Sci.*, 3, 283–293, 2017.
21. Leelananda, S.P. and Lindert, S., Computational methods in drug discovery. *Beilstein J. Org. Chem.*, 12, 2694–2718, 2016.
22. Deore, A. *et al.*, The stages of drug discovery and development process. *Asian J. Pharm. Res. Dev.*, 7, 62–67, 2019.
23. Kiriiri, G.K., Njogu, P.M., Mwangi, A.N., Exploring different approaches to improve the success of drug discovery and development projects: A review. *Future J. Pharm. Sci.*, 6, 1, 27, 2020.
24. Yu, W. and MacKerell Jr., A.D., Computer-aided drug design methods. *Methods Mol. Biol.*, 1520, 85–106, 2017.
25. Aminpour, M., Montemagno, C., Tuszynski, J.A., An overview of molecular modeling for drug discovery with specific illustrative examples of applications. *Molecules (Basel)*, 24, 9, 1693, 2019.
26. Opo, F.A.D.M. *et al.*, Structure based pharmacophore modeling, virtual screening, molecular docking and ADMET approaches for identification of natural anti-cancer agents targeting XIAP protein. *Sci. Rep.*, 11, 1, 4049, 2021.
27. Srivastava, R., Theoretical studies on the molecular properties, toxicity, and biological efficacy of 21 new chemical entities. *ACS Omega*, 6, 38, 24891–24901, 2021.
28. Lima, A.N. *et al.*, Use of machine learning approaches for novel drug discovery. *Expert Opin. Drug Discov.*, 11, 3, 225–239, 2016.
29. Allen, W.J. *et al.*, DOCK 6: Impact of new features and current docking performance. *J. Comput. Chem.*, 36, 15, 1132–56, 2015.
30. Rarey, M. *et al.*, A fast flexible docking method using an incremental construction algorithm. *J. Mol. Biol.*, 261, 3, 470–89, 1996.
31. Verdonk, M.L. *et al.*, Improved protein-ligand docking using GOLD. *Proteins*, 52, 4, 609–23, 2003.
32. Wang, D. *et al.*, Improving the virtual screening ability of target-specific scoring functions using deep learning methods. *Front. Pharmacol.*, 10, 924, 2019.
33. Schmidt, T., Bergner, A., Schwede, T., Modelling three-dimensional protein structures for applications in drug design. *Drug Discov. Today*, 19, 7, 890–897, 2014.
34. Deng, H., Jia, Y., Zhang, Y., Protein structure prediction. *Int. J. Mod. Phys. B*, 32, 18, 1840009, 2018.
35. Maia, E.H.B. *et al.*, Structure-based virtual screening: From classical to artificial intelligence. *Front. Chem.*, 8, 343, 2020.
36. Hartenfeller, M. and Schneider, G., Enabling future drug discovery by de novo design. *Wires Comput. Mol. Sci.*, 1, 742–759, 2011.
37. Schneider, P. and Schneider, G., De novo design at the edge of chaos. *J. Med. Chem.*, 59, 4077–4086, 2016.

38. Gómez-Bombarelli, R., Wei, J.N., Duvenaud, D., Hernández-Lobato, J.M., Sánchez-Lengeling, B., Sheberla, D., Aguilera-Iparraguirre, J., Hirzel, T.D., Adamsk, P., Aspuru-Guzik, A., Automatic chemical design using a data-driven continuous representation of molecules. *arXiv*, 4, 2, 268–276, 2016. arXiv:1610.02415v3. Available online: http://arxiv.org/abs/1610.02415(accessed on 5 January 2022).
39. Bickerton, G.R., Paolini, G.V., Besnard, J., Muresan, S., Hopkins, A.L., Quantifying the chemical beauty of drugs. *Nat. Chem.*, 4, 90–98, 2012.
40. Ertl, P. and Schuffenhauer, A., Estimation of synthetic accessibility score of drug-like molecules based on molecular complexity and fragment contributions. *J. Cheminformatics*, 1, 1–11, 2009.
41. Kadurin, A., Aliper, A., Kazennov, A., Mamoshina, P., Vanhaelen, Q., Kuzma, K., Zhavoronkov, A., The cornucopia of meaningful leads: Applying deep adversarial autoencoders for new molecule development in oncology. *Oncotarget*, 8, 10883–10890, 2017.
42. Bengio, Y., Learning deep architectures for AI. *Found. Trends Mach. Learn.*, 2, 1–127, 2009.
43. Struble, T.J. *et al.*, Current and future roles of artificial intelligence in medicinal chemistry synthesis. *J. Med. Chem.*, 63, 16, 8667–8682, 2020.
44. Peiretti, F. and Brunel, J.M., Artificial intelligence: The future for organic chemistry? *ACS Omega*, 3, 10, 13263–13266, 2018.
45. Plehiers, P.P. *et al.*, Artificial intelligence for computer-aided synthesis in flow: Analysis and selection of reaction components. *Front. Chem. Eng.*, 2, 2020.
46. Thakkar, A. *et al.*, Artificial intelligence and automation in computer aided synthesis planning. *React. Chem. Eng.*, 6, 1, 27–51, 2021.
47. Gams, M. *et al.*, Integrating artificial and human intelligence into tablet production process. *AAPS PharmSciTech*, 15, 1447–1453, 2014.
48. Rantanen, J. and Khinast, J., The future of pharmaceutical manufacturing sciences. *J. Pharm. Sci.*, 104, 3612–3638, 2015.
49. Aksu, B. *et al.*, A quality by design approach using artificial intelligence techniques to control the critical quality attributes of ramipril tablets manufactured by wet granulation. *Pharm. Dev. Technol.*, 18, 236–245, 2013.
50. Goh, W.Y. *et al.*, Application of a recurrent neural network to prediction of drug dissolution profiles. *Neural Comput. Appl.*, 10, 311–317, 2002.
51. Dragoi, E.N. *et al.*, On the use of artificial neural networks to monitor a pharmaceutical freeze-drying process. *Dry. Technol.*, 31, 72–81, 2013.
52. Fleming, N., How artificial intelligence is changing drug discovery. *Nature*, 557, 7706, 55, 20, 2018.
53. Wang, X., Intelligent quality management using knowledge discovery in databases, in: *2009 International Conference on Computational Intelligence and Software Engineering*, IEEE, pp. 1–4, 2009.
54. Deng, J. *et al.*, Artificial intelligence in drug discovery: Applications and techniques. *Brief. Bioinformatics*, 23, 1, 2021.

55. Hu, M. *et al.*, Micro/nanorobot: A promising targeted drug delivery system. *Pharmaceutics*, 12, 7, 665, 2020.
56. Singh, A.V. *et al.*, Emerging application of nanorobotics and artificial intelligence to cross the BBB: Advances in design, controlled maneuvering, and targeting of the barriers. *ACS Chem. Neurosci.*, 12, 11, 1835–1853, 2021.
57. Adir, O. *et al.*, Integrating artificial intelligence and nanotechnology for precision cancer medicine. *Adv. Mater.*, 32, 13, e1901989, 2020.
58. Ho, D., Wang, P., Kee, T., Artificial intelligence in nanomedicine. *Nanoscale Horiz.*, 2, 4, 365–377, 2018.
59. Kulkov, I., The role of artificial intelligence in business transformation: A case of pharmaceutical companies. *Technol. Soc.*, 66, 101629, 2021.
60. Gamalo, M., A year in review: Artificial intelligence permeates into mainstream statistics in pharmaceutical product development at a laggard pace. *J. Biopharm. Stat.*, 31, 1, 1–4, 2021.
61. Singh, J. *et al.*, Sales profession and professionals in the age of digitization and artificial intelligence technologies: Concepts, priorities, and questions. *J. Pers. Sell. Sales Manag.*, 39, 1, 2–22, 2019.
62. Abadi, M., Barham, P., Chen, J., Chen, Z., Davis, A., Dean, J., Devin, M., Ghemawat, S., Irving, G., Isard, M. *et al.*, TensorFlow: A system for large-scale machine learning. *arXiv*, 16, 265–283, 2016. arXiv:1605.08695v2.
63. Keras, The python deep learning library. Available online: https://keras.io (accessed on 04 January 2022).
64. Deepchem, Available online: https://deepchem.io (accessed on 04 January 2022).
65. Mak, K.-K. and Pichika, M.R., Artificial intelligence in drug development: Present status and future prospects. *Drug Discov. Today*, 24, 773–780, 2019.

3

Role of Bioinformatics in Peptide-Based Drug Design and Its Serum Stability

Vivek Chavda[1]*, Prashant Kshirsagar[2] and Nildip Chauhan[2†]

[1]Department of Pharmaceutics and Pharmaceutical Technology, L M College of Pharmacy, Ahmedabad, India
[2]Drug Product Development, Enzene Biosciences Limited, Pune Maharashtra, India

Abstract
Naturally occurring peptides are becoming the area of interest in peptide dug design and development now a day. Peptides stability can be increased by changing both the end of terminal amino acid using its D-form by means of glyocylation, sulfation or phosphorylation on the tyrosine residue. Pegylation is one of the powerful processes to form a conjugation of peptide which turn into reducing immunogenicity and increasing water solubility. Several approaches are made to improve peptide stability while reducing proteolytic enzyme susceptibility. One of the approaches is to identify the site of proteolytic cleavage and incorporation of chemical modification by non-natural amino acid and replacement of amide bond. Other approaches are modification of N and C terminal end, cyclization of side chain or backbone or inclusion of peptide which will provide stabilization. Here, we are also focusing on the improvement of serum stability of the same.

Keywords: Peptides, serum stability, N-terminal and C-terminal amino acids, receptor

3.1 Introduction

Peptides are made up of amino acids, when amino acids in defined ordered linked through peptide bond and form a chain. Peptide consist of 2–50

**Corresponding author*: vivek7chavda@gmail.com
[†]*Corresponding author*: nildip.chauhan@gmail.com

Vivek Chavda, Krishnan Anand and Vasso Apostolopoulos (eds.) Bioinformatics Tools for Pharmaceutical Drug Product Development, (37–54) © 2023 Scrivener Publishing LLC

amino acids and can be classified based on number of peptide bonds like dipeptide, tripeptide, oligopeptide and polypeptide [1]. Peptides which are biological and therapeutically activity can be used to treat the disease. The use of the peptides as a drug is only possible if peptides are formulated in to the dosage form which have nominal shelf life to some extent without any toxicity and immunogenicity [2]. Peptides are susceptible to chemical degradation like oxidation, hydrolysis, racemization, crosslinking etc. and physical degradation like change in conformation which ultimately may cause aggregation, precipitation or adsorption of peptide molecules [3]. To overcome above problem of chemical and physical degradation, stable formulation of peptide is necessary which can be achieved by addition of the selected excipients based on the nature of peptides and its degradation pathway [4]. In addition to normal shelf life, in use stability of the therapeutic peptide can be taken in to account and it should have several weeks or days of such stability for ease of use and handling [5]. Another serious problem linked with the use of peptides as a drug is their degradation in presence of human plasma/serum by means of various enzymes which leads to change in its therapeutic effectiveness. There are several ways to overcome the problem associated with enzymatic degradation by increasing half-life of the peptides and its bioavailability. The approach from several can be selected and can be useful if functional properties of the peptide not compromised [6].

3.2 Points to be Considered for Peptide-Based Delivery

Peptide based drug delivery system and use of peptide for different therapeutic area are now days gaining interest because of their several advantages like peptides have broad range of target, low toxicity, high diversity, high potency and selectivity to receptors, also therapeutic peptides has good efficacy, safety and tolerability [6, 7].

Besides its uses and advantages in different therapeutic area, peptides have some disadvantages also which make peptide-based drug delivery system in dilemma when it comes to formulation scientist [8]. Some of are limited bioavailability due to its short half-life and rapid clearance, poor permeability and low stability in plasma, apart from these peptides can get aggregated and exacerbate immunogenicity [9]. Another major problem is low oral bioavailability and difficulties in handling and storage [10]. Digestive enzymes designed to break down amide bonds of ingested proteins are effective at cleaving the same bonds in peptide hormones, and the high polarity and molecular weight of peptides severely limits intestinal permeability.

As oral delivery is always first preference for patients, need for injection made peptide drug less attractive and unfavourable having only option for chronic indications [11]. Serious problems associated with the use of short peptides are caused by their short lifetime in the body, due to enzymatic or chemical disintegration. Disintegration of the peptide may change the therapeutic effect of the conjugate in a deleterious way, or give misleading diagnosis [12]. The original function and benefits of the peptide and the peptide-effector conjugate might be lost if the peptide breaks down. Thus, there is a recognized need for improving the stability of functional peptides and peptide-effector conjugates. One type of peptide cyclization occurring in nature is based on a disulfide bond between two cysteine amino acids forming a cystine bridge. A cystine bridge may increase the stability against enzymatic attacks, compared to an uncyclized peptide. The disulfide bond in cystine is, however, among the chemically most reactive bonds in peptides, both *in vivo* and *in vitro* [13]. It brings chemical instability and complications to the synthesis and use of conjugates. Another well-known way of protecting peptides from enzymatic degradation, and of increasing their stability, is to cyclize the functional peptide of the conjugate produced by the solid phase synthesis [12, 14]. Figure 3.1 gives SWOT analysis of the naturally occurring peptides.

S	W	O	T
Strenght	**Weakness**	**Opportunities**	**Threats**
▪ Safety, efficacy and tolerability is good ▪ Highly selective and potent ▪ Metabolism can be predicable ▪ Shorter development time ▪ Attrition rate is low ▪ Can be synthesis easily	▪ Less chemical stability ▪ Less physical stability ▪ Prone to form aggregate ▪ faster excretion due to short half life ▪ Low membrane permeability ▪ Degradation by oral route	▪ Discover of peptide and fragment of protein ▪ Focused peptide library ▪ Optimization of sequencing ▪ Drug product formulation development	▪ Immunogenicity ▪ Competition with other advancement techniques ▪ Affordability ▪ proving Safety and efficacy of novel molecules ▪ Return of Investment

Figure 3.1 Analytical tool for analysis of its strengths, weaknesses, opportunities, and threats for naturally occurring peptides (SWOT).

3.3 Overview of Peptide-Based Drug Delivery System

The use of peptides in drug delivery has grown significantly in various therapeutic areas. Peptide either synthetic native peptide or synthetic analogue of its native form can be used for its clinical application based on their therapeutic class [15]. In 1920s first peptide insulin was isolated and used for diabetes, subsequently in 1950s structure elucidation and chemical synthesis of peptides comes in to picture and made an effort to make it possible [6]. Later in 1980s peptide are gaining interest for clinical development stage and in current decades peptides having length up to 40 amino acids can be possible to synthesise which is feasible only because of the progress in area of peptide synthesis and technology. Peptides can be classified as native, analogue, and heterogenous [15, 16]. Native peptides are manufactured synthetically or by recombinant technology but native peptides have several limitations which enables scientist to find out alternatives and focused on analogue of native peptides [17]. Analogues are modified peptides of their native form which have enhanced therapeutic effect and increase half-life. One of the examples is desmopressin which an analogue of vasopressin which has longer half-life and improved in selectivity [18]. Another example is octreotide, analogue of somatostatin with increased plasma half-life and selectivity. If we talk about Heterogenous peptide, in 1997, a 14-amino-acid peptide – romiplostim was found which acts by binding and activating TPO receptor. This is thrombopoietin mimetics peptide created by adding amino acid to C terminal end of IgG1 Fc fragment which is also term as 'peptibody' [19, 20]. Peptide conjugates also has significant role in alteration or enhancement of properties of peptides. One of the examples is pegylation of peptide using polyethylene glycol (PEG). Another advancement happened towards the determining of half-life of the peptides and creation of the library which help to get sufficient information about peptides like its name, sequence, half-life, modifications, and the experimental assay for determining half-life, biological nature and activity of the peptide. The use of such peptide libraries is useful for peptide-based drug design. The isolation of peptides and purification of adrenocorticotrophic hormone (ACTH) from pituitary glands use to treat to treat many endocrine disorder in patient [21, 22]. The genomic sciences is area of interest for industries and academic for identification and molecular characterization of receptors of many important endogenous peptides which follow novel peptide ligands for these receptors [23]. High through put screening (HTS) is one of the bioinformatic tools utilized for the peptide design and development.

The various number of platform present in modern screening libraries supported the idea which helps in identification, optimization and development of lead molecules candidate in to drug. Structural biology adds another advantage by elucidating key molecular interactions at active site of the receptor. Here one of the major challenges is the grafting of ligand binding site and specific conformational change required for signal transduction [24].

In recent advancement peptide therapeutics has emerged as potential application in broader area. Modification of amino acid or backbone modification, addition of non-structural amino acid and conjugate peptide using novel synthetic strategies modulate the pharmacokinetics properties and target specificity by improving stability and other physicochemical properties [21].

3.4 Tools for Screening of Peptide Drug Candidate

Naturally occurring peptides excels in stability and target affinity but same times it is difficult to achieve using rational peptide drug design and peptide screening libraries or peptidomimetics. Peptidomic is systematic analysis of peptide to study and identify bio-physiological properties of active peptide and their pharmacological activity. Analysis of spectrum of peptide using mass spectroscopy which is linked with advance bioinformatics technology is necessary to help in data generation.

Peptide libraries which are useful in peptide drug design and screening and reverse engineering of natural peptides are strategies used in peptidomics and are much more successful compare to earlier. More ever High through put screening of synthetic peptide chemical libraries can be possible to prepare using recent advancement in peptidomics which includes natural peptide sequences, post translation modification of peptide [25, 26].

Post-translation modification allows creating enormous libraries containing therapeutically effective peptide. Peptide libraries are widely applied as a powerful tool which provides a rapid and cost-effective screening of therapeutically active peptide. Different peptide libraries are available, one example is Alanine scanning libraries. Ala-scan is used for identification of residues which is important for activity of peptide. In this Ala scan smallest chiral natural amino acid – alanine, is substituted in to original peptide at each position and peptide activity is measured. Impact on peptide activity due to substitution of alanine is assessed and its importance of each individual residue is determined using overall peptide activity. Ala scan help in assessing *in vitro* and *in vivo* activities and reveal structure activity relationship [27].

3.5 Various Strategies to Increase Serum Stability of Peptide

Both Peptide either synthetic or recombinant undergo degradation in systemic circulation in plasma by means of enzymes present in human plasma like proteases and peptidases [28].

Proteases and peptidases are the enzymes present in human plasma which are main cause of peptide degradation and hence efficacy of the peptides are compromised [29]. When we analysed the peptide drug alone and peptide drug after addition to human plasma, it shows clear difference about main peak of peptide drug. Due to degradation of peptide in presence of plasma, intensity of the main peak and hence area is decreased significantly [30]. In short, in presence of plasma, effectiveness of peptide drug is decreases with time. To overcome these, one has to think about stability of the peptide in systemic circulation in serum and plasma. Many peptides are having stability issue in human plasma and shows only 40-50 % effectiveness compared to initial time [28].

To increase half-life and effectiveness of the peptide and peptide analogues certain modifications need to be done in peptide and before that one has to thoroughly understand the peptide chemistry [31, 32]. There are multiples way to increase effectiveness of the peptide; doing some changes in peptide which helps to increase half-life of the peptide [33]. Before starting any development for peptide-based drug delivery enormous information need to be collected related to but not limited to its structure, length, N and C terminal modification, configuration, confirmation, chirality of amino acid, amino acid sequence, origin, biological activity, degradation pathways and half-life [34, 35]. Below mentioned are some modification which will enable interest of scientist in peptide-based drug delivery for different therapeutics area [33].

3.5.1 Cyclization of Peptide

Cyclization of the peptide is a one of the techniques which enhance potency and *in vivo* efficacy of peptide by improving its conformational stability. Backbone cyclization strategies can be useful in which amide bond is formed between terminal end (N-terminal and C-terminal) of amino acid residues [36]. Also, side chain amino acid cyclization can be possible in that disulfide bond formation happens between Cysteine, lactam bridge form between glutamic/aspartic and lysine residue [37]. Forming lacton and thio lactone bridge and ether bridge between amino acid which contains functional group like hydroxyl or mercapto [38].

Cyclization of peptide slower the metabolism and increase its resistance to protease and prevent degradation of peptide which form stable peptide analogue having strong conformational and biological stability [39]. Cyclization of the peptides can be possible by creating peptide bond in-between N-terminal and C- terminal end is one way of cyclization. Other ways are amide bond and disulfide bond formation between the side chains help to maintain its conformational stability [40]. Depending upon the position of cyclization, many methods are available to form cyclic peptide for example head-tail, side chain-side chain, side chain-tail, head-side chain cyclization. Figure 3.2 illustrate various option for cyclizations. In Head-tail cyclization of peptide synthesize by formation of amide bond is formed during synthesis while side chain- side chain cyclization are form by Cys-Cys or amide bond formation. Cyclic peptide mimics the structure of biologically active peptides and bind the target *in vivo* [41, 42].

Cyclization of peptide using cys-cys Disulfide Bridge is having limited stability over the amide bonds which are chemically more stable than

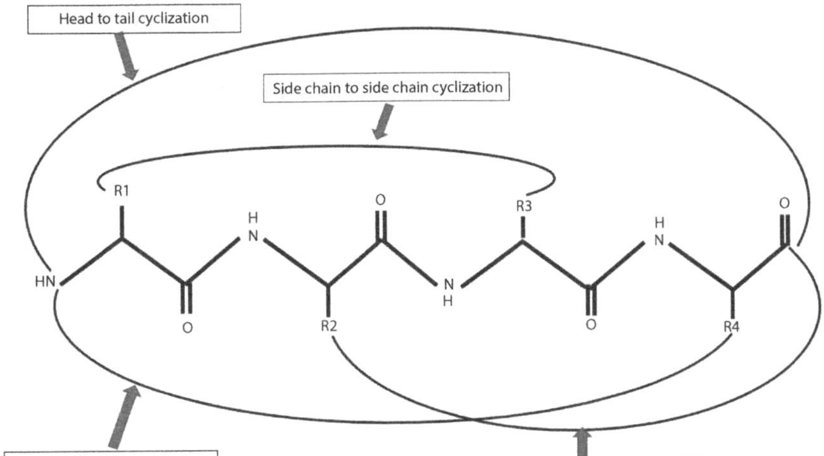

Figure 3.2 Various cyclization of peptide.

cys-cys Disulfide Bridge. Amide cyclization is also having some limitation like challenges of dimerization, undesirable side reactions such as racemization or peptide capping by coupling reagents. So, selection of the site for cyclization is very important for head-to tail cyclization (Figure 3.2) [40, 43].

3.5.2 Incorporation of D Form of Amino Acid

Incorporation of D- form of amino acid is widely used approach for protecting protease degradation of therapeutic peptides [42]. At the same time, changes in its conformation by incorporation of D-amino acid leads to change in its biological activity and effectiveness of original peptides [44].

3.5.3 Terminal Modification

N-and C-terminal of peptides are potential site for proteolytic activity by proteases and peptidases enzyme i.e. Serum amino peptidases and carboxypeptidases [45]. Different amino acids at N- and C-terminal of the peptide results in proteolytic activity and degradation of peptide. Some amino acids are more prone to degradation in plasma while some are more resistant effect in plasma [46]. So, it is always area of interest to modify the N- and/or C-terminal without compromising its affinity and targeting specificity. By doing same proteolytic degradation can be reduced to significant level and hence good amount of bioavailability can be achievable (Figure 3.3) [47]. Same way amidation at C-terminal backbone and acetylation at N-Terminal can be helpful in increasing *in vivo* stability [48].

To increase efficacy of the peptide by increasing half-life, most of the modification is done at the terminal end of the peptide i.e. N-terminal

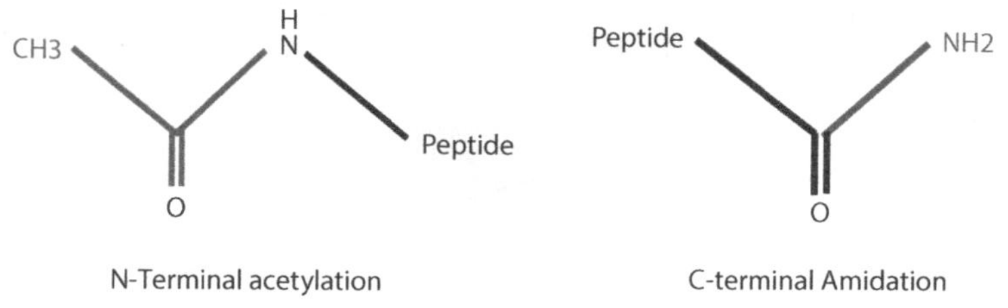

Figure 3.3 Example of terminal modification.

modification. One of the examples for N-Terminal modification is incorporation of 2, 4-dichlorophenoxyacetic acid with (CH2) spacers and subsequent acylation. Others methods used are addition of PEG, addition of HAS (human serum albumin) and hydroxylation for N-terminal modification, glycosylation, succinylation, which will help some extent in enhancing peptide half-life [49].

For C-terminal modification, amidation is the area of interest, amidation and subsequently biotinylation with polyethylene glycol (PEG) spacers is one example. There are some more C-Terminal modifications which are inclusion of serum albumin, polyethylene glycol, Fc region etc. Non terminal modification like methylation and addition of fatty acid chains, carbohydrate chains. Reducing amide or carbamate bonds and addition of amino acid which is non-natural like biphenylalanine, pyroglutamic acid, sarcosine, orthenine, nor leucine [50, 51].

Therapeutic peptides having optimal bioavailability are the area of interest for different therapeutic classes. Although half-life is directly related to bioavailability and efficacy of the peptide drug no much information is available about this. There are some bioinformatics platforms available which predict half-life of the therapeutic peptide [4]. Scientists have performed various *in vitro* and *in vivo* studies. These studies are useful in understanding the mechanism of peptide degradation and correlation between half-life of the therapeutic peptides, their structures, amino acid sequences and modifications. Bioavailability and stability of the therapeutic peptides can be determined by understanding peptide degradation by various enzymes and its pharmacokinetics. Both Enzymatic degradation and pharmacokinetics of the therapeutic peptides important roles in determining effectiveness of therapeutic peptides [52, 53].

By reducing rate of enzymatic degradation, peptide metabolism also reduces and hence stability of the peptide can be increased. Pharmacokinetic properties and proteolysis reaction can be varies based on the different organism which results in varying half-life. Variable pharmacokinetic properties of therapeutics peptides for each individual will contribute in different half-life of the peptide [54]. The factors which contributes in different half-life are amino acid sequence of peptides, N- or C-terminal modifications or chemical modification of peptides, route of administration, dose and strength of peptides [55].

Therapeutic peptides, manufactured by recombinant process or synthesised in laboratories, both have numerous challenges which hinder therapeutic advantages of peptides and is not limited to stability during storage but also having optimal *in vivo* half-life [5]. Affordability of peptide based drugs to patients is major problem for some peptides because if high production cost due to complex manufacturing set up involve in both recombinant as well synthetic peptide compare to conventional therapy [8, 9]. Peptide based drug design with optimum half-life and bioavailability remains always challenging for its therapeutic effectiveness [56, 57]. Therapeutic peptides which have optimal *in vitro* activity, with low toxicity and high selectivity for targets enters in to the development stage aiming to commercialization which benefit numbers of patients [58].

3.5.4 Substitution of Amino Acid Which is Not Natural

Amino acids which is not natural i.e. synthetic enantiomer of amino acid also area of interest to improve stability of peptide by decreasing proteolytic activity [59]. Non-natural amino acids are non-proteinogenic. These amino acids are obtained from plant or bacteria after post translation modification or, are formed by chemical synthesise. amino acids which is non-natural are extensively used either in combinatorial libraries or as chiral building blocks [48]. These modified amino acids often contribute to special biological activity, and are often incorporate into therapeutic peptidomimetic ligands which ultimately improve pharmacological properties and its biological activity and potency [57]. Several advantages of substitution of non-natural amino acids includes improvement of selectivity and receptor binding ability, modification of their agonist or antagonist activity, increase in half life and enhance transportation cross the cell membrane [35, 52].

3.5.5 Stapled Peptides

Stapled peptides are useful protein-protein interaction mimetic. Many stapled peptides show increase in both biological activity and potency (*in vivo*) [60]. α-helix peptides are highly susceptible to conformational changes and can be easily degraded by proteolysis [61]. Here, optimization is required for its therapeutics benefits. Un-optimized stapled peptides have difficulties in penetration of intact cells and hence shows reduce biological activity [62]. Significant efforts have been conducted to achieve the success in above mentioned approach. In addition, recent research indicates that stapled peptides can offer new ways to treat disease. Stapled peptides are helical peptides which will be locked using introduction of site-specific chemical linker and shows promising biological activity. Stapled peptides have ability to interact intracellularly and main elements in protein-protein interactions (PPIs) which enables novel approach for peptide therapeutics [63]. One example is α-helical peptides in which hydrocarbon is stapled which is promising candidate for drug. stapled peptide show improves in pharmacological effect, binding affinity towards the target, resistances to proteolysis and increase in cell penetration [64]. Improvement is binding affinity by use of non-native amino acids which is present in same helix to enact α-helix conformation of peptide and formation of the covalent bond between through liking together from side chain of non-native amino acid [65].

3.5.6 Synthesis of Stapled Peptides

Stapled peptide synthesis is used for various applications like analysis of binding kinetics, determination of structure, discovery of proteomics, signal transduction research, cellular analyses, imaging, and *in vivo* bioactivity studies. solid phase peptide synthesis is used for synthesis of α-helix peptides which is standard and common method used for peptide synthesis [66]. many methods are used to stabilized hydrocarbon which is linked in α-helix peptide, ring-closing metathesis, lactamization, cycloadditions, reversible reactions and thioether formation [67–69].

3.6 Method/Tools for Serum Stability Evaluation

Peptide based drug and its stability in plasma and serum should be determine in advance before the clinical stage of the development as serum stability is importance and is directly related to *in vivo* efficacy of the molecules [70]. If drug is not stable in plasma/serum it shows poor *in vivo* efficacy because of degradation of peptide drug in presence of plasma. Due to lack in stability of the drug in plasma, protein binding data results obtained from the analysis can mislead in interpretation of the data. Also, storage of the samples from pharmacokinetic study need to define very early as this can be challenging. Conformational stability of synthetic peptides is main requirement for its effectiveness as drug and hence assay to determine serum stability of peptide is first line of choice for scientist in screening of unstable peptide during development stage. One of the methods for the serum stability determination is reverse phase high performance liquid chromatography and mass spectroscopy for both *in vivo* and *in-vitro* studies. Human plasma is more relevant to access the serum stability of the peptide because both non-human and human plasma both contains different level of enzyme peptidase and has different activities. So Non-human plasma can mislead the result of peptide serum stability due to difference in peptidases level. Also, conditions of the patients with respect to disease and age also change the enzyme activity of peptidases. there are other factors also which can interfere in results like plasma prepared using EDTA which is chelating agent can exhibit peptidase inhibitor effect, immunoassay method developed are not specific for its stability. Different time interval shall be used for determination of the serum activity of the up to 1 h may be sufficient which will provide degradation profile of peptide with its degradation product which can be estimated by RP HPLC and mass spectroscopy [71].

In routine serum stability assay performed by subjecting human serum at real temperature condition following incubation for various time interval which is comparative to traditional protease assay. Protease reaction then stopped by TCA or ethanol which gives soluble peptide and peptide derivatives by precipitating large serum protein for further analysis. degradation of peptide is performed under specific condition where concentration are not rate limiting factor so reliable and reproducible results can be obtained in this case enzymatic reaction speed and enzyme concentration is rate limiting factor and are linearly dependent on serum concentration.

Supernatant undergoes protein analysis using MLADI-TOF mass spectrometry [72], or with Reverse phase HPLC under specific chromatography conditions to stability. Mass spectrometry MALDI-TOF techniques gives rare valid quantitative measurement without utilizing isotopic internal standards, on other side reverse phase chromatographic (RP-HPLC) analysis of peptides having UV detectors is directly quantitative method. In spite of it, mass spectrometry provides more insight on degradation products. It gives cleave sites or modification sites of peptides that have occur in the serum for example glycosylations, phosporylations, or degly-cosylations, dephosphorylations, etc. while taking into account many factors can cause misleading stability result for peptides [73].

It is always more relevant to perform *in vivo* testing of peptide stability rather performing *in vitro* testing. However, peptide pharmacokinetics is a better way to understand peptide stability using appropriate model can be term as *in vitro* measurement.

3.7 Conclusion

Overall, peptide-based drug design and delivery systems are gaining interest and creating space in the biotechnological field in different therapeutic areas and diseases due to their advantages such as broad range of target, low toxicity, high diversity, high potency and selectivity to receptor. Same time there are many challenges too, the efficacy of the peptide drug should not be compromised at any cost, peptides have limited bioavailability due to their short half-life, rapid clearance from systemic circulation, poor permeability and low stability in plasma. To overcome all of the problems associated with the peptide drugs till date peptide scientists have made many effectors to make peptide-based drug delivery system more efficient and available for its therapeutic use. Various approaches and strategies and numbers of in silico tools are developed in past decades for making peptide drug design faster and more stable by increasing their half-life and enhancing its serum stability. Another thing involved in peptide drug is suitable method development, its applicability for peptide and its characterization, optimized and validated methods to detect the effectiveness of peptide and their quality throughout the shelf life of the drug. Also, to make it available and viable commercially drug manufacturer has to think about its cost involve for initial set up of manufacturing facility and overall COGS per dose per individual/patient.

3.8 Future Prospects

Peptide-based drug design and delivery system have created space in different therapeutic areas for different indications. Advancement in technology, bioinformatic tools and innovative ideas for molecular target and new indications would make peptide-based drug delivery system more popular and first line of treatment in coming days by continuing research in identifying new peptides and its therapeutic use. Finally, peptide-based drug delivery system and extension of half-life approaches are the scope of area for scientists. Effort should be towards the improving oral bioavailability by means of increasing peptide drug stability in gastrointestinal tract. Also, formulation of peptide using permeability enhancers and improving availability of peptide drug at CNS will increase through conjugation and by novel technology.

References

1. Rick, S., Oral protein and peptide drug delivery, in: *Drug Delivery: Principles and Applications*, W. Binghe, S. Teruna, S. Richard, (Eds.), p. 189, Wiley Interscience, New Jersey, 2005.
2. Adessi, C. and Sotto, C., Converting a peptide into a drug: Strategies to improve stability and bioavailability. *Curr. Med. Chem.*, 9, 963–978, 2002.

3. Adessi, C. and Sotto, C., Strategies to improve stability and bioavailability of peptide drugs. *Front. Med. Chem.*, 1, 513–528, 2004.
4. Otvos, L., *Methods in Molecular Biology, Peptide-Based Drug Design E*, vol. 494, p. 1, © Humana Press, New York, NY, 2008.
5. Sayani, A.P. and Chien, Y.W., Systemic delivery of peptides and proteins across absorptive mucosae. *Crit. Rev. Ther. Drug Carrier Syst.*, 13, 85–184, 1996.
6. Lau, J.L. and Dunn, M.K., Therapeutic peptides: Historical perspectives, current development trends, and future directions. *Bioorg. Med. Chem.*, 26, 10, 2700–2707, June 1, 2018.
7. Adjei, A. and Gupta, P., Pulmonary delivery of therapeutic peptides and proteins. *J. Control. Release*, 29, 361–373, 1994.
8. Antunes, F., Andrade, F., Ferreira, D., Nielson, H.M., Sarmento, B., Models to predict intestinal absorption of therapeutic peptides and proteins. *Curr. Drug Metab.*, 14, 4–20, 2013.
9. Di, L., Strategic approaches to optimizing peptide ADME properties. *AAPS J.*, 17, 134–143, 2014.
10. Sood, A. and Panchagnula, R., Peroral route: An opportunity for protein and peptide drug delivery. *Chem. Rev.*, 101, 3275–3303, 2001.
11. Ram, I.M., Ajit, S.N., Laura, T., Duane, D.M., Emerging trends in oral delivery of peptide and protein drugs. *Crit. Rev. Ther. Drug Carrier Syst.*, 20, 153–214, 2003.
12. Lee, V.H.L., Satish, D.K., George, M.G., Werner, R., Oral route of protein and peptide drug delivery, in: *Peptide and Protein Drug Delivery*, V.H. Lee, (Ed.), pp. 691–738, Marcel Dekker, New York, 1991.
13. Saffran, M., Kumar, G., Savariar, C., Burnham, J., Williams, F., Neckers, D., A new approach to the oral administration of insulin and other peptide drugs. *Science*, 233, 1081–1084, 1986.
14. Fix, J.A., Oral controlled release technology for peptides: Status and future prospects. *Pharm. Res.*, 13, 1760–1764, 1996.
15. Kaspar, A.A. and Reichert, J.M., Future directions for peptide therapeutics development. *Drug Discovery Today*, 18, 807–817, 2013.
16. Zhang, N., Ping, Q., Huang, G., Xu, W., Cheng, Y., Han, X., Lectin-modified solid lipid nanoparticles as carriers for oral administration of insulin. *Int. J. Pharm.*, 327, 1–2, 153–159, 2006.
17. Damgé, C., Michel, C., Aprahamian, M., Couvreur, P., Devissaguet, J.P., Nanocapsules as carriers for oral peptide delivery. *J. Control. Release*, 13, 2–3, 233–239, 1990.
18. Lundin, P.D.P., Bojrup, M., Ljusberg-Wahren, H., Weström, B.R., Lundin, S., Enhancing effects of monohexanoin and two other medium-chain glyceride vehicles on intestinal absorption of desmopressin (Ddavp). *J. Pharmacol. Exp. Ther.*, 282, 2, 585–590, 1997.
19. *Romiplostim, Prescribing Information*, Amgen, Thousands Oaks, CA, August 2008, Available at: www.nplate.com Accessed October 21, 2019.

20. Burzynski, J., New options after first-line therapy for chronic immune thrombocytopenic purpura. *Am. J. Health Syst. Pharm.*, 66, 11–21, 2009.
21. Dunn, M.K., Therapeutic peptides: Historical perspectives, current development trends, and future directions. *Bioorg. Med. Chem.*, 26, 10, 2700–2707, 2018.
22. Elkinton, J.R., Hunt Jr., A.D. *et al.*, Effects of pituitary adrenocorticotropic hormone (ACTH) therapy. *J. Am. Med. Assoc.*, 141, 1273–1279, 1949.
23. Banting, F.G., Best, C.H., Collip, J.B., Campbell, W.R., Fletcher, A.A., Pancreatic extracts in the treatment of diabetes mellitus. *Can. Med. Assoc. J.*, 12, 141–146, 1922.
24. Manning, M.C. *et al.*, Stability of protein pharmaceuticals: An update. *Pharm. Res.*, 27, 544–575, 2010.
25. Andersson, L., Blomberg, L., Flegel, M., Lepsa, L., Nilsson, B., Verlander, M., Large-scale synthesis of peptides. *Biopolymers*, 55, 3, 227–250, 2000.
26. Baggerman, G., Verleyen, P., Clynen, E., Huybrechts, J., De-Loof, A., Schoofs, L., Peptidomics. *J. Chromatogr. B Analyt. Technol. Biomed. Life Sci.*, 803, 1, 3–16, Apr 15, 2004.
27. Falciani, C., Lozzi, L., Pini, A., Bracci, L., Bioactive peptides from libraries. *Chem. Biol.*, 12, 4, 417–426, 2005.
28. Jenssen, H. and Aspmo, S., Serum stability of peptides. *Methods Mol. Biol.*, 494, 177–186, 2008.
29. Neurath, H., Evolution of proteolytic enzymes. *Science*, 224, 350–7, 1984.
30. Werle, M. and Bernkop-Schnurch, A., Strategies to improve plasma half life time of peptide and protein drugs. *Amino Acids*, 30, 351–367, 2006.
31. Uhlig, T., Kyprianou, T., Martinelli, F.G., Oppici, C.A., Heiligers, D., Hills, D. *et al.*, The emergence of peptides in the pharmaceutical business: From exploration to exploitation. *EuPA Open Proteom.*, 4, 58–69, 2014.
32. Yi, J., Kim, C., Gelfand, C.A., Inhibition of intrinsic proteolytic activities moderates preanalytical variability and instability of human plasma. *J. Proteome Res.*, 6, 1768–1781, 2007.
33. Saladin, P.M., Zhang, B.D., Reichert, J.M., Current trends in the clinical development of peptide therapeutics. *IDrugs*, 12, 779–784, 2009.
34. Lax, R., The future of peptide development in the pharmaceutical industry. *PharManufacturing: Int. Pept. Rev.*, 2, 10–15, 2010.
35. Banga, A.K. and Chien, Y.W., Systemic delivery of therapeutic peptides and proteins. *Int. J. Pharm.*, 48, 15–50, 1988.
36. Gurevich, E.V. and Gurevich, V.V., Therapeutic potential of small molecules and engineered proteins, in: *Handbook of Experimental Pharmacology*, vol. 219, pp. 1–12, 2014.
37. Kontermann, R.E., Strategies for extended serum half-life of protein therapeutics. *Curr. Opin. Biotechnol.*, 22, 868–876, 2011.
38. Werner, H.M., Cabalteja, C.C., Horne, W.S., Peptide backbone composition and protease susceptibility: Impact of modification type, position, and tandem substitution. *ChemBioChem*, 17, 712–718, 2016.

39. Rezai, T., Yu, B., Millhauser, G.L., Jacobson, M.P., Lokey, R.S., Testing the conformational hypothesis of passive membrane permeability using synthetic cyclic peptide diastereomers. *J. Am. Chem. Soc.*, 128, 2510–2511, 2006.
40. Kluskens, L.D., Nelemans, S.A., Rink, R., de Vries, L., Meter-Arkema, A., Wang, Y., Walther, T., Kuipers, A., Moll, G.N., Haas, M., Angiotensin-(1-7) with thioether bridge: An angiotensin-converting enzyme-resistant, potent angiotensin-(1-7) analog. *J. Pharm. Exp. Ther.*, 328, 849–854, 2009.
41. Kale, S.S., Villequey, C., Kong, X.D., Zorzi, A., Deyle, K., Heinis, C., Cyclization of peptides with two chemical bridges affords large scaffold diversities. *Nat. Chem.*, 10, 715–723, 2018.
42. Bruno, B.J., Miller, G.D., Lim, C.S., Basics and recent advances in peptide and protein drug delivery. *Ther. Deliv.*, 4, 1443–1467, 2013.
43. Weinstock, M.T., Francis, J.N., Redman, J.S., Kay, M.S., Protease-resistant peptide design-empowering nature's fragile warriors against HIV. *Biopolymers*, 98, 431–442, 2012.
44. Werner, H.M., Cabalteja, C.C., Horne, W.S., Peptide backbone composition and protease susceptibility: Impact of modification type, position, and tandem substitution. *ChemBioChem*, 17, 712–718, 2016.
45. Puente, X.S., Gutierrez-Fernandez, A., Ordonez, G.R., Hillier, L.W., Lopez-Otin, C., Comparative genomic analysis of human and chimpanzee proteases. *Genomics*, 86, 638–647, 2005.
46. Werle, M. and Bernkop-Schnurch, A., Strategies to improve plasma half life time of peptide and protein drugs. *Amino Acids*, 30, 351–367, 2006.
47. Jambunathan, K. and Galande, A.K., Design of a serum stability tag for bioactive peptides. *Protein Pept. Lett.*, 21, 32–38, 2014.
48. Di, L., Strategic approaches to optimizing peptide ADME properties. *AAPS. J.*, 17, 134–143, 2015.
49. Corbi-Verge, C., Garton, M., Nim, S., Kim, P.M., Strategies to develop inhibitors of motif-mediated protein-protein interactions as drug leads. *Annu. Rev. Pharmacol. Toxicol.*, 57, 39–60, 2017.
50. Fosgerau, K. and Hoffmann, T., Peptide therapeutics: Current status and future directions. *Drug Discovery Today*, 20, 122–128, 2015.
51. Muttenthaler, M., King, G.F., Adams, D.J. *et al.*, Trends in peptide drug discovery. *Nat Rev Drug Discov.*, 20, 309–325, 2021. https://doi.org/10.1038/s41573-020-00135-8; And Lee, A.C., Harris, J.L., Khanna, K.K., Hong, J.H., A comprehensive review on current advances in peptide drug development and design. *Int. J. Mol. Sci.*, 20, 10, 2383, 2019. https://doi.org/10.3390/ijms20102383.
52. Lee, V., *Peptide and Protein Drug Delivery*, vol. 4, CRC Press, 1990.; Zhou, X.H. and Po, A.L.W., Peptide and protein drugs: II. Non-parenteral routes of delivery. *Int J Pharm.*, 75, 2, 117–130, 1991.
53. Lin, J.H. and Lu, A.Y., Role of pharmacokinetics and metabolism in drug discovery and development. *Pharmacol. Rev.*, 49, 403–449, 1997.

54. Werle, M. and Bernkop-Schnurch, A., Strategies to improve plasma half life time of peptide and protein drugs. *Amino Acids*, 30, 351–367, 2006.
55. Gentilucci, L., De Marco, R., Cerisoli, L., Chemical modifications designed to improve peptide stability: Incorporation of non-natural amino acids, pseudo-peptide bonds, and cyclization. *Curr. Pharm. Des.*, 16, 3185–3203, 2010.
56. Lubell, W.D., Peptide-based drug development. *Biomedicines*, 10, 8, 2037, 2022.
57. Jenssen, H. and Aspmo, S., II, Serum stability of peptides. *Methods Mol. Biol.*, 494, 177–186, 2008.
58. Fauchère, J.-L., Elements for the rational design of peptide drugs. *Adv. Drug Res.*, 15, 29–69, 1986.
59. Handelman, A., Natan, A., Rosenman, G., Structural and optical properties of short peptides: Nanotubes-to-nanofibers phase transformation. *J. Pept. Sci.*, 20, 487–493, 2014.
60. Craik, D.J., Fairlie, D.P., Liras, S., Price, D., The future of peptide-based drugs. *Chem. Biol. Drug Des.*, 81, 136–147, 2013.
61. Ruffner, H., Bauer, A., Bouwmeester, T., Human protein–protein interaction networks and the value for drug discovery. *Drug Discovery Today*, 12, 709–716, 2007.
62. Yan, C., Wu, F., Jernigan, R.L., Dobbs, D., Honavar, V., Characterization of protein-protein interfaces. *Protein J.*, 27, 59–70, 2008.
63. Bird, G.H., Irimia, A., Ofek, G., Kwong, P.D., Wilson, I.A., Walensky, L.D., Stapled HIV-1 peptides recapitulate antigenic structures and engage broadly neutralizing antibodies. *Nat. Struct. Mol. Biol.*, 21, 1058–1067, 2014.
64. Verdine, G.L. and Hilinski, G.J., Stapled peptides for intracellular drug targets, 1st ed, vol. 503, Elsevier Inc, 2012. https://doi.org/10.1016/B978-0-12-396962-0.00001-X
65. Tsomaia, N., Peptide therapeutics: Targeting the undruggable space. *Eur. J. Med. Chem.*, 94, 459–470, 2015.
66. Bird, G.H., Crannell, W.C., Walensky, L.D., Chemical synthesis of hydrocarbon-stapled peptides for protein interaction research and therapeutic targeting. *Curr. Protoc. Chem. Biol.*, 3, 99–117, 2011.
67. Chang, Y.S., Graves, B., Guerlavais, V., Tovar, C., Packman, K., To, K.-H., Stapled α-helical peptide drug development: A potent dual inhibitor of MDM2 and MDMX for p53-dependent cancer therapy. *Proc. Natl. Acad. Sci.*, 110, E3445–E3454, 2013.
68. Felix, A.M., Heimer, E.P., Wang, C.T., Lambros, T.J., Fournier, A., Mowles, T.F., Synthesis, biological activity and conformational analysis of cyclic GRF analogs. *Int. J. Pept. Protein Res.*, 32, 441–454, 1988.
69. Shepherd, N.E., Hoang, H.N., Abbenante, G., Fairlie, D.P., Single turn peptide alpha helices with exceptional stability in water. *J. Am. Chem. Soc.*, 127, 2974–2983, 2005.

70. Gilson, M.K. and Zhou, H.-X., Calculation of protein-ligand binding affinities. *Annu. Rev. Biophys. Biomol. Struct.*, 36, 21–42, 2007.
71. Böttger, R., Hoffmann, R., Knappe, D., Differential stability of therapeutic peptides with different proteolytic cleavage sites in blood, plasma and serum. *PloS One*, 12, 6, e0178943, 2017.
72. Hoffmann, R., Bulet, P., Urge, L., Otvos Jr., L., Range of activity and metabolic stability of synthetic antibacterial glycopeptides from insects. *Biochim. Biophys. Acta*, 1426, 459–467, 1999.
73. Yu, Z., Kastenmüller, G., He, Y., Belcredi, P., Möller, G., Prehn, C., Mendes, J., Wahl, S., Roemisch-Margl, W., Ceglarek, U., Polonikov, A., Dahmen, N., Prokisch, H., Xie, L., Li, Y., Wichmann, H.E., Peters, A., Kronenberg, F., Suhre, K., Adamski, J., Illig, T., Wang-Sattler, R., Differences between human plasma and serum metabolite profiles. *PLoS One,* 6, 7, e21230, 2011.

4

Data Analytics and Data Visualization for the Pharmaceutical Industry

Shalin Parikh[1], Ravi Patel[2], Dignesh Khunt[2*], Vivek P. Chavda[3] and Lalitkumar Vora[4†]

[1]Senores Pharmaceuticals Pvt. Ltd., Ahmedabad, Gujarat, India
[2]Graduate School of Pharmacy, Gujarat Technological University, Gandhinagar, Gujarat, India
[3]Department of Pharmaceutic and Pharmaceutical Technology, L M College of Pharmacy, Ahmedabad, India
[4]School of Pharmacy, Queen's University Belfast, Northern Ireland, UK

Abstract
In pharmaceutical science, multi-step drug product development processes generate an enormous amount of datasets each day as a part of chemistry, pre-clinical and clinical processes, as well as further drug product approval and pharmacovigilance. In creating useful knowledge from data and information, harnessing data analytics/visualization is a practical step for pharmaceutical researchers. In conjunction with stricter government regulation and increased competition, good data analysis is critical in the 21st century. Pharma data analytics/visualization from immense volumes of data set reveals unexpected connections and cuts through noisy data to join the correct dots to get better outcomes more quickly. A data scientist could play a knowledge bridge between the multiple departments and multidisciplinary teams in the pharmaceutical industry to speed up drug product development and reduce the economic burden. This chapter describes the importance of data analytics and visualization from drug chemistry to drug product development, valuable tools to do so, and real-time examples in the pharmaceutical and clinical world.

**Corresponding author*: digneshkhunt80@gmail.com: Orcid ID: 0000-0002-8850-7468
†*Corresponding author*: L.Vora@qub.ac.uk: Orcid ID: 0000-0001-8106-9066

Vivek Chavda, Krishnan Anand and Vasso Apostolopoulos (eds.) Bioinformatics Tools for Pharmaceutical Drug Product Development, (55–76) © 2023 Scrivener Publishing LLC

Keywords: Data analytics, data visualization, data science, product lifecycle, process

4.1 Introduction

To uncover untapped markets, pharma companies can use data science to identify potential customers and do further research. And maybe even coming up with a cure for people in need [1–4]. In the pharmaceutical industry, data science can track sales activity and provide sales-related insights. Data science is a rapidly expanding field of study for many students nowadays. Data science applies scientific techniques to gathering, analyzing, and using data [5]. Data science is unique in that it combines multiple academic fields to attain its objectives. Careers in data science need knowledge and skills from a wide range of academic disciplines, including advanced mathematics, computer science, and statistics. As a consequence, obtaining a degree in data science opens the door to an almost uncountable amount of job opportunities in a wide variety of fields that require this skill set.

Data science is an interdisciplinary subject that uses scientific methodologies, data mining, machine-learning algorithms, and large amounts of data to extract information and insights. The healthcare business creates vast databases, including valuable information on patient demographics, treatment plans, test findings, insurance, etc., [6]. Data scientists are interested in the information gathered by Internet of Things (IoT) devices. Data science offers assistance for processing, managing, analyzing, and integrating the vast amounts of scattered, organized, and unorganized data produced by healthcare systems. This data needs efficient administration and analysis to get accurate findings [7].

Before a medicine ever reaches the clinical trial phase, the screening procedure consumes the majority of the money spent by the pharmaceutical industry. This ends up being a protracted and costly procedure, as ill persons await the approval of new pharmaceuticals that potentially treat their ailment [8, 9]. Now, data science is being used to shorten and potentially reduce the cost of this hitherto lengthy procedure. Using predictive analytics, businesses may prioritize the most probable beneficial items and components in medicinal therapy. These selections will be based on a range of collected facts that will assist them in selecting from the hundreds of accessible possibilities.

To stay at the vanguard of biomedical innovation in the future decades, pharmaceutical firms must concentrate on acquiring and maintaining the greatest data science expertise available. In the past, computational scientists were often employed in the pharmaceutical sector using the same processes, criteria, and designations as experimental scientists. While this makes sense from the standpoint of equating education level and years of experience, it does not represent the increased demand for (and decreasing supply of) data scientists in the worldwide labor market [10]. Moreover, computational biologists, chemists, and biostatisticians may use their quantitative talents in other areas, such as the technology and finance sectors. As the data scientist is a fairly young career, it is crucial that pharmaceutical firms continue to develop and align themselves with international data science industry norms [11].

This manuscript covers the aspect of data analytics and data visualization for the entire path of pharmaceutical drug product development and product lifecycle.

4.2 Data Analytics

Analyzing data is referred to as "Data Analytics." It is also known as "Pharma Analytics" when it comes to drug manufacturing, identifying and developing novel drugs; targeting specific demographics; conducting clinical trials; and evaluating drug efficacy [12, 13]. Information technology, statistics, and business all come together to form a single entity known as data analytics. There are various aspects of the data analytics process that can benefit a wide range of projects. A good data analytics program will give you a clear picture of where you are, where you've been, and where you should be going by combining these components [14]. According to McKinsey, predictive analytics' potential influence in discovering and developing new breakthrough medications could increase by 45 to 70% over the next decade [15].

Big data analytics provides actionable insights at every stage of the manufacturing process through the translation of big data into actionable insights. Pharmaceutical firms can achieve greater success by leveraging the insights gained from big data. Data mining, data management, and statistical analysis are the key processes in the data analytics process [15]. It is up to the data and the purpose of the analysis to determine the relative importance and balance of these processes. The early steps in data mining are critical and time-consuming. Unstructured data sources, such as written language, raw data, or more complicated large-scale data, can all be used to get this information. Data extraction, transformation, and loading are the major processes in this process, which transform raw data into a usable and manageable format [15]. Data management entails the creation and execution of databases that make it possible to quickly access the findings of data mining projects, such as data warehouses [15]. Statistical and machine learning methods are used to decipher the data. Statistical models that highlight patterns in data can be built using large amounts of big data [15]. Predictions can be made, and decisions can be guided using these models and new data. This procedure requires statistical programming languages like R or Python [15].

Any phase of the drug development process can benefit from the use of data analytics in pharmaceutical companies. The application of pharma analytics in the R & D stage, for example, can hasten the discovery of new drugs and increase their quality. Based on market research and other variables, pharmaceutical businesses may employ cutting-edge techniques such as machine learning (ML) and artificial intelligence (AI) to do predictive analytics [15]. Batch processing software can be used by pharmaceutical companies to speed up the regulatory approval process by re-creating the entire batch procedure. To put it another way, this means that businesses can quickly ramp up to their maximum capacity [11]. Process optimization technologies can be used by pharmaceutical companies to identify areas for improvement in their day-to-day operations. When used in conjunction with process optimization technologies, pharma analytics may help manufacturers enhance resource management, quality assurance, and customer satisfaction [15]. In addition to machine learning, the internet of things (IoT) is a useful field. A great deal of data can be gleaned from these devices. Sensors in IoT devices are commonly used to gather useful information for their operation. Temperature and movement are tracked by devices like the Nest thermostat in order to control heating and cooling. Smart devices, such as this one, may learn from and predict your actions based on the data they collect. As a result, you'll have cutting-edge home automation that changes to fit your lifestyle [16].

Drug research, production, and distribution can benefit greatly from the use of data analytics, which can speed up the creation of new drugs, improve clinical trials, and enhance the ability to identify specific patients. Data analytics has an apparently limitless number of uses. Data analytics can be applied to a wider range of industries, including business, science, and everyday life, as more and more data is gathered each day [17].

4.3 Data Visualization

The goal of data visualization is to make data easier to understand and extract insights from by presenting it in a visual style such as a map or graph. Data visualization's primary purpose is to make it easier to discover patterns, trends, and outliers in massive datasets [17]. Information graphics, information visualization, and statistical graphics are all terms that can be used to describe the same thing. After data has been collected, processed, and modelled, one of the processes in the data science process specifies that it must be visualized before conclusions can be drawn. Additionally, data visualization is part of the broader field of data presentation architecture (DPA), which tries to search, locate, and modify data in the most effective manner possible before formatting and delivering it [17, 18].

Advanced data visualization technology is being increasingly used by the creators of data analytics apps to handle large volumes of data, process information, and better understand the outcomes of analytic efforts. Data analytics and business intelligence technologies must be used together to get the most out of large amounts of data. It is very important that the information is presented in a clear and concise manner [17, 19]. Data analysis is rendered meaningless if it fails to capture the substance of it. Data visualization for big data typically goes beyond traditional techniques such as pie charts, histogram plots, and business graphs. Heat maps and fever charts, on the other hand, are used as more complicated visualizations [20]. It takes sophisticated computers to collect raw data, interpret it, and create graphical representations that humans can use to swiftly make conclusions from the information. Data visualization tactics are being transformed by AI, which is a critical component in dealing with large amounts of data. Processing enormous amounts of data, frequently in real-time, from a wide range of sources, is enabled by AI. It also allows them to put more emphasis on data interpretation than analysis [20]. Future data visualization will focus on making the process more dynamic and allowing scientists to experiment with the data. Virtual reality (VR) has been used by pharmaceutical companies to see protein targets and small compounds and to examine interactions between them in a visual three-dimensional manner. VR-based solutions for drug discovery could be useful on a variety of platforms. Finding and validating pharmacological targets may be aided by systems for human genome study. Others can be used to map the dynamic 3D forms of free drug molecules, revealing previously unknown information about their behavior and physical properties [21]. Mixed reality (MR) combines features of virtual reality (VR) and augmented reality (AR). A device like Microsoft's Hololens is used in MR to create an immersive hologram that allows users to interact with virtual objects in the real world [5, 22, 23].

There are numerous ways in which data visualization tools might be used. As a reporting tool, it is its most popular use today. Using visualization technologies, dashboards may be automatically generated to monitor and visualize a company's performance across a variety of metrics. Microsoft, IBM, SAP, and SAS are just a few of the well-known manufacturers of big data software. The market for big data visualization software is dominated by the likes of Tableau, Qlik, and Tibco [24].

Drug discovery, clinical trials, marketing, sales analytics, and competitive analysis will benefit from data visualization in the pharmaceutical business. Cell culture studies, drug-target interaction studies, biochemical imaging studies, pathology studies, genomic transcriptomic metabolomics, and proteomic studies all require the appropriate tools for mining and visualizing the data they generate. Cloud and web-based solutions have revolutionized data analysis and visualization. Transform the way we see information by making it openly available through open-source data. Using machine learning and artificial intelligence, drug discovery and personalized medicine will be easier [22, 23].

4.4 Data Analytics and Data Visualization for Formulation Development

The pharmaceutical industry is distinguished by a number of peculiar characteristics, both in its organizational structure and in the nature of its commercial activities. These peculiarities are not widely known outside of the industry, but they have a significant impact on the method by which new pharmaceuticals are introduced to the market [25]. The production of a brand-new pharmaceutical requires a significant investment of time and resources, carries a significant financial burden, and entails a significant degree of risk, with only a remote possibility of yielding a fruitful result. The process of research and development is broken down here, along with all of the obstacles it presents, including those related to the environment [25].

Recently, the introduction of big data, machine learning, different analytical virtual tool, and data visualization is improved the success rate of the development of new pharmaceutical products. Not only new chemical entity (NCE) synthesis is crucial, but the development of a suitable formulation or carrier for delivery is also. Formulation development is a crucial aspect of product development that can define a pharmaceutical product's patentability, lifetime, and ultimate success [25]. Formulation success is dependent on the data integrity and their interpretation. In formulation development, data is represented as graphical or numerical. The process of analyzing data sets in order to identify patterns and arrive at inferences on the information that they hold is referred to as data analytics [26]. The analysis of data is increasingly carried out with the assistance of specialist computer systems and software. Commercial industries make extensive use of the tools and practices of data analytics in order to assist enterprises in making better-informed business decisions [26]. Analytics tools are also utilized by researchers and scientists in the scientific community in order to validate or invalidate scientific models, theories, and hypotheses. Process data analytics (also known as process analytics) refers to the methodologies deemed beneficial for analyzing data from manufacturing processes, regardless of whether the underlying phenomena are predominantly biological or chemical. In the pharmaceutical sector, process data analytics are being utilized for both chemically and biologically derived medicinal products. Using first-principles knowledge, models for chemically produced drug products, often known as small-molecule medicines, can be developed [27].

The term "data analytics" is commonly used to refer to the processes that are responsible for the fundamental data organization. It is possible to divide data analytics into four categories: descriptive, predictive, diagnostic, and prescriptive data analytics. Predictive analytics is the most dynamic strategy for data analytics out of these methodologies. It incorporates an advanced statistical methodology and algorithms based on artificial intelligence. Advanced analytics includes a subfield called predictive analytics (PA), which is widely used for making educated guesses about what might happen in the unknowable future [28].

Dong, 2021 [29] developed the PharmaSD program based on Python for the in silico formulation of stable solid dispersion. Here, their predictive analytics are used for the prediction of physical stability, dissolution type, and dissolution rate of solid dispersion independent using a regression model [29]. Figure 4.1 shows the graphical representation of the PharmaSD program. Data analytical also help to predict the drug release from various systems such as microsphere [30], Thermosensitive Chitosan Hydrogels [31].

Data visualization is a growing area of technological research and development. Massive amounts of data acquired from numerous sources must be managed, and engineering and production processes must be optimized. Data visualization approaches provide an intuitive way to learn from complex data and share knowledge with others. How to show data objects having multi-dimensional information is a critical challenge for data visualization techniques. Reduced data dimensionality is one method for visualizing multi-dimensional data in a two-dimensional (2D) or three-dimensional (3D) space [32]. Principal component analysis and partial

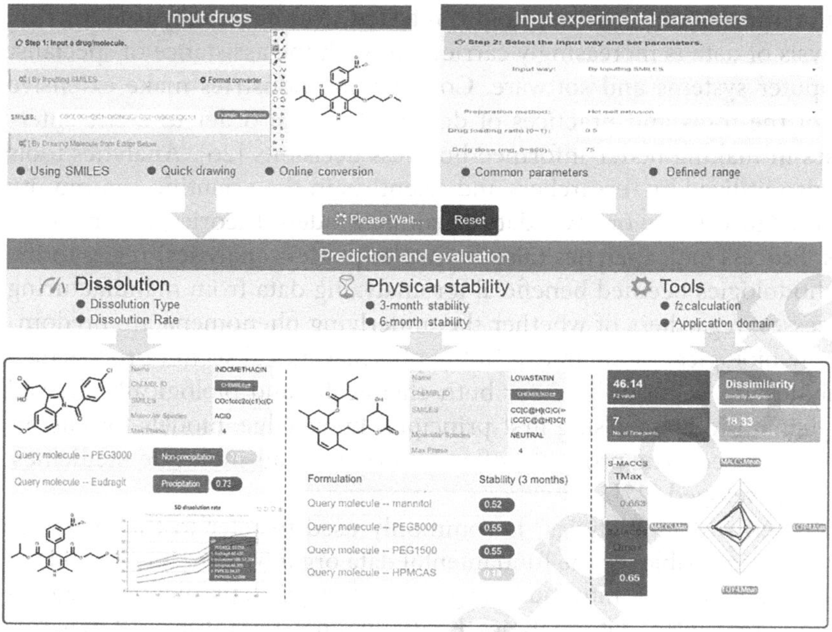

Figure 4.1 PharmaSD program for the *in silico* formulation of solid dispersion. (Reprinted with permission from Dong, 2021 [29]).

least squares approaches are common dimensionality reduction methods in which linear combinations of variables are carefully investigated to explain the greatest amount of variation in the original data set [32].

The data pertaining to the formulation is depicted in graphs, tables, and charts. A table is a methodical way of presenting statistical data in the form of vertical columns and horizontal rows, organized in accordance with some classification of the subject being discussed. The information on the tablets is intended to be presented in an organized manner that is free of clutter. Tables should not be used for numerical data if the data can be summarized simply in the text or if the relationship between the data can be clearly represented in a graph. In these cases, the data should instead be displayed in graph form. A good table is one that is not overly complicated, that focuses on a manageable number of key concepts, that is successful in presenting those concepts, and that can explain itself [33].

Figures are helpful for summarizing, explaining, or interpreting quantitative data as they use graphics to make difficult information easier to understand. If you have a modest quantity of data to present, you can utilize graphs rather than tables to do so. This is because graphs are more effective at displaying big amounts of data. A graph format that most effectively communicates the information must be selected in order to ensure that the researcher can easily comprehend the data. Examples of data visualization include drug release, drug dissolution, the impact of a process or product parameter on a critical quality attribute, and so on [33]. Graphing tools like Microsoft Excel, SPSS, STATA, SAS, and R are among the most popular options. The representation of quantitative data can take many forms, including line charts, frequency curves, histograms, scatter diagrams, and so on. The presentation of qualitative information may take the form of pie charts, bar charts, diagrams of maps, pictograms, etc.

Process capability and design space is the most commonly used parameter for the optimization of the formulation. The process capability is measured by how well it can adhere to its outlined guidelines. The capacity analysis evaluates the product specifications in light of the inherent unpredictability of a process to assess how well they match up. The part of the process variation that is due to common sources is referred to as the "inherent variability" of the process. The other kind of variability in a process is one that is brought on by particular reasons of variation [34]. The design space can be used to define the link between process inputs (material attributes and process parameters) and critical quality attributes [35]. A design space can be represented in terms of material attributes and process parameter ranges or more complicated mathematical connections. A design space can be described as a time-dependent function (for example, the temperature and pressure cycle of a lyophilization cycle) or as a mixture of variables such as components of a multivariate model. If the design space is meant to cover many operational scales, scaling factors can also be incorporated. Historical data analysis can aid in the creation of a design space. Regardless of how a design space is created, it is assumed that using it will result in a product of the specified quality [35, 36].

Other visualization techniques such as HyperDC (Hyper-Dimensionally Embedded Cuboids) were used by Yamashita 2010 [32], which was shown in Figure 4.2.

HyperDEC solves the constraint of contour plots or 3D surface plots, which cannot depict the impacts of more than two variables at the same time. N-dimensional data is mapped onto a 2D rectangular region determined by recursive slice-and-dice subdivision of the x–y plane using HyperDEC (Figure 4.2) [32]. Figure 4.1 depicts a 4-dimensional, 5-level display with x3–x4 subgraphs nested in an x1–x2 graph. Thus, in the x–y absolute coordinate system, 4-dimensional data, such as (0, 0, 2, 2), (1, 4, 2, 3), and (3, 1, 1, 3), are assigned a unique position [32].

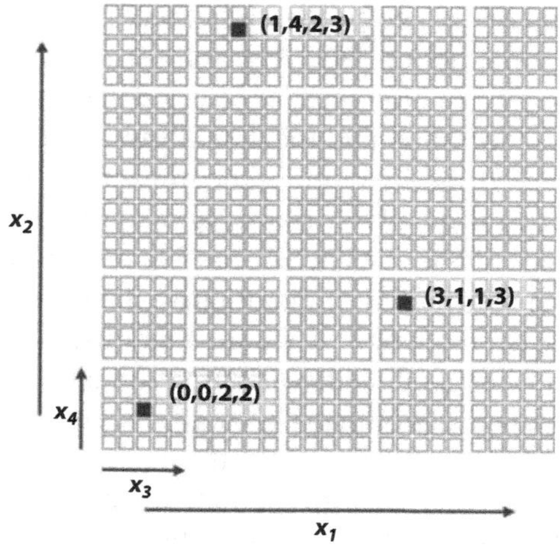

Figure 4.2 Graphical illustration of HyperDC. (Reprinted with permission from Yamashita, 2010 [32]).

The SeDeM method [37] is an innovative galenic approach that can be utilized in investigations pertaining to tablet preformulation (Figure 4.3). It describes the suitability of active substances and excipients in powder form for direct compression. The method of the SeDeM Diagram makes it possible to identify the powder properties that need to be enhanced in order to simplify the formulation of the final product for direct compression. The SeDeM Diagram approach is, therefore, also a valuable tool for examining the reproducibility of the procedure that is utilized to manufacture the

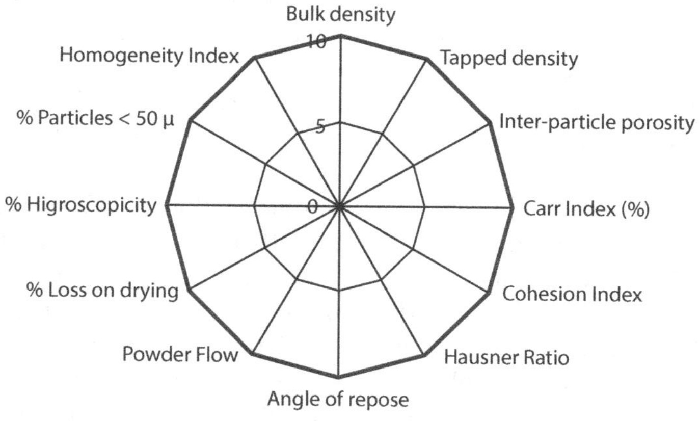

Figure 4.3 SeDem diagram. (Reprinted with permission from Suñé-Negre, 2014 [37]).

powder substance and, subsequently, for its validation. In addition to this, it has been demonstrated that it is an appropriate tool for preformulation and formulation. This is due to the fact that it characterizes the galenic properties of excipients in order to determine whether or not they are suitable for direct compression [37].

4.5 Data Analytics and Data Visualization for Drug Product Development

Pharmaceutics analytics has a wide range of applications. Pharma firms are trying to get to the top in today's dynamic and rapidly changing competitive arena while minimizing the entire cost of operations [1, 9]. It is imperative for pharmaceutical businesses to quickly adapt to new technologies like artificial intelligence and robotic process automation. Researchers in the pharmaceutical sector were able to obtain important information from Google Cloud through its COVID-19 Public Dataset Program. The pharmaceutical business has long relied on research and development (R&D). From 1, 198 in 2001 to 4, 800 in 2020, the number of pharmaceutical businesses with active R&D pipelines has increased dramatically. In response to the COVID-19 outbreak, businesses have ramped up the development of innovative new products. For the record, in 2020, there were a total of 17, 700 pharmaceuticals in the worldwide R&D pipeline [14, 15, 38]. Currently, new formulations especially Nano formulations are developed in the field of small molecules [2, 3, 39–41] as well as large molecules [4] where AI/ML helped a lot for the design of product like mRNA and DNA based vaccine for COVID-19 [42–46].

Many organizations' R&D activities have been accelerated because of the easy availability of data. The pharmaceutical industry also benefits from data in a number of other ways. In the pharmaceutical industry, data visualization is now become essential as even regulators are also supporting it [28].

This will help in summarizing the jargon of data and evaluate the same statistically to reach at some point of conclusion and help in further optimization process that will save time and cost [47, 48].

Visualization is a critical component to reaching the aim. But the type of visualization employed is essential. A couple of issues must be taken in account though. First, the tremendous amounts of data with potential interactions are not sufficient to offer a better comprehension. Second, movement in the pharmaceutical pipeline demands an awareness of numerous forms of data crossing several domains [49, 50]. Visualizations that make it possible to integrate at the analytical level are going to be of tremendous use to the pharmaceutical business [49, 51].

a. Importance of Data analytics in drug product development [9–11].

   i. Increases the accuracy of research
      COVID-19 vaccines have been developed by many businesses in less than a year, making it the quickest vaccination ever created [52]. The fact that pharmaceutical businesses, government agencies, and data analytics groups could easily share relevant data and information was a big benefit. Several processes in the R&D process can be sped up by free-flowing data exchange, as demonstrated during the pandemic response. In addition, researchers now have a clearer idea of who will be using the product thanks to the newly acquired data. Smaller sample numbers, better accuracy, reduced costs, and faster results can all be achieved with this method.
   ii. Enables the development of medical treatments that are more precise
      When, it comes to patient care, precision medicine means using information about a patient's genetic make-up, environmental circumstances, and behavioral patterns to develop diagnoses and treatments. Individuals' genes and habits can be taken into consideration in the development of tailored medicine. Patients' vulnerability to specific diseases can be better detected using this data-driven method by medicine manufacturers. In addition to reducing trial costs, precision medicine offers a greater success rate than more traditional techniques.
   iii. Real-time evaluation
      Trials will benefit immensely from the ability to obtain real-time data. With this, it's simpler to respond to difficulties in a timely manner and build more precise safety measures for trial participants, all leading to improved success rates from the R&D side. Real-world information such as medical records, insurance claims, and even social media may now be used to gather data. This information gives pharmaceutical companies a better understanding of how their products perform in the real world and across a broader range of people. The medications may now be fine-tuned and improved

because of this information. Major pharmaceutical corporations now have specialized teams gathering data from research and trials across different ailments. Their analysis of this information enables them to construct their treatments to be more powerful and effective while resisting the escalating expenses of traditional clinical trials and parallel research projects.

iv. Streamline the production process
After inventing a product, it needs to be mass-produced and disseminated. You need to know the suitable goals for the best Return on Investment. There will be a rise in this ease of production in the healthcare business and firms associated with it in the future. And with the pharmaceutical sector forecast to expand to $1.57 trillion in value, the use of data in streaming line manufacturing processes will only rise.

v. More streamlined distribution networks
Today's pharma organizations are moving away from old approaches and are embracing digital transformation and pharmaceutical data analysis on a far wider scale. As we discussed in our previous article on how to improve customer experience, this step enables them to understand and respond to the demands of both their consumers and stakeholders. You may simply validate data, spot abnormalities, benchmark operations, and get mobile and logistic reports using data analytics to increase your supply chain efficiency. Furthermore, data analytics for pharmaceutical development delivers real-time route optimization and enhanced inventory management, freeing up man-hours that would otherwise be spent watching and monitoring company operations.

b. Importance of Data visualization in drug product development [53–56].

i. Gene expression
Since microarrays were initially employed for whole organism screening, data visualization methods have been inseparable from them. Interactions are common in heat map implementations, allowing for more efficient exploration. "Brushing over a region to view gene names, conditions, and values; flipping nodes in a dendrogram to emphasize certain arrangements of interest; or adding extra columns of data

inside the same visualization help quick comprehension and further study of data."

ii. Lead discovery

In lead discovery, it's vital to identify, among a huge number of compounds, common chemical structures responsible for desirable bioactivities. One strategy is grouping the chemicals according to their spectrum of actions in biological tests of activity. Chemistry has traditionally relied on visual inspection to identify the specific properties of a chemical that are thought to be responsible for a certain property. Naturally, this technique can operate only for modest amounts of compounds. To take this form of analysis further, researchers today frequently define chemicals by a computer representation of their structure. Fast computer algorithms have been developed to swiftly produce fingerprints from hundreds of thousands of additional molecules. This strategy color codes the cell at the junction of a row and column according to some measure of importance.

iii. The intersection of biology and chemistry

Biologists often find targets, which are subsequently passed on to chemists for use in assay screening in traditional pharmaceutical processes, with minimal interaction at the interface between these realms. Because it necessitates knowledge from both fields, this intersection has been difficult to take advantage of.

iv. Toxicology and pre-clinical testing

Visualizing data from toxicological and pre-clinical research often create issues as the information is huge, scattered, in different category and quantitative that can be efficiently handled by data clustering. Enabled by such technologies, representations of toxicological and pre-clinical data can give an intuitive means for interpreting the huge amounts of data linked with these domains. The diagnosis established in pre-clinical studies is typically based on a person's subjective opinion, which is problematic.

v. Clinical

Novel techniques of displaying clinical data might give crucial insight into diagnosis and prospective therapy regimens Acute my Lloyd leukemia was the subject of a recent study in which researchers used our recent example. NSCLC is not a single illness but a class of neoplasms with distinct general defects and varying responses to therapies to elect whether successful treatments and estimate acceptable prognosis for specific patients it's therapeutically necessary to identify such genetic groupings.

4.6 Data Analytics and Data Visualization for Drug Product Life Cycle Management

Managing a product's whole lifespan, from conception to disposal, is what product lifecycle management aims to do. Product Lifecycle Management (PLM) lays the foundation for a company and its extended organization's product information. Also included are core functions such as data vaults, content management workflows, product analysis, and program management as well as the foundational technologies and standards [57, 58].

In recent years the pharmaceutical sector has encountered falling Research & Development productivity, a quickly changing healthcare landscape and severe competition from generics resulting in decreased growth and profit margins. Historically, medication development focused on clinical trials management and results. Increasingly, though, the industry is looking at more comprehensive ways to improve the delivery of new items to market, which may speed up product development while keeping operational costs to a minimum [57–59].

The heavily regulated environment necessitates complicated value chains and corporate processes, making this an uphill battle. There have been issues with pharmaceutical companies trying to adjust due to a lack of cross-functional collaboration, which is crucial in today's industry. Product Lifecycle Management, a business transformation approach for managing products and related information across the enterprise, is one key and holistic answer to today's present issues in the pharmaceutical sector. In recent years Product Lifecycle Management has offered several pharmaceutical companies with the capacity to boost their ability to deliver drugs to market quicker, assure higher regulatory compliance and efficiency while decreasing development costs [57, 58].

It's becoming increasingly important to pharmaceutical businesses to be able to observe and track all aspect of their product development process in one place. An important benefit of Agile Product Lifecycle Management is that it allows pharmaceutical businesses to make the most of their Information and Technology investments by reducing operational and production costs, shortening time to market, and meeting quality requirements like Quality by Design. Product governance may be made easier both internally and externally by enabling cross-functional teams to work together on a single, unified picture of their respective products throughout the business (i.e., compliance with regulatory agencies) [57, 58]. Several sensors monitor and review crucial system and process parameters in the pharmaceutical production process. Every products produced for the consumer contains a vast quantity of data defining every stage of the process, from arriving raw materials through process parameters, intermediate product features, and final product quality [60]. "Such manufacturing information include anything from basic laboratory analyses of incoming raw materials to complicated time series outputs for every second of the manufacturing process [61]." The information is maintained in a variety of databases and servers, and it is often only used to validate the quality of incoming raw materials, intermediate products, and finished goods. To assess the quality of data, any odd occurrences, and any needs for extra pre-processing or the entire removal of specific batches, use time series visualization. After that, do a process capability study to determine Ppk. A Ppk of more than 1 suggests a well-controlled process, which is anticipated for the chosen product. This is a highly reliable industrial method for managing product lifecycles [19].

As seen below, Product Life Cycle Management oversees the product's progress through several stages of production.

- Pharmaceutical compound creation
- Development of Novel Formulation (which comprises of container closure systems)
- Creation of experimental items and their production
- Development and finalization of a Delivery Method
- Manufacturing industry process improvement and expansion
- Analytical method Development
- Transmission of Technical Information New products are transferred across the development and production processes
- Transfers inside a production plant or between manufacturing and testing facilities for commercial items
- Commercial manufacturing
- Materials are acquired and controlled in a number of ways
- The supply of infrastructure, utilities, and equipment is a necessity
- Production and packaging

- Control and guarantee of product quality
- Storage and Distribution of Released Materials

Data analytics and visualization can be useful for various stages of drug product lifecycle management and to conclude and interpret various experiments as well as studies as below [57].

a. Study metadata
   Compounds, species, and populations are only mentioned in the study paperwork as well as other bits of data.
b. Controlled terminology
   Terminology is normally constant inside research, however among studies and throughout development programs the terminology is out of synchronization. Encoding all the various entities in a regulated method is especially critical for species, endpoints, and compounds.
c. Endpoint classification
   Endpoints may be compared across various chemicals and species using hierarchical grouping and clustering. In our approach the levels correlates to the granularity of the crucial question.
d. Treatment Effect Index Specifications
   Depending on the species, target, and illness kind, the specifics of how the Treatment Effect Index is computed may differ. With these explanations of how the baseline-controlled response and the placebo/vehicle are generated, it is clear just how important this impact is on a clinical and biological level.

4.7 Conclusion and Future Prospects

The pharmaceutical research phase of developing a new drug or pharmaceutical product is very lengthy and expensive in contrast with conventional products, so exploitation Industry 4.0-related digital technologies in the pharmaceutical development process might bring enormous benefits to industries. Industry 4.0 based new industrial revolution that employs cyber-physical technology to enhance the generation of digital and virtual data. "With the abundance of data across all aspects of the pharmaceutical industry, information visualization is promising as a vital component of discovery, development, and pharma business. Condense summaries that can offer a framework for understanding the immense volumes of data and that reveal unforeseen relationships have come to the frontline. And the capability to use these visualizations to cross domains and data types provides the ability to integrate analyses and support fast, efficient decisions [62]."

The early screening of large data sets by analytic tools during the drug discovery process will speed up the identification of lead molecules for pre-clinical and subsequent clinical development and it will create the possibility of automated drug discovery process. Cross-industry collaboration for data analytics and visualization will open the new avenue in pharmaceutical research. In the current situation of pandemic, various SARS-CoV-2 variants [63–65] emerges with many post COVID complications [66] like Omicron in this situation data analytics helps to understand the data jargon of genomic data generated that further supports in research. Data analytics and data visualization also helps in drug repurposing for COVID-19 [46, 67].

Not only that, but this may also open a new window of opportunity for the regulatory authorities to track and trace all phases of drug product development processes and that allows the timely decision or averts the delay in improving the product.

Recent development of AI and ML tools have gained considerable interest in pharmaceutical industry and these tools will play a pivotal role in coming years in transforming the newly synthesize drugs into clinical medicine in quicker and cost-effective manners. Specific emphasis will be given on artificial neural networks due to their capability to model the non-linear relations that are commonly confronted in pharmaceutical research. In coming days, AI and machine learning technologies for data analytics/visualization will be part of complete life cycle of pharmaceutical industry and regulatory body for more efficient, fast, and economical solutions.

References

1. Chavda, V., Sheta, S., Changani, D., Chavda, D., New bioinformatics platform-based approach for drug design, in: *Computation in Bioinformatics*, pp. 101–120, 2021.
2. Chavda, V.P., Patel, A.B., Mistry, K.J. *et al.*, Nano-drug delivery systems entrapping natural bioactive compounds for cancer: Recent progress and future challenges. *Front. Oncol.*, 12, 2022.
3. Chavda, V.P., Chapter 4 Nanobased nano drug delivery: A comprehensive review, in: *Micro and Nano Technologies*, S.S. Mohapatra, S. Ranjan, N. Dasgupta, R.K. Mishra, Thomas SBT-A of TND and DS (Eds.), pp. 69–92, Elsevier, 2019.

4. Chavda, V.P., Nanotherapeutics and nanobiotechnology, in: *Applications of Targeted Nano Drugs and Delivery Systems*, pp. 1–13, Elsevier, 2019.
5. Gubbi, J., Buyya, R., Marusic, S., Palaniswami, M., Internet of things (IoT): A vision, architectural elements, and future directions. *Future Gener. Comput. Syst.*, 29, 7, 1645–1660, 2013.
6. Subrahmanya, S.V.G., Shetty, D.K., Patil, V. *et al.*, The role of data science in healthcare advancements: Applications, benefits, and future prospects. *Ir. J. Med. Sci.*, 191, 1, 1473–1483, 2021.
7. Kumar, S., Tiwari, P., Zymbler, M., Internet of things is a revolutionary approach for future technology enhancement: A review. *J. Big Data*, 6, 1, 111, 2019.
8. Vivek, C., Patel, C., Bhadani, J., Metabolomics: At a glance. *RRJoDFDP*, 4, 1, 23–30, 2017.
9. Chavda, V.P., Ertas, Y.N., Walhekar, V. *et al.*, Advanced computational methodologies used in the discovery of new natural anticancer compounds. *Front. Pharmacol.*, 12, 702611, 2021.
10. Ferrero, E., Brachat, S., Jenkins, J.L. *et al.*, Ten simple rules to power drug discovery with data science. *PloS Comput. Biol.*, 16, 8, e1008126, 2020.
11. Kruchten, A.E., A curricular bioinformatics approach to teaching undergraduates to analyze metagenomic datasets using R. *Front. Microbiol.*, 11, 2020.
12. AspenTech, *Pharma Analytics*, Aspen Technol. Inc., https://www.aspentech.com/en/apm-resources/pharma-analytics. Retrieved 11 August, 2022.
13. *Master's in Data Science. What Is Data Analytics?*, 2U Inc, 2022, https://www.mastersindatascience.org/learning/what-is-data-analytics/. Retrieved 11 August, 2022.
14. Gui, H., Zheng, R., Ma, C., Fan, H., Xu, L., An architecture for healthcare big data management and analysis, in: *International Conference on Health Information Science*, pp. 154–160, Springer, 2016.
15. Darino, L., Knepp, A., Mills, N., Tinkoff, D., *How Pharma Can Accelerate Business Impact from Advanced Analytics*, McKinsey Co., 2018, https://www.mckinsey.com/industries/life-sciences/our-insights/how-pharma-can-accelerate-business-impact-from-advanced-analytics. Retrieved Aug 11, 2022.
16. Raghupathi, W. and Raghupathi, V., Big data analytics in healthcare: Promise and potential. *Health Inf. Sci. Syst.*, 2, 1, 1–10, 2014.
17. Do Nascimento, I.J.B., Marcolino, M.S., Abdulazeem, H.M. *et al.*, Impact of big data analytics on people's health: Overview of systematic reviews and recommendations for future studies. *J. Med. Internet Res.*, 23, 4, e27275, 2021.
18. Ventola, C.L., Big data and pharmacovigilance: Data mining for adverse drug events and interactions. *P. T.*, 43, 6, 340–351, 2018.
19. Zagar, J. and Mihelič, J., Big data collection in pharmaceutical manufacturing and its use for product quality predictions. *Sci. Data*, 9, 1, 99, 2022.
20. Buvailo, A., How big pharma adopts AI to boost drug discovery, *BiopharmaTrend Newsletter*. Retrieved April 27, 2020.

21. Perilla, J.R. and Schulten, K., Physical properties of the HIV-1 capsid from all-atom molecular dynamics simulations. *Nat. Commun.*, 8, 1, 1–10, 2017.
22. Bhuiyan, M.N., Rahman, M.M., Billah, M.M., Saha, D., Internet of things (IoT): A review of its enabling technologies in healthcare applications, standards protocols, security and market opportunities. *IEEE Internet Things J.*, 8, 13, 10474–10498, 2021.
23. Javaid, M. and Khan, I.H., Internet of Things (IoT) enabled healthcare helps to take the challenges of COVID-19 pandemic. *J. Oral. Biol. Craniofac. Res.*, 11, 2, 209–214, 2021.
24. Feinleib, D., The big data landscape, in: *Big Data Bootcamp*, pp. 15–34, Springer, 2014.
25. Taylor, D., The pharmaceutical industry and the future of drug development, in *Pharmaceuticals in the Environment*, 1–33, 2015.
26. Stedman, C., *Data Analytics (DA)*, TechTarget, 2020.
27. Severson, K.A., Van Antwerp, J.G., Natarajan, V., Antoniou, C., Thömmes, J., Braatz, R.D., A systematic approach to process data analytics in pharmaceutical manufacturing: The data analytics triangle and its application to the manufacturing of a monoclonal antibody, in: *Multivariate Analysis in the Pharmaceutical Industry*, pp. 295–312, Elsevier, 2018.
28. Chauhan, S., Singh, M., Aggarwal, A.K., Data science and data analytics: Artificial intelligence and machine learning integrated based approach, in: *Data Science and Data Analytics: Opportunity and Challenges*, 1, 2021.
29. Dong, J., Gao, H., Ouyang, D., PharmSD: A novel AI-based computational platform for solid dispersion formulation design. *Int. J. Pharm.*, 604, 120705, 2021.
30. Arifin, D.Y., Lee, L.Y., Wang, C.-H., Mathematical modeling and simulation of drug release from microspheres: Implications to drug delivery systems. *Adv. Drug Deliv. Rev.*, 58, 12, 1274–1325, 2006.
31. Zarzycki, R., Rogacki, G., Modrzejewska, Z., Nawrotek, K., Modeling of drug (Albumin) release from thermosensitive chitosan hydrogels. *Ind. Eng. Chem. Res.*, 50, 9, 5866–5872, 2011.
32. Yamashita, F., Itoh, T., Yoshida, S., Haidar, M.K., Hashida, M., A novel multidimensional visualization technique for understanding the design parameters of drug formulations. *Comput. Chem. Eng.*, 34, 8, 1306–1311, 2010.
33. Mistry, S., Presentation of data. *Solut. Pharm.*, 2021, https://solutionpharmacy.in/presentation-of-data/. Retrieved 11 August, 2022.
34. Vora, C., Patadia, R., Mittal, K., Mashru, R., Risk based approach for design and optimization of site specific delivery of isoniazid. *J. Pharm. Investig.*, 45, 2, 249–264, 2015.
35. Guideline ICHHT, *Pharmaceutical Development Q8 (R2) Current Step 4*, 2009.
36. Shah, B., Khunt, D., Bhatt, H., Misra, M., Padh, H., Application of quality by design approach for intranasal delivery of rivastigmine loaded solid lipid nanoparticles: Effect on formulation and characterization parameters. *Eur. J.*

Pharm. Sci., 78, 54–66, 2015. [Internet] Available from: http://www.sciencedirect.com/science/article/pii/S0928098715003231.
37. Suñé-Negre, J.M., Roig, M., Fuster, R. *et al.*, New classification of directly compressible (DC) excipients in function of the SeDeM diagarm expert system. *Int. J. Pharm.*, 470, 1, 15–27, 2014.
38. XcelPros, Importance of data & analytics in pharmaceutical product development, 2021, https://xcelpros.com/importance-of-data-analytics-in-pharmaceutical-product-development/. Retrieved 11 August, 2022.
39. Chavda, V.P., Vihol, D., Mehta, B. *et al.*, Phytochemical-loaded liposomes for anticancer therapy: An updated review. *Nanomedicine*, 17, 8, 547–568, 2022.
40. Chavda, V.P. and Shah, D., Chapter 25-Self-emulsifying delivery systems: One step ahead in improving solubility of poorly soluble drugs, in: *Micro and Nano Technologies*, A. Ficai, and Grumezescu AMBT-N for CT (Eds.), pp. 653–718, Elsevier, 2017.
41. Anand, K., Ramesh, M., Singh, T. *et al.*, One-step synthesis of picolinohydrazides from fusaric acid: DFT, structural characterization and molecular inhibitory studies on metastatic tumor-derived exosomal and non-exosomal proteins. *J. Mol. Struct.*, 1255, 132442, 2022.
42. Chavda, V.P., Hossain, M.K., Beladiya, J., Apostolopoulos, V., Nucleic acid vaccines for COVID-19: A paradigm shift in the vaccine development arena. *Biologics*, 1, 3, 337–356, 2021.
43. Chavda, V.P., Bezbaruah, R., Athalye, M. *et al.*, Replicating viral vector-based vaccines for COVID-19: Potential avenue in vaccination arena. *Viruses*, 14, 4, 759, 2022.
44. Chavda, V.P., Pandya, R., Apostolopoulos, V., DNA vaccines for SARS-CoV-2: Towards third generation vaccination era. *Expert Rev. Vaccines*, 20, 12, 1549–1560, 2021.
45. Basu, D., Chavda, V.P., Mehta, A.A., Therapeutics for COVID-19 and post COVID-19 complications: An update. *Curr. Res. Pharmacol. Drug Discovery*, 3, 100086, 2022.
46. Chavda, V.P., Kapadia, C., Soni, S. *et al.*, A global picture: Therapeutic perspectives for COVID-19. *Immunotherapy*, 14, 5, 2022.
47. Wognum, P.M. and van Drongelen, I.C.K., Process and impact of product data management implementation. *Int. J. Prod. Dev.*, 2, 1–2, 5–23, 2005.
48. Oliveira, D., *Integrating Tacit Knowledge in Product Lifecycle Management: A Holistic View of the Innovation Process*, 2022.
49. Gabrielsson, J., Dolgos, H., Gillberg, P.-G., Bredberg, U., Benthem, B., Duker, G., Early integration of pharmacokinetic and dynamic reasoning is essential for optimal development of lead compounds: Strategic considerations. *Drug Discovery Today*, 14, 7–8, 358–372, 2009.
50. Chen, E.P., Bondi, R.W., Zhang, C. *et al.*, Applications of model-based target pharmacology assessment in defining drug design and DMPK strategies: GSK experiences. *J. Med. Chem.*, 65, 9, 6926–6939, 2022.
51. Napier, C. and Wallis, R., The napiergram: A tool for visualising efficacy and safety data. *J. Pharmacol. Toxicol. Methods*, 2, 62, e12, 2010.

52. Chavda, V.P., Vora, L.K., Pandya, A.K., Patravale, V.B., Intranasal vaccines for SARS-CoV-2: From challenges to potential in COVID-19 management. *Drug Discovery Today*, 26, 11, 2619–2636, 2021.
53. Kroll, P., Hofer, A., Ulonska, S., Kager, J., Herwig, C., Model-based methods in the biopharmaceutical process lifecycle. *Pharm. Res.*, 34, 12, 2596–2613, 2017.
54. Cammarota, G., Ianiro, G., Ahern, A. *et al.*, Gut microbiome, big data and machine learning to promote precision medicine for cancer. *Nat. Rev. Gastroenterol. Hepatol.*, 17, 10, 635–648, 2020.
55. Olivera, P., Danese, S., Jay, N., Natoli, G., Peyrin-Biroulet, L., Big data in IBD: A look into the future. *Nat. Rev. Gastroenterol. Hepatol.*, 16, 5, 312–321, 2019.
56. Zand, A., Stokes, Z., Sharma, A., van Deen, W.K., Hommes, D., Artificial intelligence for inflammatory bowel diseases (IBD); Accurately predicting adverse outcomes using machine learning. *Dig. Dis. Sci.*, 1–12, 2022.
57. Stark, J., Product lifecycle management (PLM), in: *Product Lifecycle Management (Volume 1)*, pp. 1–32, Springer, 2022.
58. Mousavi, A., Mohammadzadeh, M., Zare, H., Developing a system dynamic model for product life cycle management of generic pharmaceutical products: Its relation with open innovation. *J. Open Innov. Technol. Mark. Complex.*, 8, 1, 14, 2022.
59. Szalma, S., Koka, V., Khasanova, T., Perakslis, E.D., Effective knowledge management in translational medicine. *J. Transl. Med.*, 8, 1, 1–9, 2010.
60. Su, Q., Ganesh, S., Moreno, M. *et al.*, A perspective on Quality-by-Control (QbC) in pharmaceutical continuous manufacturing. *Comput. Chem. Eng.*, 125, 216–231, 2019.
61. Zagar, J. and Mihelič, J., Creation of attribute vectors from spectra and time-series data for prediction model development. *IPSI Trans. Internet Res.*, 15, 2, 32–38, 2019.
62. Hariry, R.E., Barenji, R.V., Paradkar, A., From industry 4.0 to pharma 4.0, in: *Handbook of Smart Materials, Technologies, and Devices*, C.M. Hussain, and P. Di Sia (Eds.), Springer, Cham, 2021, https://doi.org/10.1007/978-3-030-58675-1_4-1.
63. Chavda, V.P., Patel, A.B., Vaghasiya, D.D., SARS-CoV-2 variants and vulnerability at the global level. *J. Med. Virol.*, 94, 7, 2986–3005, 2022.
64. Chavda, V.P. and Apostolopoulos, V., Is booster dose strategy sufficient for omicron variant of SARS-CoV-2? *Vaccines*, 10, 3, 367, 2022.
65. Chavda, V.P. and Apostolopoulos, V., Omicron variant (B.1.1.529) of SARS-CoV-2: Threat for the elderly? *Maturitas*, 158, 78–81, 2022.
66. Chavda, V.P. and Apostolopoulos, V., Mucormycosis–an opportunistic infection in the aged immunocompromised individual: A reason for concern in COVID-19. *Maturitas*, 58, 58–61, 2021.
67. Chavda, V.P., Gajjar, N., Shah, N., Dave, D.J., Darunavir ethanolate: Repurposing an anti-HIV drug in COVID-19 treatment. *Eur. J. Med. Chem. Rep.*, 3, 100013, 2021.

5

Mass Spectrometry, Protein Interaction and Amalgamation of Bioinformatics

Vivek Chavda[1], Kaustubh Dange[2*] and Madhav Joglekar[3]

[1]*Department of Pharmaceutic and Pharmaceutical Technology, L M College of Pharmacy, Ahmedabad, India*
[2]*Product Characterization Team, Lupin Ltd., Pune, Maharashtra, India*
[3]*Analytical Development Team, Lupin Ltd., Pune, Maharashtra, India*

Abstract
Mass spectrometry (MS) is the major and favorable analytical tool for the dynamic "-omics" technologies. It facilitates detection of thousands of proteins with its quantitation. Also, biologically active metabolites and body fluid can be analyzed in global as well as targeted way, at very trace amount level. With recent advances in MS technologies and sample handling strategies it is even possible to analyze single cells. With all advances in MS technology and Sample handling strategies, data interpretation part is still a challenging subject which are interdisciplinary, the notable domain-specific knowledge as well as sound knowledge about software platforms and mechanism behind the MS platform are needed for correct and optimal processing of data.

Keywords: Mass spectrometry, bioinformatics, protein interaction, proteomics, omics technology

5.1 Introduction

Mass spectrometry is a sensitive analytical technique in which molecule gets detected, identified and quantitated on basis of ratio of mass of ion to its charge. The development of high-throughput and quantitative MS proteomics workflows in recent time has increased the scope to understand

**Corresponding author*: kaustubhdange@gmail.com

Vivek Chavda, Krishnan Anand and Vasso Apostolopoulos (eds.) Bioinformatics Tools for Pharmaceutical Drug Product Development, (77–94) © 2023 Scrivener Publishing LLC

more about protein basic arrangement, it's function, alteration associated and global protein dynamics. Mass spectroscopy also provides qualitative information and with the help of proper controls to assay or with use of internal standards, the application further can be used for quantitative purposes (Table 5.1) [1].

Mass spectrometry plays very important role in analyzing Drug protein interactions, Protein-protein interactions, Pharmacokinetic and pharmacodynamics studies in clinical studies, Characterization of protein and peptide based new molecules and establishment of similarity between the drugs originated from chemical as well as biological origin [2].

MS coupled with LC techniques has wide range of applications. It provides valuable information about protein of interest, its structure and function relationship. The protein sample can be analyzed with 2 approaches i.e. top down and bottom up approach. Top down approach facilitates the understanding about the post translational modifications (PTMs) on the intact level and bottom down approach favors identification of PTMs by

Table 5.1 Implementation of mass spectrometry in various scientific field [1].

Field of study	Applications
Proteomics	Determination of protein structure, its function and folding pattern. Protein – protein interactions Determination of peptide fragments and post-translational changes. Relative or absolute quantitation of proteins. Monitor enzyme reactions, chemical modifications and protein digestion.
Drug Discovery	Chemical structures of medicinal synthetic compounds and their metabolites can be determined. In living organisms, look for metabolites.
Clinical Testing	Used in forensic analyses for identification of drug abuse. Also helpful in detection of disease biomarkers.
Genomics	Sequence short oligonucleotides.
Environment	Test food and beverages for impurity. Analyze soil sample pollutant.
Geology	Identify petrochemical content. Carbon mapping analysis.

digestion of the protein with various combinations of proteases and then building complete structure of protein with sequence analysis tools, also site of modification will be predicted. Commonly studied PTMs are oxidation, deamidation, acetylation, formylations etc. Apart from this MS gives information about sequence variants i.e. misincorporation of amino acid in protein sequence. Covalent interactions like disulphide bond can be studied with this approach. The quantitative analysis is now possible with new generations mass instruments coupled with different algorithm based softwares in which exact quantitation is done based on XIC. Matrix-assisted laser desorption ionization (MALDI) MS has been used to study noncovalent complexes as well [3].

Drug binding to proteins leads to changes in structural dynamics conformational modification in specimens that nullified regular protein function. Hydrogen exchange (HX) with MS causes structural modification in proteins which have higher impact on drug binding. HX MS can be used to analyze conformational changes, protein–drug binding affinity and characterize intermediates in protein folding and unfolding [4, 5]. The more explanation and brief study on HX MS have been recently carried out [6, 7].

Mass spectrometry coupled with techniques like ICP (Ion coupled plasma) and CE (Capillary electrophoresis) are gaining importance with advances in engineering filed which further helps in sensitive and accurate sample analysis. ICP-MS is used for study of metal ions by MS whereas CE-MS is where high resolution is the demand of analysis. In this chapter we will be dealing with few aspects of mass spectrometry analysis in brief.

5.2 Mass Spectrometry - Protein Interaction

In central dogma of molecular biology, proteins occupy distal strata. It is DNA where all genetic repositories reside while various RNAs and proteins (again coded by DNA) implement genetic plan. Since bulk of the cellular processes are carried out by proteins, in order to do that they interact their counterparts inside the cell, various organelles, cellular and non-cellular interfaces [8]. Cells can produce proteins of tremendous diversity and in varying abundances as per cellular requirements. To maintain a healthy order of this entire cellular symphony, proteins must interact in specific way with each other. While cells contain a large number of proteins of varied sizes and abundances, one protein virtually never serves only one purpose. A protein's exceptional capacity to fulfil several activities is common. The creation of many connections is the basic mechanism by which proteins carry out their various tasks. The nature of these interactions might be dynamic, spatially and temporally specified, steady, or transitory. One enzyme, for example, may have several substrates, and their control may have varying effects on cellular processes [9]. Similarly, one protein may be a component of numerous protein complexes, each with its own set of activities. Protein-protein interactions have become an important aspect of biological research because of their importance in cellular activities. Mass spectrometry-based proteomics allows to analyze protein expressions from which protein-protein interactions (PPI) can be judged and their interaction networks could be deduced [10].

5.2.1 The Prerequisites

PPI studies with mass can be staged in two phases. First setting affinity purification procedures and secondly mass spectrometry aided characterization of those purified complexes.

5.2.2 Finding Affinity Partner (The Bait)

Affinity purification together with mass spectrometry (AP-MS) procedure begins with identification of association partner i.e. an endogenous protein or its suitably tagged version to be used. Following are the different approaches.

5.2.3 Antibody-Based Affinity Tags

Endogenous proteins can be isolated from their host tissue wherein they express at their natural stages. Some proteins have lower endogenous levels, and their purification necessitates the availability of antibodies with high specificity and affinity in order to assure effective and clean purification.

5.2.4 Small Molecule Ligands

In most of the cases where availability of specific antibodies is a constrain, it has been proposed that small compounds, such as activity-based chemical probes or inhibitors, be covalently attached to a resin and used to isolate enzymes and their complexes. For example, histone deacetylase inhibitors were utilized in a large-scale investigation to examine their affinity for various complexes [11]. In another example, nucleic acids and engineered binding proteins were assessed for isolation of endogenous targets [12]. Small molecule ligands are advantageous for another reason for their amenability to cheaper synthetic processes and availability of versatile binding chemistries.

5.2.5 Fusion Protein-Based Affinity Tags

In this approach target protein is expressed as a fusion protein as a tag and purified using this tag specific antibodies.

5.3 MS Analysis

Once affinity purification approach has been established then isolated samples are analyzed by shotgun proteomics. It involves digestion of protein samples in to peptides [13]. These peptides are isolated and analyzed with the help of LC-MS. Mass spectroscopy measures the results based on fundamental character i.e. ratio of mass of ion to it's charge (m/z) and strength of the short chain amino acids eluting from the liquid chromatography. The selected individual peptides are fragmented of which spectra are recorded which is compared with already stored protein databases to characterize peptides and proteins [14]. This spectrometric method can be termed as qualitative as there is no direct relation between sum of peptide present and its intensity in results [15]. However, various techniques and applied science advancement have opened the door for mass spectrometry to quantify whole protein [16]. SILAC is one such approach which depends upon metabolic labelling to incorporate steady heavy isotopes into amino acid chain structure. Under some experimental settings, relative variations in small chain amino acid intensities indicate dissimilarity in protein surplus. While selection of a quantification approach is influenced by a variety of circumstances, firm isotope related technique have higher accuracy in comparison of label-free methods as in this specimen mixing with examination occurs in simultaneous steps [17].

Former technique, for example, may identify smallest modest fluctuation in sample content. For example, if a potential particular interaction is given in ample amount with prevalent impurity in research, it can be particularly saved. Spectral counts i.e., sum of number of spectra obtained per amino acid linkage is a quantitative estimation given by mass spectroscopy results is very useful tool for predicting the specificity of interactions. Obtained spectra of particular protein specimen in the tagged vs normal reveals if this interaction is specific for the selected specimen in this method or not.

5.4 Validating Specific Interactions

For quantitative protein-protein interaction measurement, a negative control is used to compare the amount of targeted specimen which co-purify simultaneously with known protein [18]. In this setup, real interaction associate possibly distinguished by particular abundance ratio, but uncertain contaminants binds without any partiality strongly in any situations, resulting in 1:1 equal proportion.

Even under modest biochemical purification conditions, this helps to screen out non-specific impurities and boosts confidence in identified interaction partners. Quantitative protein-protein interaction measurement has the benefit of being able to examine dynamic changes in protein-protein interactions after disruption. To detect modification-dependent interactions, researchers employed immobilized peptides with certain post-translational changes and their unchanged equivalent [19].

Precipitation of proteinous antigen or epitope fused biotechnological recombinant protein has also been performed before and after stimulation [20]. Finally, quantification reveals alterations in the partners in interaction of wild-type proteins in addition to its variants linked with disease [21]. If mutations occur to a protein having unspecified role, an affinity purification depended on MS can give useful idea with regards to known activities of established interactions.

Relative quantification is exemplified by the methods given above. As a result, they may be utilized to identify particular interaction couples from unwanted specimen, as well as to give justification in terms of quantity for difference occurring in interactions when they are perturbed. These approaches can only examine the same protein under different circumstances, and they rarely give any indication of interaction stoichiometry. To prove this, one method is to employ synthetic isotope-labeled reference peptides injected in standards to determine absolute abundances of suspected proteins [22]. This is arduous and costly for a proteome-scale task with a high number of proteins. As a result, the SH-quant technique includes an extra standard peptide in the affinity part [23]. This makes it easier to quantify the bait as well as the proteins of interest, in case they were employed as known proteins in further research. This tie up quantification may be used to determine peptide complex relationship and absolute protein complex content. An amalgam of affinity purification and quantification on basis of peak intensity possibly used to identify the chemistry of protein structure [24]. This method has the benefit of being simple to implement and does not need the tagging of several proteins. It's also worth noting that the same protein can be found in several different protein complexes. As a result, not all proteins that purify along with bait belong to the same complex. The separate pull-down of all components is required to distinguish between these distinct complexes.

5.5 Mass Spectrometry – Qualitative and Quantitative Analysis

Analysis using mass spectrometry is indispensable and irreplaceable tool nowadays. Initially, due to technological constrained, quantification analysis was not possible for protein specimen. But with current advance instrument setups, it is possible to perform semi quantitative and quantitative analysis. We will be discussing about qualitative and quantitative analysis with the help of software.

5.6 Challenges Associated with Mass Analysis

Traditionally, with various mass spectrometers and ionizations techniques are used to get information about the molecular mass, any type of modification in the parent structure of analyte, presence of any impurity qualitatively. As its scope increases to quantitative analysis there are issues associated with instrument categories and ionization techniques (Table 5.2). Nevertheless, sample preparation also play important role in analysis. Before heading to the quantitative analysis these issues should be considered and appropriately addressed. The various mass spectrometers help in quantitative analysis which are frequently used in protein structure based studies are time-of-flight, quadrupole, ion trap, ion cyclotron resonance, or orbitrap [24–27].

The ion velocity is evaluated in time of flight analyzer to identify particle size. Quadruple analysis is used to study how an ion moves in an electric field, and an ion trap is a sort of quadrupole that traps ions using current and oscillating electric fields.

Quantitative capabilities of MS can be affected by some parameters (Table 5.2). These can be divided into 2 parts: instrument based and sample based. The characteristics of the ion source, its transmission and detection ability and contamination of spectrometry parts covered under instrument-based problems. Ionization power, degradation rate and concentration of analytes, sample preparation, signal stability, ionization with

Table 5.2 Identified hurdles in various steps of mass spectrometry [28].

Aspect	Challenges
Sample preparation	Sample matrix interferences in analysis.
Sample homogeneity	Quantitative analysis is not appropriate for inhomogeneous samples. As a result, analysing dry samples or matrix deposits is time-consuming.
Labelling	For labelling purposes, there is a restricted spectrum of derivatizing agents for the target molecules of interest.
Internal standards	Internal standards with identical ionisation efficiencies to those of the analytes are difficult to come by in many circumstances. Occasionally synthesized internal standards can be used.
Interfacing samples	Before or during the ionisation of analyte molecules, samples in the solid or liquid phases must be introduced to the gas phase.
Ion suppression	Different sample matrix components restrict analyte ionisation to varying degrees. Depending on the operating conditions, the level of ion suppression may vary.
Separation	Analyte separation using liquid or gas chromatography, capillary electrophoresis, ion mobility spectroscopy, or other methods can decrease sample matrix interferences, but it complicates analytical procedures and restricts sample throughput.
Detection	Various ions with varying m/z values have different detection efficiency.
Spectral interferences	Some ions originating from the sample matrix and/or the ionisation matrix may overlap with the analyte ions.
Concentration/ mass calibration	Over a wide range, signal–quantity relationships are not linear. The calibration equation parameters may vary over time.
Automation	Sample handling equipment that is automated can enhance reproducibility, but it is expensive.
Data processing and interpretation	To transform the raw data collected by a mass spectrometer into understandable results and scientifically valid conclusions, expert expertise is necessary.

detection interference are all sample based problems [28]. The way mass spectrometers are handled, it is possibly a source of artefacts, reducing the capabilities of its operations. But we may expect many fewer consequences of human mistakes than in the past, given to significant advancements in software and hardware, as well as increased knowledge of correct sample management. Also sample preparation is the one of the important measures. Separation procedures are used to reduce sample matrices interferences and increase mass spectrometric systems' quantitative abilities.

5.7 Relative vs. Absolute Quantification

There can be large amount of deviation in MS results due to various physical or chemical properties so it's used in quantitative identification is not justifiable [29]. Also, due to its mechanism and functioning, minute amount of peptide in sample is present for ionization. This leads to desire to carryout relative and absolute proteomic quantification [30, 31].

Relative quantification which is generally based on analysis of specimens by MS and comparison of respective spectra peaks, compare the levels of peptides in a sample with having same levels experimentally treated peptide chain [30, 32].

The other option is absolute quantification which involves use of internal standards. The XIC (extract ion chromatogram) based analysis is performed to get correlation between analyte and internal standard to derive the quantification. However selection of the internal standard becomes crucial part in this type of analysis and this also involves impact of parameters mentioned in Table 5.2. Also in addition to that LC (liquid chromatography) part can be used for quantitation and MS part can be used as qualitative part. This type of semi quantitation by mass can be used where it serve the purpose [30, 33]. With this all approached to qualitative and quantitative analysis let us go through some of the researches which depict remarkable contribution MS analysis.

The demonstration of biosimilarity is important factor in approval of biosimilar, which includes analytical evaluation of the biosimilar product. In addition to demonstrating biosimilarity, product-related impurities must be extensively evaluated and control measures applied. Due to the process pegylation certain obstacles are created for structural evaluation such as heterogeneity of PEG, Number of joined pegylated moieties, and location of addition. Peptide mapping was used for studying this complex molecule attribute using Liquid Chromatography - Mass Spectrometry. This approach also used to demonstrate product related impurities like deamidated, oxidized, in addition to reduced. With the use of MS these impurities are identified [34, 35]. This approach further can be coupled with softwares for getting quantitative data on XIC based analysis.

Post translation modification in protein is one of the key area in which MS analysis is unavoidable. These modifications have direct impact on the biological activity of proteins and peptides. With high sensitivities in instruments modifications with very small mass range, up to 1 Dalton can be figured out. Hence this has wide applications in PTM analysis, determination of protein sequence variants and amino acid sequencing. These studies are carried out by multiple enzymatic digestion approach so that maximum sequence coverage obtained by ionization of all the peptides generated by digestion [36, 37].

One study demonstrates the identification of additional oxidation site other than methionine, i.e. Tryptophan (Trp) in monoclonal antibodies and quantification of the same is carried out with LC-MS. This type of oxidative degradation is studied by many authors. There are reports of decrease in binding and in biological activity due to photo oxidation induction of the Trytophan amino acid oxidation in complementary determining region (CDRs) of monoclonal antibody. Hence this Trp oxidation is studied quantitatively here. The XIC based quantitation is done for the same by comparing modified peptide with its native peptide [38].

Currently application of MS also play important role in analysis of molecular attribute like disulphide linkages. This tool is also explored for the identification and further quantification of the product related impurities like Host cell protein (HCP) [39, 40].

5.8 Mass Spectrometry – Lipidomics and Metabolomics

MS also has very significant application in field of Lipidomics and metabolomics. High resolution mass spectrometry now a days allows for the study of cellular proteins and metabolites that are responsible for physiological homeostasis and disease pathogenesis [41].

Lipidomics is the analysis of lipids and their interactions. Lipids occur in small quantities. Often they are most important molecule to sustain important process of the body for example in diagnosis and in identification of pathology of particular disorder. Detection of lipid and its pathways involves identification of disease like tumor, diabetes mellitus, obesity, Cardiac diseases, joint related diseases such as rheumatoid arthritis, lung diseases, IBD and many more. While degraded forms of lipids might be associated with diseases like Alzheimer's [42–44].

Direct infusion is the technique which can be used for analysis of lipids. For this lipids might be extracted with solid phase extraction techniques. Lipid profiling can be done by chromatographic separation follows by mass analysis. This approach can be explored for quantitative analysis of lipids as well. Various softwares and data bases are available for identification and analysis of lipids.

Metabolomics can be defined as study of metabolomes which are molecular end products of cellular pathways that have defining function in physiology of the body. Metabolites are very small moiety as compared to peptide chains sometimes also tiny sized than majority of lipids. Lipids are classified as sub division of metabolites. But in case of mass analysis, they behave differently, hence in analysis front they must be treated differently [45]. With chromatographic separation metabolites can be analysed with MS both qualitative and quantitatively. This technique is used in identifying disease conditions or identification of biomarkers in case of diseases.

5.9 Mass Spectrometry - Drug Discovery

High resolution mass spectroscopy (HRMS) has significant contribution in drug discovery at various stages of drug development cycle. High sensitivity and resolution leads to accurate identification and quantitation simultaneously, when it is need of analysis. Figure 5.1 provides information of various stages of product cycle where MS is used widely [46].

Thus applications of MS are throughout early stage development to late stage development i.e. pre-formulation and formulation studies. It scope also extends to clinical studies which includes pharmacokinetic and pharmacodynamics studies (PKPD).

The target product profile (TPP) which brief about the ideal characteristics of the drug attributes with their specialized justification gives confidence to drug developers by diminishing the chances of development failures at ending stages, and also provides safety and efficacy data at needed intervals. The TPP contains a description of drug product related qualities such as physical and chemical characteristics, amino acid sequence and post-translational modifications (PTMs). In initial stages, the product attributes need to be checked for effect on biological activity, safety, ADMET (absorption, distribution, metabolism, excretion, and toxicity) properties immunogenicity risk, and potential critical quality attributes (CQAs) are decided. Testing starts in later stage discovery, generally before

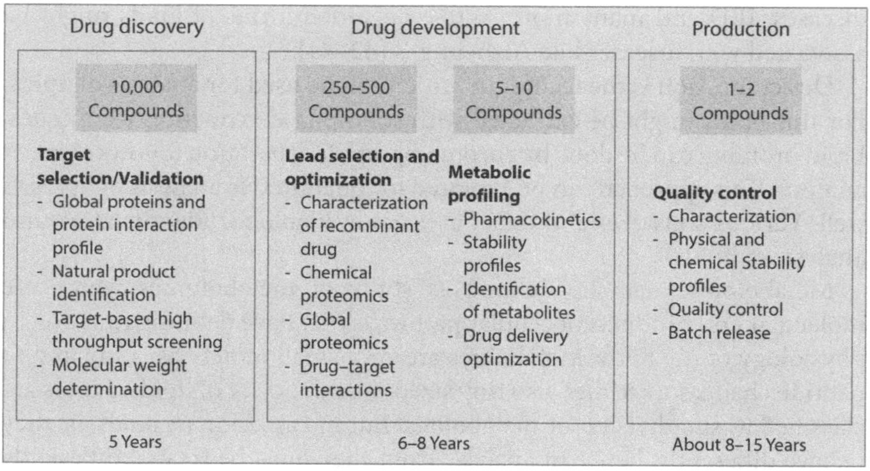

Figure 5.1 Implementation of mass spectrometry in drug discovery, development and production process.

candidate selection in clinical trials. The product profile then rectified and modified throughout the product development process resulting into the quality target product profile (QTPP) [47].

In clinical studies, quantification of drug moiety from the serum or plasma samples is carryout by MS after separation techniques like solid phase extraction (SPE) and chromatography [48].

5.10 Conclusion and Future Scope

The integration of proteomics and metabolomics workflows, from the very first step of sample preparation to the final step of data acquisition and network-based computational analysis, offers comprehensive understanding of complex biological systems. The MS technology is advancing in fast pace and as a result of which we can target higher sensitivity and resolution in analysis, leading to lower detection limits and accurate mass identification. With change in technology MS instruments are also changing in dimensions. Now a days MS detector equivalent to size of UV/PDA detectors are available, which can be used for basic and on line screening information. Many advances are done to create bench top models of technologies like TOF. With all these advantages and new technologies MS will serve its purpose as it have done for last few decades.

5.11 Resources and Software

With advances in technology and more and more researchers working in MS throughout the globe there are various resources where MS related knowledge is available. Every make of the mass instruments has unique features and technological differences. These can be studied for the knowledge bases of manufactures. Few examples are Planet orbitrap, where all information related to applications of various models is provided. It also consists of various application notes. Similar information centers are also available with other makers like Sciex and Waters [49, 50].

With enormous amount of data produced by MS, to save time processing softwares are indivisible part of analysis to interpret the generated data. Every make has its own processing software package compatible with their file system. The information about the same is available at knowledge centers. Some third party softwares like 'Protein Metrics software package' are also available, which has advantage to analyze raw data generated by various different instruments with single software. For gaining basic information about MS ionizations, detectors etc. websites like 'IonSource' serves the purpose.

Acknowledgement

The authors would like to acknowledge Sagar Popat (Research & Development, Amneal Pharmaceuticals Pvt. Ltd., Ahmedabad - 382213, Gujarat, India) for contributing in editing of chapter.

References

1. Thermo Scientific Application Note, Overview of mass spectrometry for protein analysis. 1–2.
2. Aebersold, R. and Mann, M., Mass spectrometry-based proteomics. *Nature*, 422, 198–207, 2003.
3. Farmer, T.B. and Caprioli, R.M., Determination of protein-protein interactions by matrix-assisted laser desorption/ionization mass spectrometry. *J. Mass. Spectrom.*, 33, 8, 697–704, 1998.
4. Katta, V., Carr, S., Chait, B.T., Conformational changes in proteins probed by hydrogenexchange electrospray-ionization mass spectrometry. *Rapid Commun. Mass Spectrom.*, 5, 214–217, 1991.

5. Ramanathan, R., Gross, M.L., Zielinski, W.L., Layloff, T.P., Monitoring recombinant protein drugs: A study of insulin by H/D exchange and electrospray ionization mass spectrometry. *Anal. Chem.*, 69, 5142–5145, 1997.
6. Engen, J.R. and Smith, D.L., Investigating protein structure and dynamics by hydrogen exchange MS. *Anal. Chem.*, 73, 256A–265A, 2001.
7. Hoofnagle, A.N., Resing, K.A., Ahn, N.G., Protein analysis by hydrogen exchange mass spectrometry. *Annu. Rev. Biophys. Biomol. Struct.*, 32, 1–25, 2003.
8. Pandey, A. and Mann, M., Proteomics to study genes and genomes. *Nature*, 405, 837–846, 2000.
9. Aebersold, R. and Goodlett, D.R., Mass spectrometry in proteomics. *Chem. Rev.*, 101, 269–295, 2001.
10. Aebersold, R. and Mann, M., Mass spectrometry-based proteomics. *Nature*, 422, 198–207, 2003.
11. Bantscheff, M. *et al.*, Chemoproteomics profiling of HDAC inhibitors reveals selective targeting of HDAC complexes. *Nat. Biotechnol.*, 29, 3, 255–265, 2011.
12. Ruigrok, V.J. *et al.*, Alternative affinity tools: More attractive than antibodies. *Biochem. J.*, 436, 1, 1–13, 2011.
13. Aebersold, R. and Mann, M., Mass spectrometry-based proteomics. *Nature*, 422, 6928, 198–207, 2003.
14. Eng, J.K., Searle, B.C., Clauser, K.R., Tabb, D.L., A face in the crowd: Recognizing peptides through data base search. *Mol. Cell. Proteomics*, 10, 11, R111.009522, 2011.
15. Ong, S.E. and Mann, M., Mass spectrometry-based proteomics turns quantitative. *Nat. Chem. Biol.*, 1, 5, 252–262, 2005.
16. Cox, J. and Mann, M., Quantitative, high-resolution proteomics for data-driven systems biology. *Annu. Rev. Biochem.*, 80, 273–299, 2011.
17. Lau, H.T., Suh, H.W., Golkowski, M., Ong, S.E., Comparing SILAC- and stable isotope dimethyl-labeling approaches for quantitative proteomics. *J. Proteome Res.*, 13, 9, 4164–4174, 2014.
18. Vermeulen, M., Hubner, N.C., Mann, M., High confidence determination of specific protein–protein interactions using quantitative mass spectrometry. *Curr. Opin. Biotechnol.*, 19, 4, 331–337, 2008.
19. Selbach, M. and Mann, M., Protein interaction screening by quantitative immunoprecipitation combined with knockdown (QUICK). *Nat. Methods*, 3, 12, 981–983, 2006.
20. Sury, M.D., Mcshane, E., Hernandez-Miranda, L.R., Birchmeier, C., Selbach, M., Quantitative proteomics reveals dynamic interaction of c-Jun N-terminal kinase (JNK) with RNA transport granule proteins splicing factor proline and glutamine-rich (Sfpq) and non POU domain containing octamer binding protein (Nono) during neuronal differentiation. *Mol. Cell. Proteomics*, 14, 1, 50–65, 2015.

21. Hosp, F., Vossfeldt, H., Heinig, M., Vasiljevic, D., Arumughan, A., Wyler, E. *et al.*, Quantitative interaction proteomics of neurodegenerative disease proteins. *Cell Rep.*, 11, 7, 1134–1146, 2015.
22. Schmidt, C., Lenz, C., Grote, M., Luhrmann, R., Urlaub, H., Determination of protein stoichiometry within protein complexes using absolute quantification and multiple reaction monitoring. *Anal. Chem.*, 82, 7, 2784–2796, 2010.
23. Wepf, A., Glatter, T., Schmidt, A., Aebersold, R., Gstaiger, M., Quantitative interaction proteomics using mass spectrometry. *Nat. Methods*, 6, 203–205, 2009.
24. Schwanhausser, B., Busse, D., Li, N., Dittmar, G., Schuchhardt, J., Wolf, J. *et al.*, Global quantification of mammalian gene expression control. *Nature*, 473, 337–342, 2011.
25. Glish, G.L. and Burinsky, D.J., Hybrid mass spectrometers for tandem mass spectrometry. *J. Am. Soc. Mass Spectrom.*, 19, 2, 161–172, 2008.
26. Scigelova, M., Hornshaw, M., Giannakopulos, A., Makarov, A., Fourier transform mass spectrometry. *Mol. Cell. Proteomics*, 10, 7, M111.009431, 2011.
27. Lucitt, M.B., Price, T.S., Pizarro, A., Wu, W., Yocum, A.K., Seiler, C. *et al.*, Analysis of the zebrafish proteome during embryonic development. *Mol. Cell. Proteomics*, 7, 5, 981–994, 2008.
28. Urban, P.L., Chen, Y.-C., Wang, Y.-S., *Time-Resolved Mass Spectrometry: From Concept to Applications*, pp. 217–228, Wiley, Chichester, UK, 2016.
29. Zhu, H., Pan, S., Gu, S., Bradbury, E.M., Chen, X., Amino acid residue specific stable isotope labeling for quantitative proteomics. *Rapid Commun. Mass Spectrom.*, 16, 2115–2123, 2002.
30. Urban, P.L., Chen, Y.-C., Wang, Y.-S., *Quantitative Measurement by Mass Spectrumetry*, pp. 11–43, Wiley, Chichester, UK, 2016.
31. Oda, Y., Huang, K., Cross, F.R., Cowburn, D., Chait, B.T., Accurate quantitation of protein expression and site-specific phosphorylation. *Proc. Natl. Acad. Sci. U.S.A.*, 96, 6591–6596, 1999.
32. Ong, S.E., Blagoev, B., Kratchmarova, I., Kristensen, D.B., Steen, H., Pandey, A., Mann, M., Stable isotope labeling by amino acids in cell culture, SILAC, as a simple and accurate approach to expression proteomics. *Mol. Cell Proteomics*, 1, 376–386, 2002.
33. Berger, S.J., Lee, S.W., Anderson, G.A., Pasa-Tolic, L., Tolic, N., Shen, Y., Zhao, R., Smith, R.D., High-throughput global peptide proteomic analysis by combining stable isotope amino acid labeling and data-dependent multiplexed-MS/MS. *Anal. Chem.*, 74, 4994–5000, 2002.
34. Shekhawat, R., Shah, C.K., Patel, A., Srinivasan, S., Kapoor, P., Patel, S. *et al.*, Structural similarity, characterization of poly ethylene glycol linkage and identification of product related variants in biosimilar pegfilgrastim. *PloS One*, 14, 3, e0212622, 2019.
35. Krijgsveld, J., Ketting, R.F., Mahmoudi, T., Johansen, J., Artal-Sanz, M., Verrijzer, C.P., Plasterk, R.H., Heck, A.J., Metabolic labeling of C. elegans and

D. melanogaster for quantitative proteomics. *Nat. Biotechnol.*, 21, 927–931, 2003.

36. Thompson, A., Schäfer, J., Kuhn, K., Kienle, S., Schwarz, J., Schmidt, G., Neumann, T., Johnstone, R., Mohammed, A.K., Hamon, C., Tandem mass tags: A novel quantification strategy for comparative analysis of complex protein mixtures by MS/MS. *Anal. Chem.*, 75, 1895–1904, 2003.
37. Ong, S.E. and Mann, M., Mass spectrometry-based proteomics turns quantitative. *Nat. Chem. Biol.*, 1, 252–262, 2005.
38. Hensel, M., Steurer, R., Fichtl, J., Elger, C., Wedekind, F. *et al.*, Identification of potential sites for tryptophan oxidation in recombinant antibodies using tert-butylhydroperoxide and quantitative LC-MS. *PloS One*, 6, 3, e17708, 2011.
39. Sechi, S. and Oda, Y., Quantitative proteomics using mass spectrometry. *Curr. Opin. Chem. Biol.*, 7, 70–77, 2003.
40. Ong, S.E., Foster, L.J., Mann, M., Mass spectrometric-based approaches in quantitative proteomics. *Methods.*, 29, 124–130, 2003.
41. Blum, B., Mousavic, F., Emili, A., Single-platform 'multi-omic' profiling: Unified mass spectrometry and computational workflows for integrative proteomics–metabolomics analysis. *Mol. Omics*, 14, 307, 2018.
42. Fahy, E., Subramaniam, S., Murphy, R.C., Nishijima, M., Raetz, C.R. *et al.*, Update of the LIPID MAPS comprehensive classification system for lipids. *J. Lipid Res.*, 50, Supplement, 9–14, 2009.
43. Kraegen, E.W., Cooney, G.J., Ye, J.M., Thompson, A.L., Furler, S.M., The role of lipids in the pathogenesis of muscle insulin resistance and beta cell faiture in type II diabetes and obesity. *Exp. Clin. Endocrinol. Diabetes*, 109, Suppl 2, 189–201, 2001.
44. Morris, M. and Watkins, S.M., Focused metabolomic profiling in the drug development process: Advances from lipid profiling. *Curr. Opin. Chem. Biol.*, 9, 4, 407–412, 2005.
45. Smith, R., Mathis, A.D., Ventura, D. *et al.*, Proteomics, lipidomics, metabolomics: A mass spectrometry tutorial from a computer scientist's point of view. *BMC Bioinf.*, 15, S9, 2014.
46. Leurs, U., Mistarz, U.H., Rand, K.D., Applications of mass spectrometry in drug development science. In: Müllertz, A., Perrie, Y., Rades, T. (eds), *Analytical Techniques in the Pharmaceutical Sciences. Advances in Delivery Science and Technology*. Springer, New York, NY, 2016. https://doi.org/10.1007/978-1-4939-4029-5_7
47. USFDA, *Target Product Profile–A Strategic Development Process Tool*, USFDA, 2007, https://www.fda.gov/downloads/drugs/guidancecomplianceregulatory information/guidances/ucm080593.pdf.
48. Cravatt, B.F., Simon, G.M., Yates III, J.R., The biological impact of mass-spectrometry-based proteomics. *Nature*, 450, 991–1000, 2007.

49. Mueller, L.N., Brusniak, M.Y., Mani, D.R., Aebersold, R., An assessment of software solutions for the analysis of mass spectrometry based quantitative proteomics data. *J. Proteome Res.*, 7, 51–61, 2008.
50. Bantscheff, M., Schirle, M., Sweetman, G., Rick, J., Kuster, B., Quantitative mass spectrometry in proteomics: A critical review. *Anal. Bioanal. Chem.*, 389, 1017–1031, 2007.

6

Applications of Bioinformatics Tools in Medicinal Biology and Biotechnology

Harshil Shah[1†], Vivek Chavda[2†] and Moinuddin M. Soniwala[3*]

[1]Formulation and Development Department, Cadila Healthcare Limited, Ahmedabad, Gujarat, India
[2]Department of Pharmaceutics and Pharmaceutical Technology, L M College of Pharmacy, Ahmedabad, Gujarat, India
[3]Department of Pharmaceutics, B K Mody Government Pharmacy College Rajkot, Gujarat, India

Abstract
Development of modern medicine necessitates the collection, integration and interpretation of molecular, genomic, and cellular data, together with clinical data. Hence, it produces a significant amount of challenges to bioinformatics. For the investigation and understanding of biological complexity, a variety of methods and software have been created. To speed up biotech development, bioinformatics technologies like as sequence analysis and matching, molecular modelling, docking, indexing, and simulation techniques are used. Numerous upcoming bioinformatics breakthroughs are predicted to promote the study of large amounts of biomedical information. Consequently, bioinformatics plays a critical role in analyzing different types of data created by high-throughput research methods, such as genomic, transcriptomic, and proteomic datasets, and then arranging the knowledge gathered from traditional biomedicine. Bioinformatics has progressed from sequence data to high - throughput sequencing whole genome or transcriptome understandings, and is now focusing on contemporary fields of integrative and translational genetics, with a view to customized treatment in the future. This chapter encompasses all the above mentioned possibilities with various applicabilities of such bioinformatics advances.

Keywords: Bioinformatics, medical diagnosis, cancer, drug discovery, molecular medicine, personalized medicine

**Corresponding author*: moinhani@gmail.com
†Contributed equally and shared the first authorship

Vivek Chavda, Krishnan Anand and Vasso Apostolopoulos (eds.) Bioinformatics Tools for Pharmaceutical Drug Product Development, (95–116) © 2023 Scrivener Publishing LLC

6.1 Introduction

"Bioinformatics is brief form for Biological Informatics. This is considered to be an amalgam of biological sciences and computer science and some researchers synonymously use the term, computational biology. This branch of science advanced further when the human genome project came into existence. Bioinformatics merges branches like biology, computer science and information technology to form a single discipline." The main intention of the field is to facilitate the finding of new biological acumens as well as to generate a global outlook from which coalescing ethics in biology can be acknowledged.

Bioinformaticians are often indulge in designing new algorithms, software, developing rationalized databases which all support in decoding numerous biological complications [1]. For improving the understanding of biological intricacy, to store and analyze the biological data, many data base, bioinformatics tools, and software are available. Thus, it reduces time, cost and wet lab practice. Researchers on realizing the significance of databases sequencing just after insulin peptides sequences became available, the first protein sequence database was generated in 1956 [2].

The human body is made up of billions (rather trillions) of cells, which are convoluted in several difficult methods. The cells are organized by DNA (Deoxy Ribo Nucleic Acid - the central processing machinery). Understanding of DNA can expose a lot about the organism and equally the risks of diseases can be higher in the future [3].

Chronic diseases are rapidly growing all over the world. The conventional drug discovery process and drugs are not working as efficiently as they have to. According to a study circulated in Nature, the top 10 maximum earning drugs recommended in the US help merely a lesser percentage (<25%) of the patients. Further in case of cholesterol drugs, the success rate is very lower side (about 2% of patients). So the possibility of success is very minor when compared with the expenses made on research, approval, and marketing activities [4]. Therefore, the associated costs of healthcare are growing at a stellar rate. For this reasons the world needs personalized treatments tailor-made to the genetics of increasingly diverse patient populations, isolated by factors like clinical & family history, life style & diet, environmental and several parameters. For this massive amount of data collection, integration, processing, and analysis.

Current technologies like Next Generation Sequencing (NGS), genome sequencing, microarray profiling have generated a large amount of data. Bioinformatics can be a precise, dominant & effective device where the big data which is produced from Genome, Transcriptome, Proteome, and Metabolome need to be systematized into databases and examined [5]. The results of analysis of these large data are applied in healthcare, preventive medicine, and drug discovery [6].

6.2 Bioinformatics Tools

Computer software programs and internet are the vital tools for data scientist. An essential activity is proteins and DNA sequential analysis utilizing numerous programs and databases. Anybody, from clinicians to molecular biologists, by applying fundamental bioinformatics tools to understand the large molecules [7]. This in no sense infer that it's easy to handle and examine of raw genomic data for retrieving, arranging out, analyzing, calculating, and storing DNA and protein sequence data [8]. There is need of data scientists in the pharmaceutical industry to evaluate the multifactorial data [9]. The progress of bioinformatics has been a worldwide project, which creates computer networks that have endorsed easy right to use to biological data and allowed the enlargement of softwares for easy scrutiny [8]. Several multinational information intended to provide gene-protein database are accessible spontaneously online to the entire scientific fraternity [9].

6.3 The Genetic Basis of Diseases

Bioinformatics exhibits enormous character in the areas of "structural, functional and nutritional genomics" [10]. "Genomics is an interdisciplinary field of science concentrating on the structure, function, evolution, mapping, and editing of genomes" [11]. A genome is an organism's complete set of DNA, which covers all of its genes. Each genome comprises entire information which is desire to form and preserve that organism (Figure 6.1) [12].

Don't confuse between genomics and genetics. "Genetics is the learning of particular genes and their roles in inheritance. In contrast, genomics targets at the mutual characterization and quantification of genes, which direct the production of proteins with the help of certain enzymes and messenger molecules" [13, 14]. "The field of genomics produces a huge volume of data from gene sequences, their interrelation, and roles. Bioinformatics plays a very significant part to deal with this massive data. Bioinformatics delivers both theoretical bases and practical methods for identifying systemic

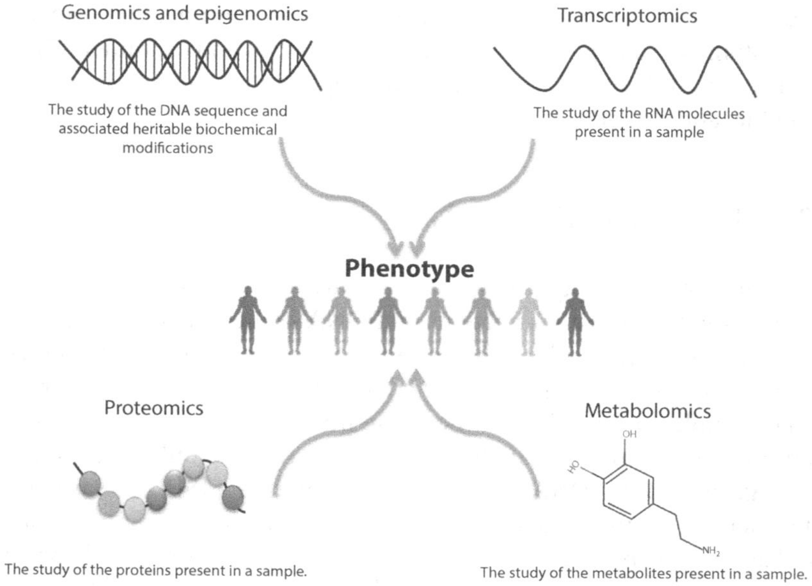

Figure 6.1 Functional Genomics is the study of how the genome, transcripts (genes), proteins and metabolites work together to produce a particular phenotype.

well-designed activities of the cell and the organism" [15]. Currently, There are numerous assets for estimation of candidate genes (G2D, TOM, SUSPECTS Gene Seeker etc.) and functional single nucleotide polymorphisms [SNPs (LS-SNP, PANTHER, SIFT, SNAP etc.)] [16].

Furthermore, during the last decade, substantial bioinformatics effort has gone to empirical ways to depict precise variations in order to detect the molecular impacts of these genetic modifications. Bioinformatics initiatives have centered on two main categories, in relation to genomic experimental investigations. First, researchers compared genetic variation data with molecular properties to see how they could impact function. Second, statistical approaches for predicting mutations that may have a molecular impact have been developed. Approaches for studying the molecular activities of SNPs and mutations are explored and identified in this protocol document.

6.4 Proteomics

"Proteomics has developed from genomics plus mapping and successful sequencing of the genomes of a wide variety of organisms including humans [17]; Proteomics is the higher level learning of proteins. It insurances developing scientific research and the examination of proteomes from the overall level of intracellular protein composition (protein profiles), protein structure, protein-protein interaction, and unique activity patterns (e.g. post-translational modifications)" (Figure 6.2) [18, 19]. Proteomics is a vital constituent of functional genomics, genetics, biochemistry, and molecular biology. Proteomics involves well-organized, high-throughput approach to protein expression analysis of a cell or an organism [20].

Typical results of proteomics studies are accounts of the protein content of differentially expressed proteins across numerous conditions [5]. This can be accomplished by arranging peptide mass finger printing and peptide fragmentation fingerprinting, gel technology, HPLC, and mass spectrometry. The vast protein data (proteomics results) can be accomplished and access effortlessly by applying bioinformatics tools, software, and databases [21, 22].

Though the exhaustive description of a biological system is inadequate, advancement in genomic sequencing has significantly boosted the perception to the intricacy of life. Concentrating the focus on proteomics has developed another massive platform for enlightening the interpretation of life sciences. Experimentation with proteomics can be utilized for various features like medical and health sciences plus identification of drug target, food technology and biomarker discovery.

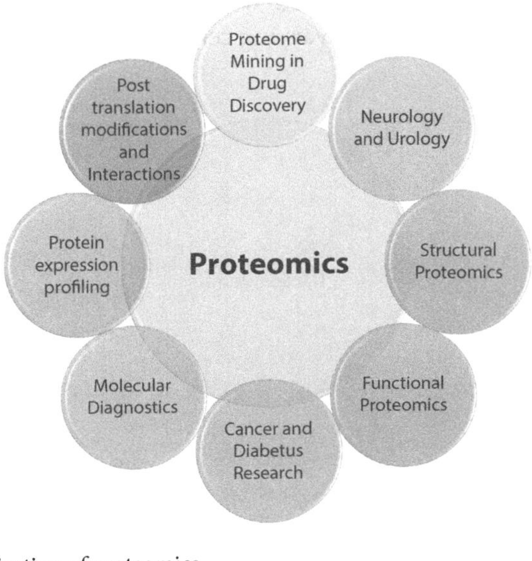

Figure 6.2 Application of proteomics.

Hence proteins are crucial ingredients of foods, proteomic technology can display and discriminate protein content of foods and throughout production process their transformation. Research in proteomic biomarkers is progressive in various ailments like carcinomas, HIV infections, cardiac and renal function complications that deliver non-invasive systems by the usage of body fluids like urine and plasma. By using various proteomic networks like chemical proteomics and protein interaction it can also use in identification of drug targets. Over the last decade, growth and application of proteomics has enhanced significantly. The expansion in proteomics methods can produce many encouraging newer methods that helps in novel diagnostics as well as therapeutic findings [23].

6.5 Transcriptomic

"The study of sets of all messenger RNA molecules formed by the genome in the cell is termed as transcriptomics [24]. It can also be named as Expression Profiling where DNA microarray is used to define the expression level of mRNA in a given cell population" (Figure 6.3). The microarray technique generates huge volume of numbers, single run produces thousands of data value and hundreds of runs required by experiment [25].

Many software packages are used to analyze such a huge data [26]. It is used to examine the constantly varying cellular transcriptome [27].

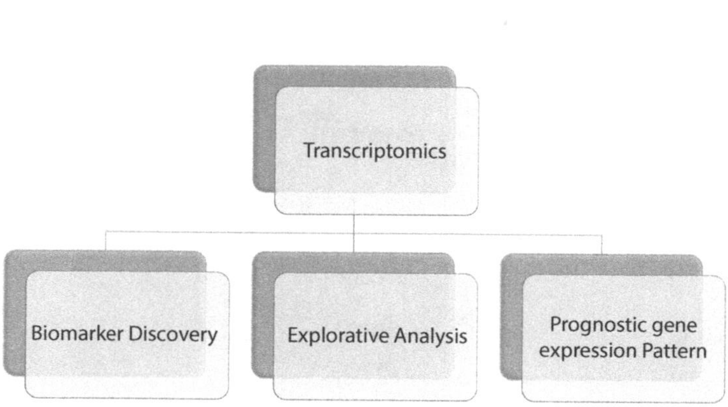

Figure 6.3 Application of transcriptomics.

6.6 Cancer

One of the most frequent reasons of patient's death is malignancy and it is a multifarious disease which can happen in any of the body organ or tissue. There are numerous reasons of deprived prognoses, diagnoses and therapies of this ailment ranging from variation in severities, sensitivity, affected tissues/organs, and drug resistance, cell differentiation and origin, and ambiguity in perception of development of disease. There are certain evidences which proves that the interaction between proteins and genes play avital role in investigation molecular mechanism in the progress of cancer. It's essential key to put forward novel concepts and methods in investigation in malignancy and medical treatment, to assimilate systems biology, medical knowledge, and advanced computing to expand early detection of cancer its precise investigation and treatment of diseases [28].

Cancer bioinformatics is unique path to distillate bioinformatics techniques in cancer, with respect to the type of cancer, signaling, metabolic rate, progress, and spread of cancerous cells. Clinical bioinformatics is an important branch which can address appropriately the obstacles in clinical prognosis and explore possible novel therapies for cancerous patient. It also combines clinical and medical information with information technology, mathematics, and omics science [29]. To give response to the specific questions of cancer it is essential to established specific methods or presents certain newer tools of bioinformatics. For instance, the Semantic Web technology which was repossessed from Corvus was utilized to recognize information from medical sciences and established semantic models, a store room for data which delivers a even edge to several forms of Omics data, created on methodical knowledge of biology and by implementation of SPARQL endpoint [30]. Semantic models were smeared for the interplay among molecular level of a cell and its response to anticancer treatment. This model also contains genomic, transcriptomic and epigenomic data from cancerous samples with gene oncology data and regulatory networks made from information of binding of transcription factor. Multivariate assays is a method to exemplify error introduced in the assay that results from the intrinsic error during sample preparation and other factors which contributes to errors, were used to assist and guide the doctors [31].

Cancer bioinformatics is anticipated to have significant part in the recognition and analysis of biomarkers, precise to clinical phenotype associated to early detection of disease, dimensions to observe growth of the ailment, the therapeutic responses and predictions to enhance the quality of patient's life. Certain variables in the genes, proteins, peptides, chemicals or the base of physics in malignancy, biomarkers are been scrutinized from a sole one to multiple biomarkers with respect to their expressions and functionality as well as from the network to dynamic network. Network biomarkers as a unique type of markers with interaction between protein-protein explored and incorporation of information on protein annotation, interactions and signaling pathway [28]. Dynamic network biomarkers can be defined as when changes of network biomarkers can be examined and assessed at several parts and time points during the expansion of illnesses. It can be linked with clinical informatics which also includes patient's objections, record, treatments, clinical signs, imaging reports, doctor's reviews, biochemical and other tests [32]. In short, clinical specimen gathered from human studies under unblemished and stringent standards are gathered with an entire outline of medical informatics. Gene and protein profiles of specimen can be scrutinized and relations between genes/proteins can be reckoned out by bioinformatics and medical sciences [33].

Novel treatments to the malignancy have been anticipated as a newer idea in the direction of realization to predict, prevent, personalize and participatory (P4) medicine [33, 34]. The cluster of huge data produced from high throughput technology from the patients could be untangled, which can include one or multiple illness perturbed networks in the cells in the affected organ by the disease [35]. Molecular networks perturbed due to cancer may show the abnormality in initial signals and working, to optimize P4 treatment in this disease. Clinical bioinformatics involved in cancerous treatment is an significant path to touch systems clinical medicine by merging medical interpretations with malignancy generated bioinformatics, evaluating medical indications and symptoms, mode of advancement and progress of disease, with clinical investigations, pathology, biochemical tests, MRIs and the therapeutic policies [12, 36]. The prognosis to treat tamoxifen treated recurrent primary breast cancer with alternative endocrine therapies or chemotherapy can be made feasible with the early diagnosis using gene expression signature [37]. Focus of pharmacogenomics in the oncology is to envisage therapeutic response as well as toxicity to drugs to assist the individualization of patient treatment [38].

6.7 Diagnosis

Better understanding of protein expression have appreciably widened the understanding of the ailments at molecular level and now it is feasible to some extent to explain the concealed mechanisms of physiological disorders like diabetes, cancer, autoimmune disorders etc. Microarray technology is a probable technique which can enable quick and complete surveillance of gene expression profile of the sick person. Collection of vast amounts of relevant data can result in well-established correlations which could be utilized for the diagnosis or even for the preventive treatment of the disease reducing the vulnerability to ailments or allergies. The differential expression of genes in healthy and sick tissues is frequently highly distinguishable. For the quick and precise analysis of variation in gene expression for the moto of diagnosis, the target gene is plotted in the co-ordinates of the two dimensional system in accord with the relative abundance of the genes in the healthy and sick tissues. The constituents of plasma, peptides along with other intact or fragmented biomacromolecules are very revealing diagnostic source. To identify these nucleic acid/proteins mass spectrometry appears to be more useful than microarray assay.

Gene chips also permits precise and unambiguous recognition of invading microbe nuclear material in a patient, preventing the pain staking task of trying to cultivate the microorganism in laboratory and then identifying it phenotype.

6.8 Drug Discovery and Testing

Bioinformatics plays a highly essential role in approximately entire features of discovery of drug, its evaluation and progress. This increasing importance of bioinformatics is not only as it handles huge bulk of data, but in the usefulness of bioinformatics tools to forecast, examine and help interpret clinical and preclinical findings [39]. Conventionally, pharmacology and chemistry based drug discovery methods faces numerous problems in searching of novel drugs. Prominent attention in bioinformatics is due to its propensity to produce more new drugs in a minimum time interval with little threat or side effects. Drug development and discovery consist of recognizing the target accountable for the ailment. Once the target is known researchers attempt to identify novel or existing molecules that interact with the therapeutic target. In fact, now there has been developed a new distinct arena recognized as "Computer Aided Drug Design (CADD)" helps in the novel molecule design and development [40]. The conventional approaches are not showing to be very active in searching novel drugs and/or accomplishing anticipated treatment result (Figure 6.4).

A fruitful and dependable drug design procedure suggestively decrease the duration and rate of the drug discovery & development process. Computational methods and bioinformatics tools are used to forecast the

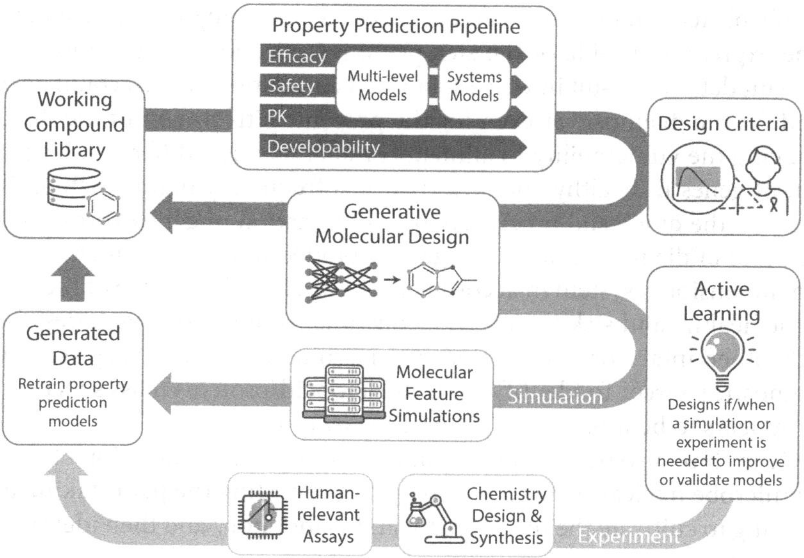

Figure 6.4 *In silico* drug design platform approach (Accelerating Therapeutics for Opportunities in Medicine).

drug-likeness. It principally means the identification and removal of candidate molecules that are doubtful to endure the advanced phases of discovery and development. Moreover, bioinformatics is also putting the base for the development of the arena of Computation Synthetic Biology (CSB). Cellular proteins instead of existing as a lone protein, binds with other proteins forming the multi-protein assemblies which controls normal as well as abnormal functions including reaction to allergens, interior and exterior signals, response to hormones etc. Information regarding network of these interactions are needed to recognize the proteins that can act as most appropriate treatment targets. There is a need to unfold a concrete map of the cell which allows analysis of the data masses obtained through mining techniques and will assist training predictive procedures to calculate pathways and how to integrate them collectively. Afterwards by incorporating the molecular aspects of active sites, the most appropriate biologically valid drug targets can be identified and subjected to more stringent evaluation (Figure 6.5).

The pharmaceutical bioinformatics deals with scientific computer based technologies for drug development, designing and discovery coupled with studies of drug pharmacokinetics, mechanism of action, drug interactions,

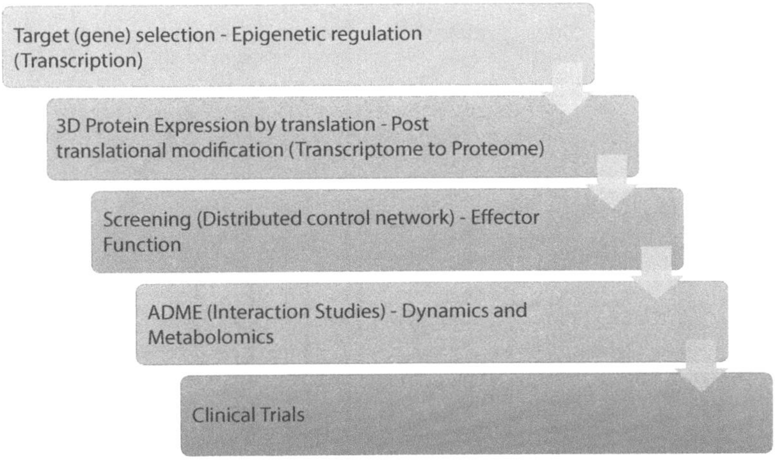

Figure 6.5 Stages of protein drug discovery and development.

and other aspects of pharmacology along with knowledge of drug formulation. Target drugs can be designed to precisely act on specific genes and their associated protein accountable for particular disease condition [37, 41].

6.9 Molecular Medicines

The incorporation of clinical techniques into clinical practice is required for the research of illness genetic pathways. Current medicine is based only on the foundations of clinical techniques, which are often helpful on a gene-by-gene basis. Many of illnesses will be linked by biomarkers supplied by high-throughput genotyping and effective genomic, proteomic, and metabolomic research in the post-genomic age. Clinical medicine based on molecularly orientated diagnostics will be linked to illness detection and diagnosis via such a platform (Figure 6.6) [42].

To attain this mission, enormous and genome wise biological and clinical data must be integrated with biostatistics and bioinformatics analyses to model biological systems. Gathering classified and linked data from molecular studies, and the succeeding development of assumptions, generates the essentials of systems biology. This extremely multifaceted analytical process replicates a newer scientific model known as integrative genomics [43].

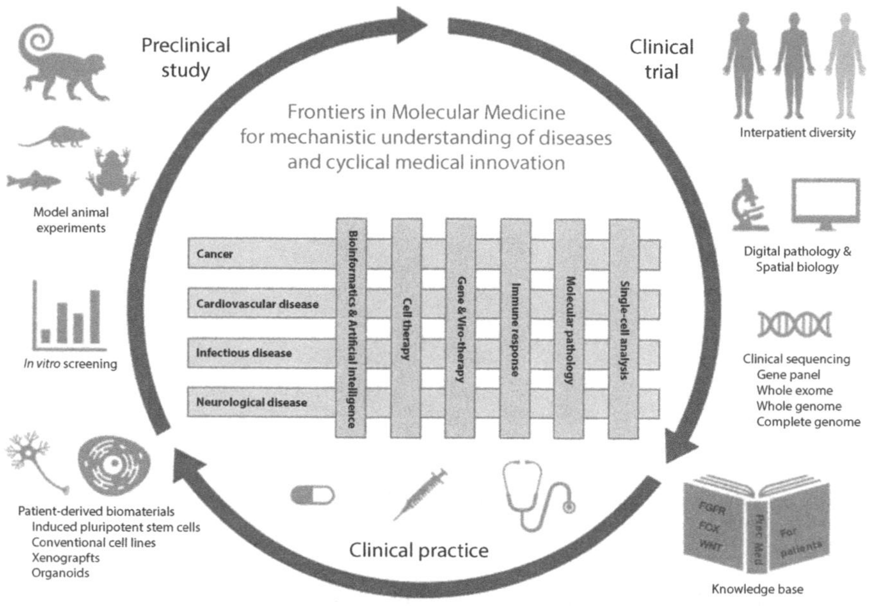

Figure 6.6 Structure of molecular medicine.

6.10 Personalized (Precision) Medicines

"Precision medicine is composed to have an influence on patients, health-care delivery systems and research participants' means that were only made-up 15 years ago while the human genome was first sequenced. While innovation using genome-based technologies has enhanced, these have only initiated to be accepted into clinical medicine" [44]. Personalized medicine is medical care modified to every patient's genetic makeup. Drugs are often given in amalgamation in order to enlarge the therapy accomplishment percentage [45]. The association among the molecular data relating to a patient and their disease phenotype are multifaceted and cannot be determined automatically [46].

Bioinformatics is a necessary constituent in elementary research, in the progress of new perceptions for diagnosis and therapy as well as in clinical practice [47]. Bioinformatics can produce a dominant role in inferring the molecular data and as an instrument for producing references for the practicing physician. Undertaking gene therapy clearly needs information of the genome [48]. A major challenge is the perplexity to introduce the target DNA/RNA into the host cell from an external source.

The emphasis for the future effort must be to increase weightage on the precision medicine to have an impact not only on individuals but also populations and hence the name "precision public health" [48]. In current years, dissertations around "personalized," "stratified," and "precision" medicine have flourished. The meanings and usages of the ideas are, however, plural, disputed and categorized by varied thoughts about the types of futures that are anticipated and wanted [49].

Personalized medicine generally considers phenotypic variations for the treatment (Figure 6.7) [50]. According to Knochelmann HM, "The accessibility of current biomedical technologies such as DNA sequencing, proteomics, and wireless monitoring devices, has allowed the identification of this difference, fundamentally revealing the necessity for the personalization of medicine at particular stage. The upcoming tasks related with this truth will be to not only advance the competence in the way in which individuals are considered, but also in the way in personalized medicines are made and examined to show their usefulness. This is not to say that interferences that work universally (i.e., the old-style single agent 'block buster' drugs) should be overlooked if recognized, but rather that they might be very stiff to classify going advancing" [51]. Auspiciously, this matter is not unavoidably exclusive to healthcare [52]. Moreover, emerging more

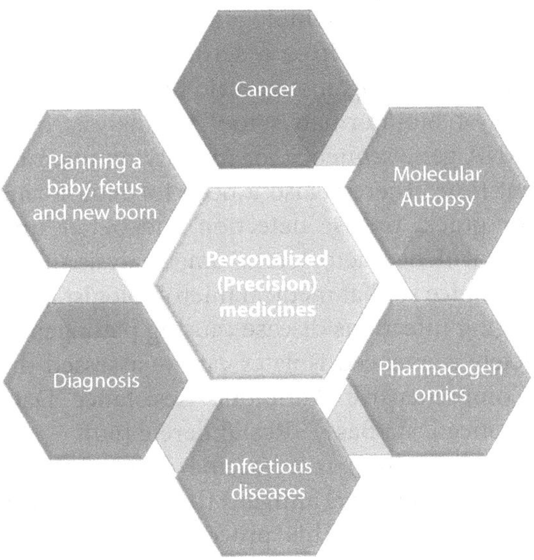

Figure 6.7 Application of personalized (precision) medicines.

effectual ways of evolving personalized medicines [53]. Finally, enhanced techniques of teaching and training medical workers about personalized therapy must be developed and deployed in order for many participants to adopt personalized medicine [52].

6.11 Vaccine Development and Drug Discovery in Infectious Diseases and COVID-19 Pandemic

During the extensive global war against the devastating disease of COVID-19, the significance of bioinformatics in research of vaccine and drug discovery have never been so crucial to combat against infectious diseases [54]. Various online platforms like CoVex have been developed to predict novel drug targets and drug repurposing candidates by integrating "SARS-CoV (severe acute respiratory syndrome coronavirus)", SARS-CoV-2 human virus protein interactions, antigenic epitopes, peptide-protein docking, antibody structures, simulate antigen-antibody reactions and to integrate it all into a large scale interactome. This permits scientists to identify already approved drugs to repurpose for COVID-19, which could be faster than developing new drugs from conventional processes [55–57]. *In-silico* method offers methodical and rapid ways to yield repurposed drugs. When the drug targets linked with a particular disease is identified, and the protein structure or its homologs are accessible, by using structural bioinformatics it is feasible to virtually scrutinize the collection of prevailing drugs for its application against the said disease [58, 59].

The utilization of bioinformatics tool in analysis of whole genome sequence and rRNA gene sequence for identifying microbes is becoming popular in recent time. There is also a need for bioinformatics resources and database for quick, precise detection and better understanding of resistance factors, virulence factors, resistome analysis and mechanisms for antimicrobial resistance so that medical microbiologist and physicians can control the emerging infectious disease causing pathogens. Antimicrobial genes in completely sequenced isolates can be assessed through services like "CARD (Comprehensive Antibiotic Resistance Database), ARDB (Antibiotic Resistance Data Base)", ResFinderetc [60].

"Reverse vaccinology (RV) is a vaccine development process which involves the recognition of novel antigens through analysis of the genomic information of an organism. This process depends on bioinformatics tools such as the VaxiJen server to identify target allergens using genetic makeup information of the pathogen and determine various antigenic and physico-chemical properties associated with the antigenic epitopes. RV can disclose the genes that encode proteins that could lead to good epitopes" [61, 62]. Reverse vaccinology saves the time as well as cost effective than the traditional drug design approach. It has been utilized in the invention of multiepitope chimeric vaccines against the SARS-COV-2 [63].

"Immunoinformatics involves the scrutiny of the total information on an organism's immunomics and using the generated data to make prediction of immune response against specific molecule. Immuno informatics have been utilized in recognition of the humoral and cellular immune cells epitopes on SARS-CoV-2" [64].

6.12 Prognosis of Ailments

Prostate cancer is one of the most lethal malignancies in males and researchers are now attempting to track its biomarker. As molecular interaction networks has developed for human, network level biomarker develops as a hopeful method that can aid in prognosis and diagnosis of human prostate cancer [65].

microRNA (miRNA) plays a key role in the regulation of the different biological processes which in turn can be studies for the prognosis and diagnosis of various diseases [66]. Obstructive sleep apnea (OSA) is a common chronic obstructive sleep disorder. MicroT-CDS and Target Scan databases were used to predict target genes of the differentially expressed microRNAs between OSA patients and healthy controls and regulatory co-expression network was built with Cytoscape software and functional scrutiny was conducted using FunRich. The outcome of this type of study can provide a basis for the prevention diagnosis pathogenesis and treatment of OSA [67].

The miRNA and transcription factors regulation network of hub genes in gastric cancer and colorectal cancer may assist understanding of the molecular level pathophysiology for these malignancies and provide potential targets for its prognosis, diagnosis and treatment [68, 69].

Similar outcome is also derived by exploiting the homeobox (HOX) genes specifically HOXC13, a class of transcription factors for the prognosis of breast cancer and mRNA - protein expression of hub genes like IGF1, ACADL, CYP2C9, and G6PDmay serve as targets for the prognosis and treatment of hepatocellular carcinoma developed in obese individuals [70, 71]. Execution of metabolic data information will enable application of advanced data integration and models to integrate biological and biomedical data, construction of systems functional structure model, organized design of experiment to permit accurate analysis, recognition of anomalous metabolic pathways, predict metabolic disorders, prognosis of genetic predisposition, diagnosis, drug development, and toxicology [72]. Different miRNAs, along with their target genes are involved in the intricate pathophysiology of type 2 diabetes mellitus. miRNAs play significant role in metabolic homeostasis via regulation of various genes and have attracted considerable scientific attention as prognostic and diagnostic biomarkers in type 2 diabetes mellitus [73]. The specified miRNAs exhibit significant changes reasonably before the severe and irrevocable cerebral damage, they can potentially identify patients at risk and allow early stroke diagnosis before they develops an acute stroke [74].

6.13 Concluding Remarks and Future Prospects

Clinical bioinformatics delivers biological and medical evidence to permit for personalized healthcare. The statistics achieved from using microarray is tremendously complex. The selection of suitable software to examine the microarray data for medicinal verdict makes it vital. Proteomics strategy tools frequently emphasis on similarity searches, structure prediction, and protein modeling. To reveal the purpose, the proteomic data must be used in conjugation with clinical data in clinical bioinformatics. In pharmacogenomics, clinical bioinformatics comprises elaborate study of bioinformatics and several evidences of proteomics associated with drug target recognition and medical validation [75]. By applying clinical bioinformatics, scientists relate computational and high throughput investigational methods to research in malignancy and systems biology. For now, bioinformatics and medicinal investigators have combined clinical bioinformatics to widen the scope of healthcare system, using biological and clinical information. Clinical bioinformatics by exploring huge amount biological data, will give improvement in the practice of the healthcare system. It can be considered that clinical bioinformatics offers assistances to improve healthcare, prevent evolution of disease and maintenance of health as the society move ahead in the tenure of personalized medicine.

Next Generation Sequencing (NGS) technology, frequently perceived as the base of precision medicines, has been efficaciously used in prognosis, diagnosis and immunotherapy of cancer and auto immune diseases. With the development in gene diagnostics and immunotherapy, there are certainly probabilities to inhibit the tumor growth and improve the life quality of patients which go through chemotherapy. To stimulate interpretation of precision medicine from bench to bedside and from use of genetic testing to personalized medicine, newer analytical techniques for NGS and genetic data certainly needed to establish. For instance, the NGS panel is relatively altered from whole genome sequencing (WGS), which only concentrating on lesser genes or regions still it involves higher accuracy and proficiency. For multifarious illnesses, such as malignancies, the main genes are frequently a gene clusters in a regulatory network. Graph theories, similar to shortest path analysis and random walk algorithms, will assistance dissect genome wide interactions into key modules or paths whose dysfunction is related with progress of disease [76]. The exercise of studying genetic disease is varying from examination of single genes in separation to find out cellular networks of genes, understanding their multifaceted interactions, and recognizing their role in illness [77]. As an outcome of this, an entire newer phase of independently tailored medicine will appear. Bioinformatics will direct and assistance molecular biologists and clinical researchers to exploit on the advantages gave by computational biology. The clinical research teams that will be supreme successful in the approaching years will be those that can move easily among the laboratory bench, clinical practice, by using of these sophisticated computational functions [78].

Acknowledgement

Figure 6.1 is adopted from https://www.ebi.ac.uk/training/online/courses/functional-genomics-i-introduction-and-design/what-is-functional-genomics/ while figure 6.4 is adopted from Hinkson IV, Madej B and Stahlberg EA (2020) Accelerating Therapeutics for Opportunities in Medicine: A Paradigm Shift in Drug Discovery. Front. Pharmacol. 11:770. doi: 10.3389/fphar.2020.00770 under Creative Commons Attribution 4.0 International (CC BY 4.0) license. Figure 6.6 is adopted under Creative Commons Attribution 4.0 International (CC BY 4.0) license from Katoh M and Katoh M (2021) Grand Challenges in Molecular Medicine for Disease Prevention and Treatment through Cyclical Innovation. *Front. Mol. Med.* 1:720577. doi: 10.3389/fmmed.2021.720577.

References

1. Bhat, P., Mattarollo, S.R., Gosmann, C., Frazer, I.H., Leggatt, G.R., Regulation of immune responses to HPV infection and during HPV-directed immunotherapy. *Immunol. Rev.*, 239, 1, 85–98, 2011.

2. Gildener-Leapman, N., Ferris, R.L., Bauman, J.E., Promising systemic immunotherapies in head and neck squamous cell carcinoma. *Oral. Oncol.*, 49, 12, 1089–1096, 2013.
3. Leibowitz, M.S., Filho, P.A.A., Ferrone, S., Ferris, R.L., Deficiency of activated STAT1 in head and neck cancer cells mediates TAP1-dependent escape from cytotoxic T lymphocytes. *Cancer Immunol. Immunother.*, 60, 4, 525–535, 2011.
4. Leibowitz, M.S., Srivastava, R.M., Filho, P.A.A. *et al.*, SHP2 is overexpressed and inhibits pSTAT1-mediated APM component expression, T-cell attracting chemokine secretion, and CTL recognition in head and neck cancer cells. *Clin. Cancer Res.*, 19, 4, 798–808, 2013.
5. Cheng, F., Wang, H.-W., Cuenca, A. *et al.*, A critical role for Stat3 signaling in immune tolerance. *Immunity*, 19, 3, 425–436, 2003.
6. Moutsopoulos, N.M., Wen, J., Wahl, S.M., TGF-β and tumors—An ill-fated alliance. *Curr. Opin. Immunol.*, 20, 2, 234–240, 2008.
7. Herberman, R.B. and Holden, H.T., Natural cell-mediated immunity. *Adv. Cancer Res.*, 27, 305–377, 1978.
8. Bayat, A., Bioinformatics. *BMJ*, 324, 7344, 1018–1022, 2002.
9. Teufel, A., Krupp, M., Weinmann, A., Galle, P.R., Current bioinformatics tools in genomic biomedical research (review). *Int. J. Mol. Med.*, 17, 6, 967–973, 2006.
10. Dunn, G.P., Bruce, A.T., Ikeda, H., Old, L.J., Schreiber, R.D., Cancer immunoediting: From immunosurveillance to tumor escape. *Nat. Immunol.*, 3, 11, 991–998, 2002.
11. Russell, J.H. and Ley, T.J., Lymphocyte-mediated cytotoxicity. *Annu. Rev. Immunol.*, 20, 1, 323–370, 2002.
12. Komohara, Y., Jinushi, M., Takeya, M., Clinical significance of macrophage heterogeneity in human malignant tumors. *Cancer Sci.*, 105, 1, 1–8, 2014.
13. O'Brien, P.M. and Campo, M.S., Evasion of host immunity directed by papillomavirus-encoded proteins. *Virus Res.*, 88, 1–2, 103–117, 2002.
14. Allen, C.T., Ricker, J.L., Chen, Z., Van Waes, C., Role of activated nuclear factor-κB in the pathogenesis and therapy of squamous cell carcinoma of the head and neck. *Head Neck: J. Sci. Spec. Head Neck*, 29, 10, 959–971, 2007.
15. Kammertoens, T., Schüler, T., Blankenstein, T., Immunotherapy: Target the stroma to hit the tumor. *Trends Mol. Med.*, 11, 5, 225–231, 2005.
16. Mooney, S.D., Krishnan, V.G., Evani, U.S., Bioinformatic tools for identifying disease gene and SNP candidates. *Methods Mol. Biol.*, 628, 307–319, 2010.
17. Camacho, M., León, X., Fernández-Figueras, M.T., Quer, M., Vila, L., Prostaglandin E2 pathway in head and neck squamous cell carcinoma. *Head Neck: J. Sci. Spec. Head Neck*, 30, 9, 1175–1181, 2008.
18. Johnson, B.F., Clay, T.M., Hobeika, A.C., Lyerly, H.K., Morse, M.A., Vascular endothelial growth factor and immunosuppression in cancer: Current knowledge and potential for new therapy. *Expert Opin. Biol. Ther.*, 7, 4, 449–460, 2007.

19. Ralainirina, N., Poli, A., Michel, T. *et al.*, Control of NK cell functions by CD4+ CD25+ regulatory T cells. *J. Leukoc. Biol.*, 81, 1, 144–153, 2007.
20. Callahan, M.K. and Wolchok, J.D., At the bedside: CTLA-4-and PD-1-blocking antibodies in cancer immunotherapy. *J. Leukoc. Biol.*, 94, 1, 41–53, 2013.
21. Quezada, S. and Peggs, K., Exploiting CTLA-4, PD-1 and PD-L1 to reactivate the host immune response against cancer. *Br. J. Cancer*, 108, 8, 1560–1565, 2013.
22. Lyford-Pike, S., Peng, S., Young, G.D. *et al.*, Evidence for a role of the PD-1: PD-L1 pathway in immune resistance of HPV-associated head and neck squamous cell carcinoma. *Cancer Res.*, 73, 6, 1733–1741, 2013.
23. Amiri-Dashatan, N., Koushki, M., Abbaszadeh, H.-A., Rostami-Nejad, M., Rezaei-Tavirania, M., Proteomics applications in health: Biomarker and drug discovery and food industry. *Iran J. Pharm. Res.*, 17, 4, 1523–1536, 2018.
24. Ferris, R.L., Lu, B., Kane, L.P., Too much of a good thing? Tim-3 and TCR signaling in T cell exhaustion. *J. Immunol.*, 193, 4, 1525–1530, 2014.
25. Pak, A.S., Wright, M.A., Matthews, J.P., Collins, S.L., Petruzzelli, G.J., Young, M., Mechanisms of immune suppression in patients with head and neck cancer: Presence of CD34 (+) cells which suppress immune functions within cancers that secrete granulocyte-macrophage colony-stimulating factor. *Clin. Cancer Res.*, 1, 1, 95–103, 1995.
26. Ferris, R.L., Immunology and immunotherapy of head and neck cancer. *J. Clin. Oncol.*, 33, 29, 3293, 2015.
27. Ostrand-Rosenberg, S., Ostrand-Rosenberg, S., Sinha, P., Myeloid-derived suppressor cells: Linking inflammation and cancer. *J. Immunol.*, 182, 4499–4506, 2009.
28. Wu, D., Rice, C.M., Wang, X., Cancer bioinformatics: A new approach to systems clinical medicine. *BMC Bioinf.*, 13, 71, 2012.
29. Lemmon, M.A., Schlessinger, J., Ferguson, K.M., The EGFR family: Not so prototypical receptor tyrosine kinases. *Cold Spring Harb. Perspect. Biol.*, 6, 4, a020768, 2014.
30. Lemmon, M.A. and Schlessinger, J., Cell signaling by receptor tyrosine kinases. *Cell*, 141, 7, 1117–1134, 2010.
31. Specenier, P. and Vermorken, J.B., Cetuximab in the treatment of squamous cell carcinoma of the head and neck. *Expert Rev. Anticancer Ther.*, 11, 4, 511–524, 2011.
32. Zhang, X., Gureasko, J., Shen, K., Cole, P.A., Kuriyan, J., An allosteric mechanism for activation of the kinase domain of epidermal growth factor receptor. *Cell*, 125, 6, 1137–1149, 2006.
33. Schlessinger, J., Receptor tyrosine kinases: Legacy of the first two decades. *Cold Spring Harb. Perspect. Biol.*, 6, 3, a008912, 2014.
34. Yarden, Y. and Pines, G., The ERBB network: At last, cancer therapy meets systems biology. *Nat. Rev. Cancer*, 12, 8, 553–563, 2012.

35. Sega, E.I., Leveson-Gower, D.B., Florek, M., Schneidawind, D., Luong, R.H., Negrin, R.S., Role of lymphocyte activation gene-3 (Lag-3) in conventional and regulatory T cell function in allogeneic transplantation. *PloS One*, 9, 1, e86551, 2014.
36. Schuler, P.J., Harasymczuk, M., Visus, C. *et al.*, Phase I dendritic cell p53 peptide vaccine for head and neck cancer. *Clin. Cancer Res.*, 20, 9, 2433–2444, 2014.
37. Chanrion, M., Negre, V., Fontaine, H. *et al.*, A gene expression signature that can predict the recurrence of tamoxifen-treated primary breast cancer. *Clin. Cancer Res.*, 14, 6, 1744–1752, 2008.
38. Bandrés, E., Zárate, R., Ramirez, N., Abajo, A., Bitarte, N., García-Foncillas, J., Pharmacogenomics in colorectal cancer: The first step for individualized-therapy. *World J. Gastroenterol.*, 13, 44, 5888, 2007.
39. Goddard, E.T., Bozic, I., Riddell, S.R., Ghajar, C.M., Dormant tumour cells, their niches and the influence of immunity. *Nat. Cell Biol.*, 20, 11, 1240–1249, 2018.
40. Jain, A., Reyes, J., Kashyap, R. *et al.*, What have we learned about primary liver transplantation under tacrolimus immunosuppression?: Long-term follow-up of the first 1000 patients. *Ann. Surg.*, 230, 3, 441, 1999.
41. Mbah, C. and Okorie, N., Pharmaceutical bioinformatics: Its relevance to drug metabolism. *Madridge J. Bioinform. Syst. Biol.*, 1, 1, 19–26, 2018.
42. Gannon, F., Molecular medicine: Trendy title or new reality? *EMBO Rep.*, 4, 8, 733, 2003.
43. Ostrowski, J. and Wyrwicz, L.S., Integrating genomics, proteomics and bioinformatics in translational studies of molecular medicine. *Expert Rev. Mol. Diagn.*, 9, 6, 623–630, 2009.
44. Chang, S.-H., Ho, H.-Y., Zang, C.-Z. *et al.*, Screening of nitrosamine impurities in sartan pharmaceuticals by GC-MS/MS. *Mass Spectrom. Lett.*, 12, 2, 31–40, 2021.
45. Shaikh, T., Gosar, A., Sayyed, H., Nitrosamine impurities in drug substances and drug products. *JAPP*, 2, 48–57, 2020.
46. O'Donnell, J.S., Teng, M.W., Smyth, M.J., Cancer immunoediting and resistance to T cell-based immunotherapy. *Nat. Rev. Clin. Oncol.*, 16, 3, 151–167, 2019.
47. Xing, D.T., Khor, R., Gan, H., Wada, M., Ermongkonchai, T., Ng, S.P., Recent research on combination of radiotherapy with targeted therapy or immunotherapy in head and neck squamous cell carcinoma: A review for radiation oncologists. *Cancers*, 13, 22, 5716, 2021.
48. Shibata, H., Saito, S., Uppaluri, R., Immunotherapy for head and neck cancer: A paradigm shift from induction chemotherapy to neoadjuvant immunotherapy. *Front. Oncol.*, 11, 3533, 2021.
49. Erikainen, S. and Chan, S., Contested futures: Envisioning "personalized," "stratified," and "precision" medicine. *New Genet. Soc.*, 38, 3, 308–330, 2019.

50. Amin, N., Maroun, C.A., El Asmar, M. *et al.*, Neoadjuvant immunotherapy prior to surgery for mucosal head and neck squamous cell carcinoma: Systematic review. *Head Neck*, 44, 2, 562–571, 2022.
51. Knochelmann, H.M., Horton, J.D., Liu, S. *et al.*, Neoadjuvant presurgical PD-1 inhibition in oral cavity squamous cell carcinoma. *Cell Rep. Med.*, 2, 10, 100426, 2021.
52. Goetz, L. and Schork, N., Personalized medicine: Motivation, Challenges and progress. *Fertil. Steril.*, 109, 6, 952–963, 2018.
53. Everett, C., Desai, A.M., Cavanaugh, M.E. *et al.*, Neoadjuvant and adjuvant nivolumab and lirilumab in patients with recurrent, resectable squamous cell carcinoma of the head and neck. *Clin. Cancer Res.*, 28, 3, 468–478, 2022.
54. Chukwudozie, O.S., Duru, V.C., Ndiribe, C.C., Aborode, A.T., Oyebanji, V.O., Emikpe, B.O., The relevance of bioinformatics applications in the discovery of vaccine candidates and potential drugs for COVID-19 treatment. *Bioinform. Biol. Insights*, 15, 11779322211002168, 2021.
55. Jin, Z., Du, X., Xu, Y., Deng, Y., Liu, M., Zhao, Y., Zhang, B., Li, X., Zhang, L., Peng, C., Duan, Y. *et al.*, Structure of Mpro from SARS-CoV-2 and discovery of its inhibitors. *Nature*, 582, 289–293, 2020.
56. Wang, J., Fast identification of possible drug treatment of coronavirus disease-19 (COVID-19) through computational drug repurposing study. *J. Chem. Inf. Model.*, 60, 6, 3277–3286, 2020.
57. Parikesit, A.A. and Nurdiansyah, R., Drug repurposing option for COVID-19 with structural bioinformatics of chemical interactions approach. *Cermin Dunia Kedokteran*, 47, 3, 222–226, 2020.
58. Lee, C.H. and Koohy, H., *In silico* identification of vaccine targets for 2019-nCoV. *F1000Res.*, 25, 9, 145, 2020.
59. Enayatkhani, M., Hasaniazad, M., Faezi, S. *et al.*, Reverse vaccinology approach to design a novel multi-epitope vaccine candidate against COVID-19: An in silico study. *J. Biomol. Struct. Dyn.*, 39, 8, 2857–2872, 2021.
60. Saeb, A.T., Current bioinformatics resources in combating infectious diseases. *Bioinformation*, 14, 1, 31, 2018.
61. Ullah, M.A., Sarkar, B., Islam, S.S., Exploiting the reverse vaccinology approach to design novel subunit vaccines against Ebola virus. *Immunobiology*, 225, 3, 151949, 2020.
62. Sanami, S., Zandi, M., Pourhossein, B. *et al.*, Design of a multi-epitope vaccine against SARS-CoV-2 using immunoinformatics approach. *Int. J. Biol. Macromol.*, 164, 871–883, 2020.
63. María, R., Arturo, C., Alicia, J.A., Paulina, M., Gerardo, A.O., The impact of bioinformatics on vaccine design and development. *Vaccines*, 2, 3–6, 2017.
64. Srivastava, S., Verma, S., Kamthania, M. *et al.*, Structural basis for designing multiepitope vaccines against COVID-19 infection: *In silico* vaccine design and validation. *JMIR Bioinf. Biotechnol.*, 1, 1, e19371, 2020.

65. Chen, J. and Shen, B., Network biomarkers for diagnosis and prognosis of human prostate cancer, in: *Bioinformatics for Diagnosis, Prognosis and Treatment of Complex Diseases*, pp. 207–220, Springer, NY, 2013.
66. Mani, I., Role of bioinformatics in microRNA analysis, in: *Advances in Bioinformatics*, pp. 365–373, Springer, NY, 2021.
67. Li, K., Wei, P., Qin, Y., Wei, Y., MicroRNA expression profiling and bioinformatics analysis of dysregulated microRNAs in obstructive sleep apnea patients. *Medicine*, 96, 34, e7917, 2017.
68. Li, T., Gao, X., Han, L., Yu, J., Li, H., Identification of hub genes with prognostic values in gastric cancer by bioinformatics analysis. *World J. Surg. Oncol.*, 16, 1, 1–12, 2018.
69. Gong, B., Kao, Y., Zhang, C., Sun, F., Gong, Z., Chen, J., Identification of hub genes related to carcinogenesis and prognosis in colorectal cancer based on integrated bioinformatics. *Mediators Inflamm.*, 2020, 5934821, 14, 2020.
70. Li, C., Cui, J., Zou, L., Zhu, L., Wei, W., Bioinformatics analysis of the expression of HOXC13 and its role in the prognosis of breast cancer. *Oncol. Lett.*, 19, 1, 899–907, 2020.
71. Ceylan, H., Identification of hub genes associated with obesity-induced hepatocellular carcinoma risk based on integrated bioinformatics analysis. *Med. Oncol.*, 38, 6, 1–11, 2021.
72. Chen, M. and Hofestädt, R., A medical bioinformatics approach for metabolic disorders: Biomedical data prediction, modeling, and systematic analysis. *J. Biomed. Inform.*, 39, 2, 147–159, 2006.
73. Pordzik, J., Jakubik, D., Jarosz-Popek, J. *et al.*, Significance of circulating microRNAs in diabetes mellitus type 2 and platelet reactivity: Bioinformatic analysis and review. *Cardiovasc. Diabetol.*, 18, 1, 1–19, 2019.
74. Eyileten, C., Wicik, Z., De Rosa, S. *et al.*, MicroRNAs as diagnostic and prognostic biomarkers in ischemic stroke—A comprehensive review and bioinformatic analysis. *Cells*, 7, 12, 249, 2018.
75. Chang, P.L., Clinical bioinformatics. *Chang Gung Med. J.*, 28, 4, 201–211, 2005.
76. Cai, Y., Huang, T., Yang, J., Applications of bioinformatics and systems biology in precision medicine and immunooncology. *BioMed. Res. Int.*, 2018, 1–2, 2018.
77. Debouk, C. and Metcalf, B., The impact of genomics on drug discovery. *Annu. Rev. Pharmacol. Toxicol.*, 40, 193–208, 2000.
78. Butler, D., Are you ready for the revolution? *Nature*, 409, 758–760, 2001.

7

Clinical Applications of "Omics" Technology as a Bioinformatic Tool

Vivek Chavda[1]*, Rajashri Bezbaruah[2], Disha Valu[3], Sanjay Desai[4], Nildip Chauhan[5], Swati Marwadi[6], Gitima Deka[7] and Zhiyong Ding[8]†

[1]Department of Pharmaceutics and Pharmaceutical Technology, L.M. College of Pharmacy, Ahmedabad, Gujarat, India
[2]Department of Pharmaceutical Sciences, Faculty of Science and Engineering, Dibrugarh University, Dibrugarh, Assam, India
[3]Drug Product Development Lab, Intas Pharmaceutical Ltd. (Biopharma division), Ahmedabad, Gujarat, India
[4]Analytical Development Lab, Sun Pharma Advanced Research Centre, Vadodara, Gujarat, India
[5]Drug Product Development, Enzene Biosciences Limited, Pune, India
[6]Department of Biotechnology, Sinhgad College of Engineering, Pune, India
[7]College of Pharmacy, Yeungnam University, Gyeonsan, Republic of Korea
[8]Mills Institute for Personalized Cancer Care, Fynn Biotechnologies Ltd., Gangxing 3rd Rd, High-Tech and Innovation Zone, Jinan City, Shandong Province, P. R. China

Abstract

In the new era of scientific research, the word 'Omics' has been the most significant term. This term comes up with the ideology of studying and analyzing almost all the aspects of biological systems, which specifically concentrate on a complex system of life. It also includes high-throughput molecular biology techniques used by computational drug discovery tools. The use of this technology is mainly to study, analyze and interpret the data of the entire human genomic sequence, which is the most significant achievement in the discipline of biomedical and bio-informational scientific research. Comprehensive data analysis is accomplished using a multidisciplinary approach such as microarrays and other bioinformatics tools, so it becomes easier for researchers to examine

**Corresponding author*: vivek7chavda@gmail.com
†*Corresponding author*: zhiyong.ding@fynnbio.com

Vivek Chavda, Krishnan Anand and Vasso Apostolopoulos (eds.) Bioinformatics Tools for Pharmaceutical Drug Product Development, (117–146) © 2023 Scrivener Publishing LLC

the biological activity of 30,000 human genes and polymorphism on large scale beyond 20 lakhs numbers. Polymorphism is relatively common, known for its dynamic functions and interaction, which affects the human species, nowadays it is considered rare, but the vast majority of them are single nucleotide polymorphisms. As "Omics" techniques are used to expose the network among gene products, as humans are genetically similar, they could aid greatly in disease diagnosis and treatment by monitoring and analyzing the interaction of biomolecules in living systems.

Keywords: Omics technology, genomics, proteomics, metabolomics, lipomics, etc.

Abbreviations

COVID-19	The Coronavirus Disease
SARS-CoV-2	Severe acute respiratory syndrome coronavirus 2
m/z	mass to-charge ratio
DNA	Deoxyribonucleic acid
RNA	Ribonucleic acid
MS	Mass Spectrometry
ELISA	Enzyme-linked immunosorbent assay
SILAC	Stable Isotope Labeling by/with Amino acids in Cell culture
ITRAQ	Multiplexed Isobaric Tagging Technology for Relative Quantitation
SDS-PAGE	Sodium dodecyl-sulfate polyacrylamide gel electrophoresis
2D-PAGE	Two-dimensional gel electrophoresis
2D-DIQE	Two-dimensional difference gel electrophoresis
NMR Spectroscopy	Nuclear Magnetic Resonance Spectroscopy
TGP	Toxicogenomics Project

7.1 Introduction

Informational science is the experimental study of biological data, which is nothing but the collection of information of the biotic system. As it is the interdisciplinary field of science, which has the foundation of appropriate computational tools and procedures to assemble, understand, analyze as well as provide measurable and accurate biological data [1]. Nowadays, more and more biological research is relying on information science. Indeed, to obtain beneficial information of network within the human biological living system, as it has many practical applications in informational science, that has provided us parallel opportunity to apply new technological approaches to get a better understanding of highly multiplexed sequencing methods with the power of computational tools and algorithms [2]. Rapid progress in biochemistry and genetic research with aid of computational tools has generated a huge volume of genetic and protein sequence data [3]. But nowadays, as this field is explored in molecular biology, it becomes difficult to do research using high-throughput technologies to study complex biotic systems and quantify the data as the unavailability of such multidisciplinary-oriented trained manpower and appropriate computational procedures. The development of a new biological research paradigm and preciseness of work in the biological field using software tools in the future will be beneficial to study the genome, which would help accomplish all these tasks starting from drug discovery to biomarker finding. Also, a few years back there is a high demand for biomedical research and genetics, the focus of scientists to study human biology is to identify the sequencing of thousands of genomes, which mostly show diversity in their gene products, as this data will provide fundamental insight into human biology [4, 5]. Currently, these pathways of using computational tools in the biological field bring primary challenges to researchers and scientists, which face various problems in bioinformatics [6]. COVID-19 is currently having a terrible influence on mankind owing to its infectious and quick dissemination. Although SARS-CoV-2 vaccines have been created, the treatment requires the identification of proven, effective, and targeted medicinal compounds. Throughout these attempts, the whole-genome sequencing of SARS-CoV-2 has provided a roadmap for investigating omics systems and techniques to combat this global health crisis. Sequence investigations of the genome, proteome, and metagenome have aided in identifying virus nature, which has aided in understanding the molecular mechanism, anatomical understanding, and clinical progression [7, 8].

7.2 Execution Method

The discovery of biomolecule, biomarker, and its development has been vast in biomedical research and informational science, through complex technologies that aim to evaluate what type of sample should be used and sample preparation for biomarker discovery [9]. However, the identification of biomarkers should be a systematic approach; it must be economical, quick, consistent, and compatible in biological fluids so that it could be evaluated easily. To obtain accurate and reliable data, that should be safe and easy to measure, rigorous reproducible steps in a standardized manner are essential. In addition, samples must be collected, stored, and translocated systematically [10].

Biomarkers may provide crucial information about the metabolic profile in drug development [11]. The biological samples harvested by biopsy are needed in such a case which helps to maintain the efficacy and safety. 'Omics' experiments include the necessary step of sample preparation that should be reproducible. For the chemical analysis of proteomics and metabolomics, high-throughput technology i.e. mass spectrometry is used [12]. This strategy usually includes the process of creating ions from neutral proteins, peptides, or metabolites via chemical ionization or electron impact, and the chemical separation of the molecules occurs as per their mass-to-charge ratio (m/z) and is identified using an analytical method such as mass spectrum analysis, which is defining feature of the molecular mass and/or structure [13]. Interestingly, the comprehensive analysis of metabolomics in biomedical research using various technological approaches, required that are well versed with many multi-omics experiments [14]. Metabolomics provides some useful guidelines for better understanding of sampling, handling, and processing, as well as multi-omics experiments performed by other scientists, that help in enhancement of data assessment and this data (integrated-omics data, Figure 7.1) with the metadata, will be crucial under circumstances being taken for studies. Here, we are having

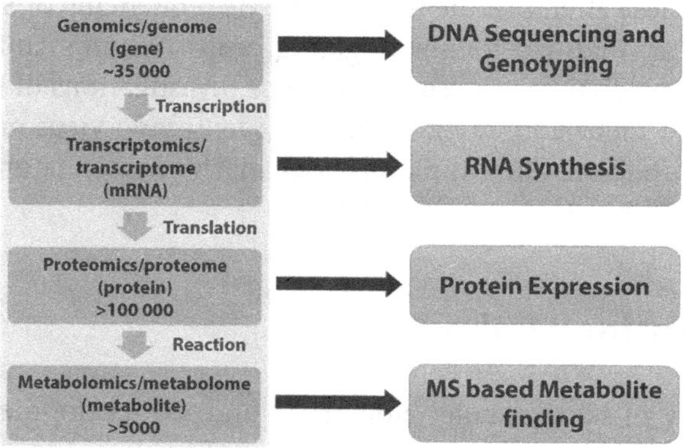

Figure 7.1 Omics science and their interaction.

the presence of a community of microbes i.e. host-associated microbiomes, based on recent research will have an idea about the mechanistic bases of their associations, as data from this microbiome can now also be integrated with exometabolomic data [15, 16].

7.3 Overview of Omics Technology

In today's world of scientific research, the word 'Omics' technology referred to the computational tools and high throughput techniques, which aim to interpret the meaningful biological data in biomedical and genetics research, that must be accurate and reliable (Figure 7.2). This technology has been able to focus on analysis and integration of the data associated with the biomolecule in a wide spectrum. Although, this technology in the area of bioinformatics was able to regulate the network of the biological systems and their evaluation on large scale [17, 18]. On the contrary, with regards to explorative analysis, researchers have pa problems in extracting the relevant data related to 'Omics' technology [19].

Although 'Omics' technology is the latest technology, which provides data on large scale in a relatively short time, it has several issues that refer to a biomolecule in an 'Omic' experiment, wherefrom the statistical point of view the recognition of similar features regarding a phenotype which is susceptible to error in the data analysis [20, 21]. Here, concerning obtaining meaningful and useful data from 'Omics', bioinformatics is an important tool. Furthermore, Omics data overview and its evaluation is done using 'Omics' technology in bioinformatics [22–24]. Table 7.1 summarizes the overall overview of omics arms and their applicability, and Figure 7.3 depicts the integrated workflow of the same.

Since this technique incorporates the use of high-throughput omics strategies, which provide a preferentially more effective and manageable framework for understanding data in biomedical research and agriculture, it also develops appropriate treatment of these illnesses such as the plethora of chronic conditions, including chronic disorders like adult-onset diabetes and obesity, and aids in explaining the relation between genetics and nutrition for recognizing the food constituents in the diet [16]. Moreover, qualitative or semi-quantitative data have been produced in more than 20 years with the aid of this technology in bioinformatics. Here, the differentiation that is unsupported by the data across platforms is the qualitative data. Advancement of this technology has to be done to generate precise data, measurement of various platforms over a stipulated period. Moreover, a smaller number of assays of proteomics and genomics are translated,

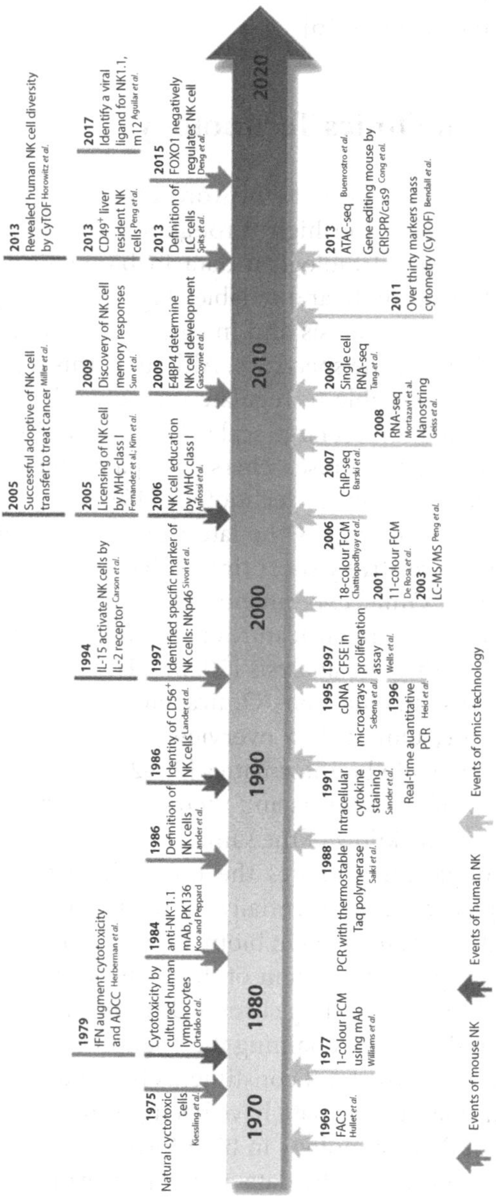

Figure 7.2 Evolution of omics technology.

Table 7.1 Overview of the omics arms and their applicability.

"Omics" technology	Definition	Evaluate	Remark
Nutrigenomics	"Study of the effects of foods and food constituents on gene expression"	DNA/genes	• Nutritional optimization • Helps in the management of severe disease related to nutritional imbalance or deficiency
Transcriptomics	"Study of the complete set of RNA transcripts that are produced by the genome"	RNA/mRNA	• Helps in molecular understanding of some of the diseases • Helps in disease profiling • As a diagnostic tool
Proteomics	"A large-scale study of the set of proteins produced in an organism"	Proteins	• As a diagnostic tool • Disease management • Identification of disease biomarkers
Metabolomics	"A large-scale study of metabolites within cells or organisms"	Metabolites	• As a diagnostic tool • Molecular understanding of disease pathophysiology • Disease management • Identification of disease biomarkers
Ayurgenomics	Ayurgenomics combines Ayurvedic concepts such as Prakriti with modern genetics research.	"Tridoshas (*vata, pitta, and kapha*) and *Prakriti*"	• In Personalized care • Biomarker identification • Therapeutic management

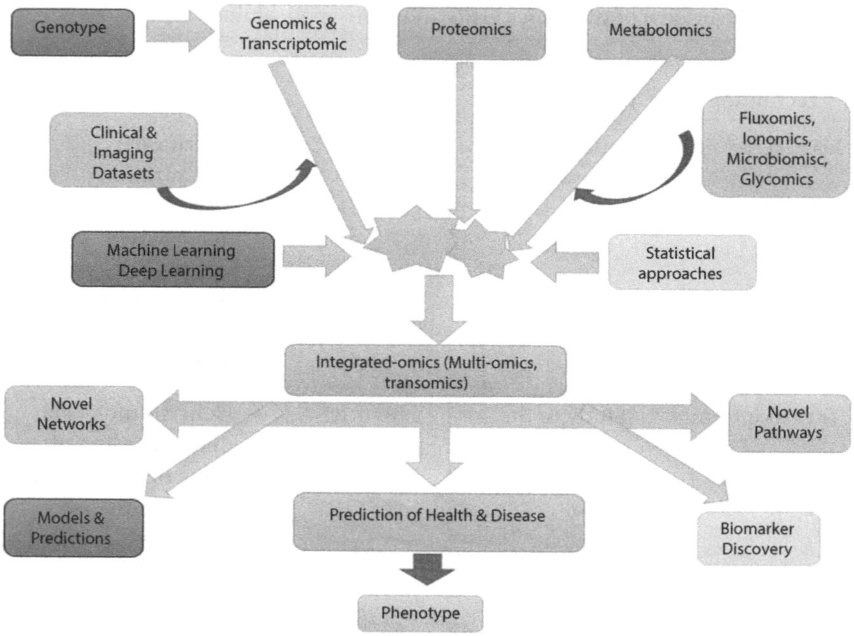

Figure 7.3 Workflow for the integrated omics.

because of a lack of measurement of data Nutrigenomics: The Genome–Food Interface [12, 19]. In addition to the advancement in this technology, the development of about 75,000 genetic tests has been possible with the aid of quantitative genotyping. Also, several chemical tests that have been enabled by quantitative measurement are greater than 300 [25–28].

Likewise, massive information can be generated and interpreted in most other forms facilitating such an approach that will be useful for scientists over a stipulated period at any platform in bioinformatics. So, implementation of publicly valuable data is most significant where standards have been followed. The comprehensive analysis and quantification of 'Omics' data in any format, makes it easier with the use of ontologies [29].

7.4 Genomics

Genomic technology includes genome sequencing techniques and genotype analysis [30]. DNA sequences from genes and other regions can use genome sequencing technology be emanated while genotype analysis detects sequence variation between individual genes in individuals [31].

In earlier days genome sequencing was an impressive task and faster growth in sequencing technology has increased output surprisingly with a decrease in cost. Genome technology now beats all the standard technology used for Human genome projects [32]. Extremely, by using genome sequencing and Genotyping technology it can be possible now to analyze whole genome sequences of individuals. Simultaneously genotyping technology assesses the multiple variants of the whole genome in a large group of the population instead of one or multiple gene polymorphisms (Figure 7.4) [33, 34].

a) The application of genomic technology in gene discovery and medicinal biology in the diagnosis of genetic diseases
Genomics technology has been widely used in the identification of genetic abnormalities [35]. Additionally, research scientists can now discover a new biological unit, i.e., gene, which is responsible for causing the genetic disease with great success [33]. In a recent year, more than 4000 genetic disorders and diseases are identified which have a single common genetic cause which was around 50 in the past decades during the 1990s which proves its vast applicability in the genomic field [36, 37].
b) Identification and diagnosis of genetic factors contributing to common disease
Common genetic factors and the rate of the disease progression can easily be understood by genetic technology which is primarily involved in the

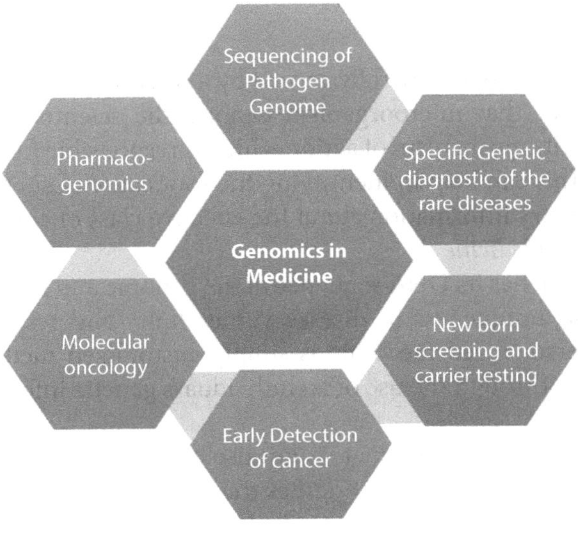

Figure 7.4 Application of genomics in medicines.

development of common diseases like hypertension, cancer, neurological disorders, and other lifestyle disease [38].

c) Pharmacogenetic and target therapy

The genetic information of individuals will give a fair idea about the response of the specific drug to the individuals, its effectiveness in getting a response, and its adverse effect associated with that drug [39]. All this information together helps doctors in choosing the right medicine in the right ways and hence better treatment for the patients. For example, in target therapy, cancer-causing genetic factors and their target can easily be identified and drugs specific to bind with that target can be selected which ultimately act accordingly in the defined pathway.

d) Prenatal diagnosis and testing

Children at an early age are most susceptible to genetic disorders and diseases which may overwhelm and lead to major disability and fatality. The use of prenatal diagnostic during pregnancy or at birth is significantly useful for parents and treatment based on the diagnosis of the genetic disorder can be possible [40]. The earlier prenatal diagnostic was used but not that effective, which puts pregnancy and the life of the fetus at risk. Improved technology and advancements in diagnostic tools, such as non-invasive prenatal testing using genomic technology, make prenatal testing much more secure, and the risk associated with it is significantly reduced by knowing the fetus's DNA. The use of Next-generation sequencing and genetic method which is based on chromosomal microarray analysis for prenatal samples enhance the diagnostic results up to the level during pregnancy [40, 41].

e) Infectious disease

An infectious disease is generally caused by a microorganism. Sequencing the genomes of that microorganism enables the scientist to know the organism and its mechanism of action which is responsible for symptom of the disease. This can help in identifying the root cause of such spread and provide necessary information about the effective class of antibiotics [42].

e) Personalized medicine

Every individual has its DNA sequence of the genome and is unique. Every individual has uniqueness in disease vulnerability and response for the treatment. Personalized medicine is simply customized medicine that is made available through the use of an individual's genetic information [43].

f) Gene therapy

Gene therapy is a technique that makes use of a gene product that serves the abnormalities observed or modifies the expression of genes. Here, the compensation of abnormal genes can be beneficial by the inception of biological gene products into the cells [44].

g) Genome editing
Genome modification can be possible by genome editing using molecular techniques. Section of DNA sequence can be added in, cut us, or replace by genome editing [45].

7.5 Nutrigenomics

Nutrigenomics enables to alteration of the diet based on the individual genetic makeup [46]. Here, the significance in the documentation of target genes, metabolic imbalance, and genetic variations in the DNA sequence is offered by the project, which provides useful genetic data for humans and its research involved with, nitrogenic tests library to assess in clinic, ethnopharmacology, phytopharmaceuticals therapy, and nutrition supplements are the primary evidence of the interaction between nutrients and botanicals with the genome, which can lead to genome modification (Figure 7.5) [47].

All these are the major driving force to develop bio-medicinal food which is non-toxic that try to find out a way to improve health for individual genetic profile [48–50]. The ongoing large-scale nutrition intervention studies allow for the validation of nutrigenomic concepts in specific genes. Which will continue to add new tests in this genomic bio-medicinal panel [51, 52]. The idea of the nutrigenomic concept gives some options to

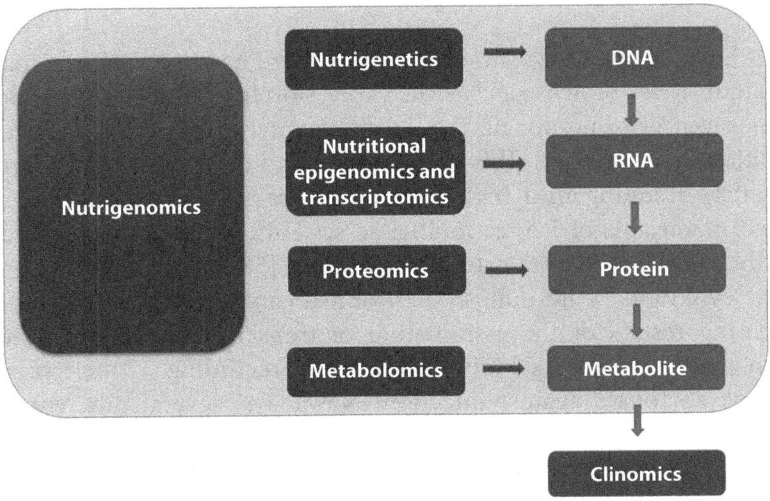

Figure 7.5 Applications of nutrigenomics.

avoid the risk associated with metabolic problems and prevention of health problems. Nutrigenomics helps to know the gene which affects the diet-related disease and provides a solution that triggers genetic predisposition [53]. personal diet plans based on a person's nutritional requirement can be determined by genetic makeup which can clarify the etiological perception of chronic lifestyle diseases like type-2 diabetes, cancer, obesity, heart disease such as CVD [54, 55]. Nutrigenomics can also be used to identify genes associated with diet, gene interactions, and polymorphism. Diet-gene interplay can have significant ramifications and impact environmental factors on gene regulation [56]. By making the use of nutritional genetic tool diet gene interaction studies are showing proof on which gene-specific dietary intervention trials are planned to get the confirmed results. Additional knowledge of biological function can be obtained by nutrigenomics research. However, the use of information by physicians in preventing chronic disease has not yet been accepted for treatment and prevention, but it may be possible to use such type of information in a large group the population at the same time feasibility and applicability can be determined, so principles of nutrigenomics shall be applied and more targeted interventions are expected. Collaborative scientific research and efforts shall be much required and should be implemented and followed in creating experimental design analysis and storage of nutritional research which can ultimately help clinicians and dietitians [57].

7.6 Transcriptomics

Using high throughput technologies which are based on the microarray technique, these omics examine the expression level of mRNAs produced in the given cell line during the developmental stage or under different conditions (Figure 7.6). This technology has been constantly improved ultimately resulting in a high level of accuracy in examining the data related to variants of RNAs, multigene systems, and also in interpreting their response to different external conditions [58].

The evolutionary immune system of fish can be better understood by evaluating results of the assimilation of transcriptomic and proteoses, which involves complex biotic systems and recording of their primary immune responses against infection. Nowadays, several different computational approaches are available to examine and interpret the results of unrevealed variations in the expression of the biological product and regulatory processes which are relevant to the biomedical field, and also to uncover the relationship amongst complex biotic systems. These high

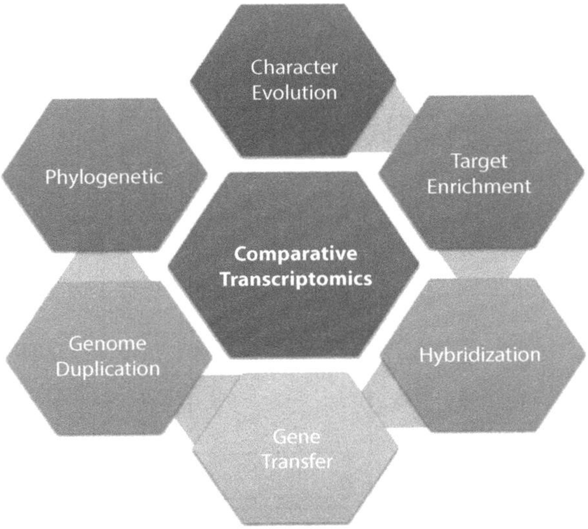

Figure 7.6 Applications of comparative transcriptomics.

throughput multidimensional techniques enabled the generation of vast amounts of information about various cell stages and the lineage of complex biotic systems. For example, by sequencing every transcript in primary tissue under a microscope while maintaining spatial information about the location of each transcript within each cell [59–62].

7.7 Proteomics

This omic technology makes the use of high throughput multidimensional computational technologies such as mass spectrometry (MS) and microarray technologies. As the protein is a very delicate bio-molecule and also its structure is very complex because the concentration of protein present differs in each cell of the organism it becomes difficult to interpret the data related to the complex biotic system (Figure 7.7 and 7.8). Hence, using these methods of informational science, complete analysis of the constituents of complex protein mixtures has been possible in biological science [63, 64]. There are several different advantages of this technology in the field of biomedical science for the diagnosis of a particular disease, which makes the use of computational software, algorithms a target for new drug discovery, where the most number of drug targets are proteins [65]. Alternately, scientists and researchers are trying to study this complex

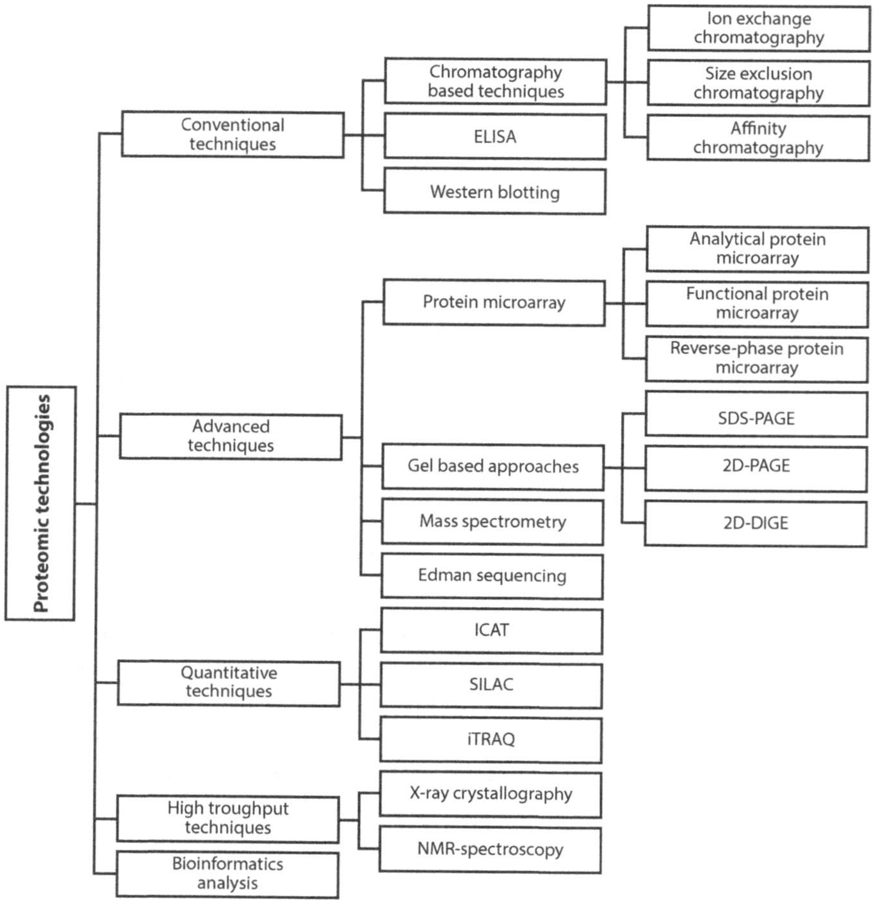

Figure 7.7 Proteomics technologies at a glance.

biomolecule and developing the most effective drug that can be beneficial for individual treatment [66, 67].

7.8 Metabolomics

In the current world, it is the most emerging area of omics technology in informational science, which is used for the systematic recognition and quantification of dynamic changes or the metabolic reaction of biologically relevant small molecules of the given biofluids in the biotic system [68]. Because the metabolic process's chemical molecules bounce back

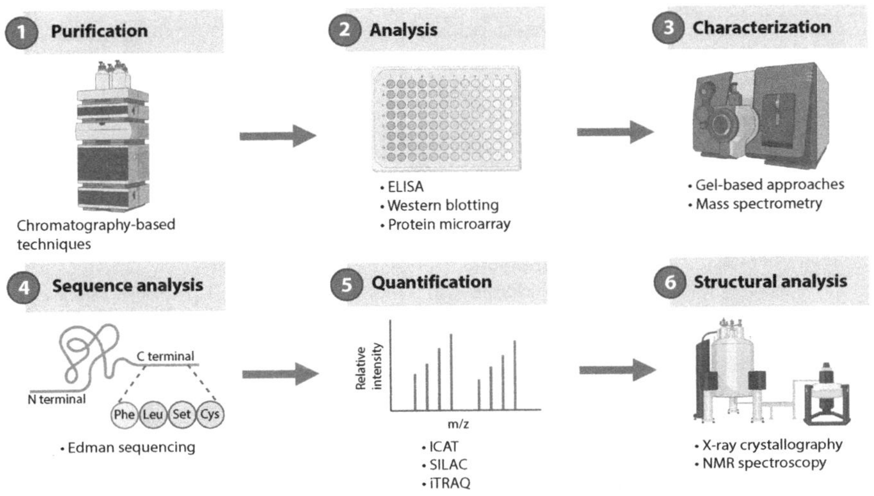

Figure 7.8 Standard proteomics study template. (Created with Biorender.com using Template).

the functionality of these complex biomolecules and biological products that encode them. This technology is very efficient and impartial, which involves the separation, combination, and detection techniques to simultaneously recognize and quantify the chemical molecules. As this area is expanding, there are also some restrictions in producing the data related to simultaneous measurement of as many as small chemical molecules in the biotic system. Immensely, this technology is used in the characterization of disease models which is a key strength among various approaches as well as it represents the endpoint of the biological and pathophysiological processes. In addition, integrated applications with genomics, transcriptomics, and proteomics provide a greater understanding of global system biology [69]. Also, this technology measures the changes in nuclear magnetism of thousands of small molecules in the given compartment of cell or tissue at a time with aid of such high throughput multidimensional NMR spectroscopy and MS techniques. As in all the areas of research, this omics technology needs computational software which has access to searchable databases and approaches for multivariate screening such as in newborn screening so that it will assimilate more with the biotic systems to enhance the knowledge for biological research. Moreover, in the case of clinical application, many genetic diseases include disease of small molecule metabolisms such as atherosclerosis, diabetes, Alzheimer's, cancer, and this can be uncovered by this omics technology [70].

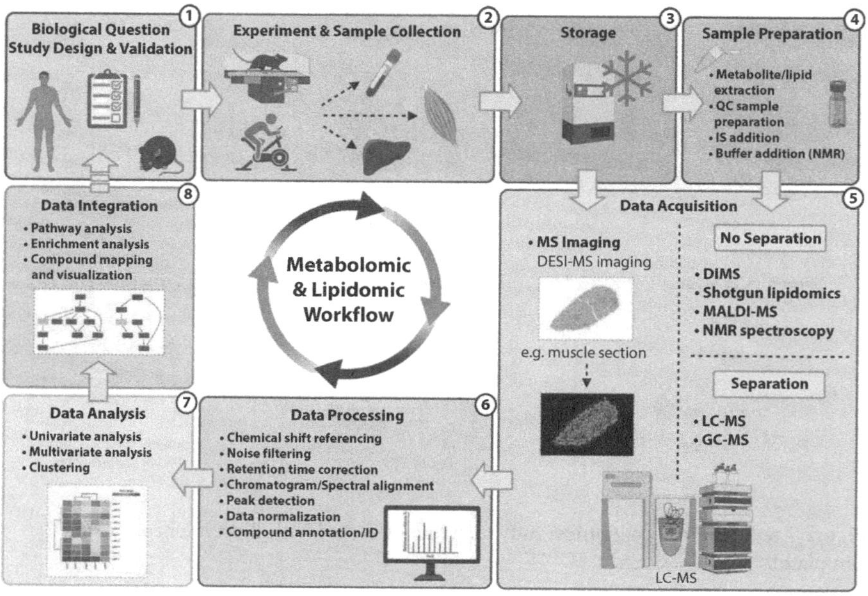

Figure 7.9 Typical metabolomics/lipidomics workflow: (1) after establishing a given biological question, appropriate and optimized study design is a critical step to answer this biological question with minimal bias and noise (i.e., investigation induced variability). (2) Sample collection before/during/after the experiment also requires particular attention and care to avoid introducing potential biases. Therefore, consistency of collection timing, materials and reagents is important. Metabolic reactions are rapid and must be stopped as soon as possible following collection by snap freezing or placing the sample on ice. (3) Samples are then prepared accordingly (e.g., centrifugation of whole blood to collect plasma or serum) for storage until planned sample preparation or direct data acquisition. (4) Sample preparation depends on the analytical platforms utilized and the molecular species to be extracted (e.g., lipids or other metabolites). During this step, QC samples are usually prepared and added to all aliquots to screen and correct platform-related shifts and enhance reproducibility. (5) Samples are analyzed and data are acquired using one or multiple analytical platforms. (6) Acquired raw data are then processed through multiple steps to eventually allow accurate compound identification/annotation. (7) Multiple statistical tests are performed on the identified/annotated compounds to determine potential differences between samples and/or groups in line with the biological question and experimental design. (8) Finally, data are placed into biological context using pathway/enrichment analysis and visualization tools, which also help inform future biological research questions and experimental designs, therefore leading back to step one of the workflow. Alternatively, targeted validation of metabolites/lipids of interest within the dataset may be performed following data integration.

These discoveries have led to the identification of previously unknown therapeutic targets as well as novel potential therapeutic strategies. Earlier metabolomics was not that much developed accessible to the researchers but nowadays it is emerging as a rapidly growing omics technology in informational science. Hence, the computational methods and techniques it comprises aid of which huge amount of data related to many small compounds in the biotic system can be interpreted (Figure 7.9) [71]. However, it is also able to manage the amount of time required for the drug for moving through the development pipeline within a short period. Through the development of personalized phenotyping and individualized drug-response monitoring, metabolomics is beginning to play a role in precision medicine. In addition, this technology has immense knowledge in the biomedical and biological fields of scientific research which has the potential to extract information about thousands of chemical constituents of an abiotic system for the early diagnosis of disease [72]. It can also be used in designing and processing cancer therapies and treating tumors [73].

7.9 Lipomics or Lipidomics

This term in omics technology has been used for studying the lipid, which are the constituents of cellular membrane they have an immense advantage in biomedical and informational science. Currently, this lipomics involve comprehensive knowledge of lipid and determining the relationship among the lipids by making the use of computational high throughput methods to pathology [74]. However, the unproper functioning of this lipomics leads to several diseases as well as important in harmful drug reactions. Although, this omics technology has an immense advantage in a variety of disease states and in obtaining information on disease pathology, but also causes several diseases, which are unrecognizable aid of using biomarker analyses. Here, this change in lipid metabolomics represents shifting in the concentration of chemical molecules simultaneously, which makes them undetectable [75].

Now the recent advances in the biomedical and biological area, related to lipomics involves the progression of high throughput multidimensional assay also accessible standardized database has started extracting the knowledge of lipids and their relationship to pathology (Figure 7.9). These analytical tools and knowledge will allow drug discovery, development, and testing to be conducted with a better understanding of their effects on lipid metabolism [76].

7.10 Ayurgenomics

The combination of genomics and Ayurveda, provided new insights into research i.e., Ayurgenomics [77]. Ayurveda is a complementary medical solution that offers significant evidence for a theoretical-level examination of all facets of life. Unlike modern medicine, Ayurveda is based on the "tri-doshas (vata, pitta, and kapha) and Prakriti" [78]. It has been demonstrated that geo-climatic regions, familial characteristics, and ethnicity all influence phenotypic variability. Prakriti-based treatments can help change the current situation in healthcare by successfully coordinating 'omics'. The approaches and methods of Ayurveda are composed of three Prakriti aspects: aushadhi (medication), vihara (lifestyle), and ahara (diet). These ayurvedic attributes can be used to lay the groundwork for Prakriti-based medicine, preventative medicine, and the enhancement of life quality and longevity [79]. According to Huang and other researchers, "Ayurgenomics forges a new link between modern and traditional medicine by providing a scientific understanding of fundamental concepts while also incorporating ayurvedic practical prophylactic techniques into modern care. This ground-breaking system aims to shift the emphasis from a disease-focused system to a patient-focused wellness system. It is closely related to other emerging areas of medicine such as personalized, integrative, preventive, lifestyle, and functional medicine [80–82]."

7.11 Pharmacogenomics

Currently, this term in omics technology possesses vast knowledge on variations in the biological product at the genome level in genetic and pharmaceutical science which affects the drug product life cycle. Developing an efficient and safe vaccine also improves the accuracy in determining the drug dosage, scanning, and screening of certain diseases this technology has an immense effect to deliver beneficial medical care to the patients (Figure 7.10). These advances in genomic science are associated with several different disorders. The number of populations that have been targeted associated with the disorder related to phenotype, this omics technology will affect the target selection and there will be a rise in efficacy during clinical development. Finally, it will affect patient care which contributes benefit to the physicians' ability to deliver better medical care to patients. This, omics technology in today's world has a tremendous application in informational science in making the profile related to the sensitivity of

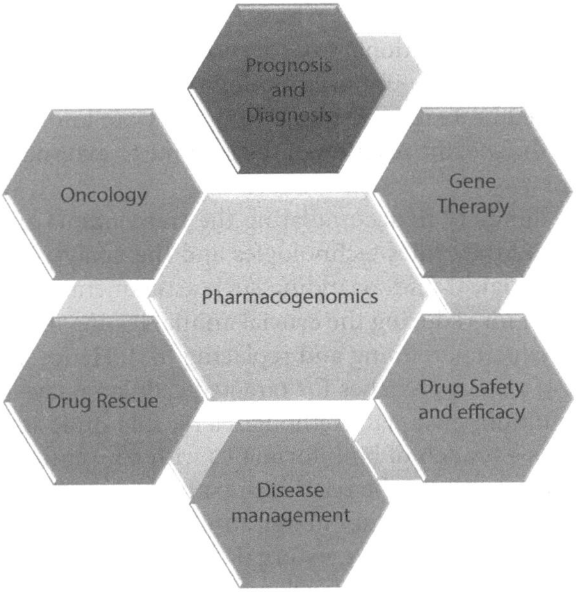

Figure 7.10 Applications of pharmacogenomics.

all the pharmaceuticals, biomarkers, and data related to laboratory tests and also in making the design of drugs using high throughput methods which requires knowledge related to genomics in drug development. Furthermore, the ideology behind drug discovery is to characterize disease risk, contribute to novel therapeutics, and provide insights into the optimal medication regime based on a combination of clinically as well as genetically defined diseases [83–85].

Conventional animal toxicological studies are time-consuming, low-capacity, costly, and only analyses a restricted number of endpoints. Such methods are inadequate to cope with the expanding number of substances detected in the environment for which no toxicity data exists. Mechanism-centered high-throughput testing is a novel way to address this pressing demand, but it is limited by our present understanding of toxicity processes [86].

7.12 Toxicogenomic

The involvement of this 'Omics' technology in the medicinal and bioinformational discipline has an immense effect on modern scientific technologies and methodologies which makes this field distinguished in information science. Functional toxicogenomic, basically have an important role in recognizing the important cellular constituents and network of channels involved in toxicity response [87]. They are known for their role in monitoring the specific reaction of the genome to external environmental stress factors.

As there is difficulty in accumulating the tremendous amount of data obtained from all the omics technologies and the analysis of this statistical data into biological understanding such assessment of toxicogenomic take deep insight for reducing the crucial animal testing making the use of series of R as reducing, refining and replacing [88]. Hence, facilitating the development of new approaches for targeted cellular assays requires high throughput multidimensional methods. Here, this omic technology can be referred to as a branch of bioinformatics with conventional toxicology, which involves the study of the relationship among harmful biological factors and genome as well as these effects caused by several exogenous agents such as toxins, chemicals, drugs, external stressors. In addition, gathering and representing this data as well as accumulation of information related to a biomolecule and biological product in response to external stress factors [89, 90].

In the past recent years, this technology came up with the ideology of using high throughput computational techniques for the global evaluation of biological products regulation following treatment with several external stress factors. Indeed, to obtain beneficial information of biological product and its expression profiling and also changes in reaction to harmful external stress factors of variant classes [91, 92].

As it has many practical applications in informational science that has provided us a parallel opportunity to apply new technological approaches to get a better understanding of highly multiplexed sequencing methods with the power of computational tools and algorithms. In addition, to uncover the biological marker for large-scale stress factors i.e. toxicants this expression profiling method has been used on large scale to interpret the data in informational science [93, 94], Which can be used to inform the selection of mechanism-based assays, and thus are an important starting point to the identification of toxicity endpoints for cellular assays. However, there is a big challenge that remains for industry and researchers in the investigation, of difficulty in mining, accumulating the tremendous amount of data obtained from all the omics technologies, and the analysis of this statistical data into biological understanding.

"Several large-scale projects and the creation of minable databases are currently underway to collect all of this omics data on a large scale, including the Japanese Toxicogenomics Project (TGP) [95], the European Innomed PredTox [96], and the Liver Toxicity Biomarker Study. Similarly, all other omics technologies (e.g., proteomics, metabolomics) are being used to investigate toxicity pathways and have been examined extensively elsewhere [97, 98]. While these omic technologies are useful, one limitation is that they are correlative and do not evaluate the functionality of a gene for the cellular response to a toxic substance. As a consequence, there has been much discourse on the need for quantifiable "phenotypic anchors" to link altered gene/protein/metabolite expression patterns to specific parameters of well-defined toxicity indices [99]. In contrast to other omic approaches, functional toxicogenomics can provide a direct link between genes and toxicants."

Definition of functional genomics is "the application and development of global (genome-wide or system-wide) experimental techniques to evaluate gene function by utilizing the knowledge and reagents furnished by physical genome mapping and sequencing" [100, 101]. This functional data is gained by monitoring collections of cells/organisms that are deficient in either genes (due to deletion) or proteins (through blocking translation by using technologies such as RNAi). Functional toxicogenomics, which is capable of providing a better understanding of an increased mechanistic of toxicant-induced phenotypes, was recognized for providing a better understanding of an increased mechanistic of toxicant-induced phenotypes (Figure 7.11) [102]. Table 7.2 summarizes pros and cons of the omics technology.

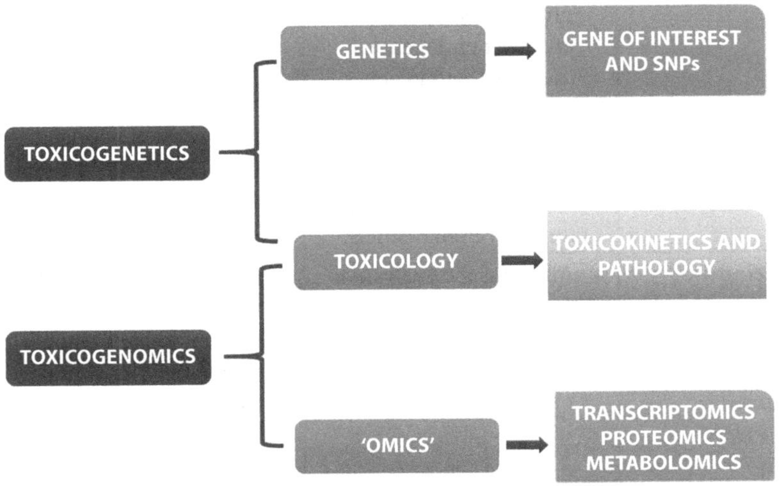

Figure 7.11 Relationship of toxicogenetic and toxicogenomic.

Table 7.2 Pros and cons of different omics approaches.

Technique	Pros	Cons
Genomics	• SNP identification provides valuable information for early disease diagnosis, prevention, and treatment. • Individual susceptibility to some drugs and different responses among individuals is demonstrated by studies on gene polymorphisms, particularly on metabolizing enzymes.	• Because of post-transcriptional and post-translational changes, as well as epigenetics, it is difficult to anticipate the final biological effect of DNA using only genome analysis.
Transcriptomics	• The major pathways involved in drug response and toxicity are identified. • Reproducibility is high for interlaboratory studies.	• Due to post-translational modifications, data is insufficient. • Modifications in the transcriptome cannot cause a change in the pattern of "endproducts."
Metabolomics technologies	• Metabolomics is advantageous to genomics and proteomics. As there are fewer endogenous metabolites than genes, transcripts, and proteins, there are fewer data to interpret. • Finding genetic markers for diseases like cancer.	• Expensive • Different outcomes as a result of a post-translational modification.
Proteomics	• Allow for the analysis of low-abundance proteins in complex samples.	• Expensive, fairly insensitive to low copy proteins, and not applicable to the entire proteome. • Isoelectric point precipitation (pI) • Different outcomes as a result of post-translational modification

7.13 Conclusion and Future Prospects

Each omic technology has a specific use, Omic technology is used for diagnosis and treatment of disease due to any modification related to genes, RNA, protein, and metabolites. It is specific toward the treatment of disease; even they provide a link between genes and toxins. Hence, one can conclude that it is a highly specific technology but the disadvantage of this technology are cost, still, several companies started their new project based on omic technology to give specific treatment for diseases like cancer, cardiac and brain-related (i.e., autoimmune disorder and disease due to toxin intercalating with genes). So, we can say a new era started for this technology and in the upcoming year it may be successful technology in their respective field.

Acknowledgement

Figure 7.2 is adopted from, "Zhou Y, Xu X, Tian Z and Wei H (2017) "Multi-Omics" Analyses of the Development and Function of Natural Killer Cells. Front. Immunol. 8:1095. doi: 10.3389/fimmu.2017.01095" under the terms of the Creative Commons Attribution License (CC BY). Figure 7.9 is adopted from, "Belhaj MR, Lawler NG, Hoffman NJ. Metabolomics and Lipidomics: Expanding the Molecular Landscape of Exercise Biology. Metabolites. 2021 Mar 7;11(3):151. doi: 10.3390/metabo11030151. PMID: 33799958; PMCID: PMC8001908." under the terms of the Creative Commons Attribution License (CC BY).

References

1. Shaheen, T., Iqbal, M.A., Zafar, Y., Bioinformatics: A way forward to explore "plant omics", in: *Bioinformatics-Updated Features and Applications*, pp. 204–226, IntechOpen, Croatia, 2016.
2. Stein, L., Genome annotation: From sequence to biology. *Nat. Rev. Genet.*, 2, 7, 493–503, 2001.
3. Maggio, E.T. and Ramnarayan, K., Recent developments in computational proteomics. *Trends Biotechnol.*, 19, 7, 266–272, 2001.
4. Hampel, H., Nisticò, R., Seyfried, N.T. *et al.*, Omics sciences for systems biology in Alzheimer's disease: State-of-the-art of the evidence. *Ageing Res. Rev.*, 69, 101346, 2021.

5. Reel, P.S., Reel, S., Pearson, E., Trucco, E., Jefferson, E., Using machine learning approaches for multi-omics data analysis: A review. *Biotechnol. Adv.*, 49, 107739, 2021.
6. Can, T., Introduction to bioinformatics, in: *miRNomics: MicroRNA Biology and Computational Analysis*, pp. 51–71, Springer, Humana Press, Totowa, NJ, 2014.
7. Chavda, V.P., Kapadia, C., Soni, S. *et al.*, A global picture: Therapeutic perspectives for COVID-19. *Immunotherapy*, 14, 5, 351–371, 2022.
8. Chavda, V.P., Feehan, J., Apostolopoulos, V., A veterinary vaccine for SARS-CoV-2: The first COVID-19 vaccine for animals. *Vaccines*, 9, 6, 631, 2021.
9. Westerhoff, H.V. and Palsson, B.O., The evolution of molecular biology into systems biology. *Nat. Biotechnol.*, 22, 10, 1249–1252, 2004.
10. Subramanian, I., Verma, S., Kumar, S., Jere, A., Anamika, K., Multi-omics data integration, interpretation, and its application. *Bioinform. Biol. Insights*, 14, 1177932219899051, 2020.
11. Saigusa, D., Matsukawa, N., Hishinuma, E., Koshiba, S., Identification of biomarkers to diagnose diseases and find adverse drug reactions by metabolomics. *Drug Metab. Pharmacokinet.*, 37, 100373, 2021.
12. Kell, D.B., Systems biology, metabolic modelling and metabolomics in drug discovery and development. *Drug Discovery Today*, 11, 23–24, 1085–1092, 2006.
13. Theodorescu, D. and Mischak, H., Mass spectrometry based proteomics in urine biomarker discovery. *World J. Urol.*, 25, 5, 435–443, 2007.
14. Koh, H.W., Fermin, D., Choi, K.P., Ewing, R., Choi, H., iOmicsPASS: A novel method for integration of multi-omics data over biological networks and discovery of predictive subnetworks. *bioRxiv*, 374520, 2018.
15. Schloss, P.D., Identifying and overcoming threats to reproducibility, replicability, robustness, and generalizability in microbiome research. *MBio*, 9, 3, e00525-18, 2018.
16. Pinu, F.R., Beale, D.J., Paten, A.M. *et al.*, Systems biology and multi-omics integration: Viewpoints from the metabolomics research community. *Metabolites*, 9, 4, 76, 2019.
17. Mayer, G., Heinze, G., Mischak, H. *et al.*, Omics-bioinformatics in the context of clinical data, in: *Bioinformatics for Omics Data*, pp. 479–497, Springer, Humana Press, 2011.
18. Strom, S.P., Fundamentals of RNA analysis on biobanked specimens, in: *Biobanking*, pp. 345–357, 2019.
19. Bogyo, M. and Rudd, P.M., New technologies and their impact on 'omics' research Editorial overview. *Curr. Opin. Chem. Biol.*, 17, 1–3, 2013.
20. Mallick, H., Ma, S., Franzosa, E.A., Vatanen, T., Morgan, X.C., Huttenhower, C., Experimental design and quantitative analysis of microbial community multiomics. *Genome Biol.*, 18, 1, 1–16, 2017.

21. Cattaneo, A. and Pariante, C.M., Integrating 'omics' approaches to prioritize new pathogenetic mechanisms for mental disorders. *Neuropsychopharmacology*, 43, 1, 227–228, 2017.
22. Srivastava, V., Obudulu, O., Bygdell, J. *et al.*, On PLS integration of transcriptomic, proteomic and metabolomic data shows multi-level oxidative stress responses in the cambium of transgenic hipI-superoxide dismutase populus plants. *BMC Genom.*, 14, 1, 1–16, 2013.
23. Santiago-Rodriguez, T.M. and Hollister, E.B., Multi 'omic data integration: A review of concepts, considerations, and approaches. *Semin. Perinatol.*, 45, 6, 151456, 2021.
24. Tuck, M., Blanc, L., Touti, R. *et al.*, Multimodal imaging based on vibrational spectroscopies and mass spectrometry imaging applied to biological tissue: A multiscale and multiomics review. *Anal. Chem.*, 93, 1, 445–477, 2021.
25. Casamassimi, A., Federico, A., Rienzo, M., Esposito, S., Ciccodicola, A., Transcriptome profiling in human diseases: New advances and perspectives. *Int. J. Mol. Sci.*, 18, 8, 1652, 2017.
26. Diamandis, E.P., Cancer biomarkers: Can we turn recent failures into success? *J. Natl. Cancer Inst.*, 102, 19, 1462–1467, 2010.
27. Trivedi, D.K., Hollywood, K.A., Goodacre, R., Metabolomics for the masses: The future of metabolomics in a personalized world. *New Horiz. Transl. Med.*, 3, 6, 294–305, 2017.
28. Phillips, K.A., Deverka, P.A., Hooker, G.W., Douglas, M.P., Genetic test availability and spending: Where are we now? Where are we going? *Health Aff.*, 37, 5, 710–716, 2018.
29. Yurkovich, J.T. and Palsson, B.O., Quantitative-omic data empowers bottom-up systems biology. *Curr. Opin. Biotechnol.*, 51, 130–136, 2018.
30. Varshney, R.K., Terauchi, R., McCouch, S.R., Harvesting the promising fruits of genomics: Applying genome sequencing technologies to crop breeding. *PloS Biol.*, 12, 6, e1001883, 2014.
31. Wambugu, P.W., Ndjiondjop, M.-N., Henry, R.J., Role of genomics in promoting the utilization of plant genetic resources in genebanks. *Brief. Funct. Genomics*, 17, 3, 198–206, 2018.
32. Pettersson, E., Lundeberg, J., Ahmadian, A., Generations of sequencing technologies. *Genomics*, 93, 2, 105–111, 2009.
33. Collins, F.S., Green, E.D., Guttmacher, A.E., Guyer, M.S., A vision for the future of genomics research. *Nature*, 422, 6934, 835–847, 2003.
34. Frazer, K.A., Murray, S.S., Schork, N.J., Topol, E.J., Human genetic variation and its contribution to complex traits. *Nat. Rev. Genet.*, 10, 4, 241–251, 2009.
35. Hofker, M.H., Fu, J., Wijmenga, C., The genome revolution and its role in understanding complex diseases. *Biochim. Biophys. Acta Mol. Basis Dis.*, 1842, 10, 1889–1895, 2014.
36. Collins, F.S. and Fink, L., The human genome project. *Alcohol Health Res. World*, 19, 3, 190–195, 1995.

37. Macken, W.L., Vandrovcova, J., Hanna, M.G., Pitceathly, R.D.S., Applying genomic and transcriptomic advances to mitochondrial medicine. *Nat. Rev. Neurol.*, 17, 4, 215–230, 2021.
38. Claussnitzer, M., Cho, J.H., Collins, R. *et al.*, A brief history of human disease genetics. *Nature*, 577, 7789, 179–189, 2020.
39. Goetz, L.H. and Schork, N.J., Personalized medicine: Motivation, challenges, and progress. *Fertil. Steril.*, 109, 6, 952–963, 2018.
40. Wieacker, P. and Steinhard, J., The prenatal diagnosis of genetic diseases. *Dtsch.* Ärztebl. *Int.*, 107, 48, 857, 2010.
41. Levy, B. and Wapner, R., Prenatal diagnosis by chromosomal microarray analysis. *Fertil. Steril.*, 109, 2, 201–212, 2018.
42. Relman, D.A., Microbial genomics and infectious diseases. *N. Engl. J. Med.*, 365, 4, 347–357, 2011.
43. Ginsburg, G.S. and Willard, H.F., Genomic and personalized medicine: Foundations and applications. *Transl. Res.*, 154, 6, 277–287, 2009.
44. Dunbar, C.E., High, K.A., Joung, J.K., Kohn, D.B., Ozawa, K., Sadelain, M., Gene therapy comes of age. *Science*, 359, 6372, eaan4672, 2018.
45. Doudna, J.A., The promise and challenge of therapeutic genome editing. *Nature*, 578, 7794, 229–236, 2020.
46. Subbiah, M.R., Understanding the nutrigenomic definitions and concepts at the food–genome junction. *Omics J. Integr. Biol.*, 12, 4, 229–235, 2008.
47. Marcum, J.A., Nutrigenetics/nutrigenomics, personalized nutrition, and precision healthcare. *Curr. Nutr. Rep.*, 9, 4, 338–345, 2020.
48. Stover, P.J., Influence of human genetic variation on nutritional requirements. *Am. J. Clin. Nutr.*, 83, 2, 436S–442S, 2006.
49. Fenech, M., Genome health nutrigenomics and nutrigenetics–diagnosis and nutritional treatment of genome damage on an individual basis. *Food Chem. Toxicol.*, 46, 4, 1365–1370, 2008.
50. Gad, S.C., Recent developments in replacing, reducing, and refining animal use in toxicologic research and testing. *Fundam. Appl. Toxicol.*, 15, 1, 8–16, 1990.
51. Bakker, G.C., Van Erk, M.J., Pellis, L. *et al.*, An anti-inflammatory dietary mix modulates inflammation and oxidative and metabolic stress in overweight men: A nutrigenomics approach. *Am. J. Clin. Nutr.*, 91, 4, 1044–1059, 2010.
52. Mizoguchi, T., Takehara, I., Masuzawa, T., Saito, T., Naoki, Y., Nutrigenomic studies of effects of Chlorella on subjects with high-risk factors for lifestyle-related disease. *J. Med. Food.*, 11, 3, 395–404, 2008.
53. Kaput, J., Developing the promise of nutrigenomics through complete science and international collaborations. *Nutr. Oppor. Asia.*, 60, 209–223, 2007.
54. Miggiano, G.A. and De Sanctis, R., Nutritional genomics: Toward a personalized diet. *Clin. Ter.*, 157, 4, 355–361, 2006.
55. Davidson, N. and Harris, P., Nutrition and welfare, in: *The Welfare of Horses*, pp. 45–76, Springer, Dordrecht, 2007.

56. Debusk, R.M., Fogarty, C.P., Ordovas, J.M., Kornman, K.S., Nutritional genomics in practice: Where do we begin? *J. Am. Diet. Assoc.*, 105, 4, 589–598, 2005.
57. Mead, M.N., Nutrigenomics: The genome–food interface. *Environ. Health Perspect.*, 115, 12, A582–A589, 2007.
58. Lowe, R., Shirley, N., Bleackley, M., Dolan, S., Shafee, T., Transcriptomics technologies. *PloS Comput. Biol.*, 13, 5, e1005457, 2017.
59. Junker, J.P., Noël, E.S., Guryev, V. *et al.*, Genome-wide RNA tomography in the zebrafish embryo. *Cell J.*, 159, 3, 662–675, 2014.
60. Lee, J.H., Daugharthy, E.R., Scheiman, J. *et al.*, Highly multiplexed subcellular RNA sequencing in situ. *Science*, 343, 6177, 1360–1363, 2014.
61. Crosetto, N., Bienko, M., Van Oudenaarden, A., Spatially resolved transcriptomics and beyond. *Nat. Rev. Genet.*, 16, 1, 57–66, 2015.
62. Dong, Z. and Chen, Y., Transcriptomics: Advances and approaches. *Sci. China Life Sci.*, 56, 10, 960–967, 2013.
63. Monti, M., Orru, S., Pagnozzi, D., Pucci, P., Interaction proteomics. *Biosci. Rep.*, 25, 1, 45–56, 2005.
64. Paša-Tolić, L., Masselon, C., Barry, R.C., Shen, Y., Smith, R.D., Proteomic analyses using an accurate mass and time tag strategy. *Biotechniques*, 37, 4, 621–639, 2004.
65. Yokota, H., Applications of proteomics in pharmaceutical research and development. *Biochim. Biophys. Acta Proteins Proteom.*, 1867, 1, 17–21, 2019.
66. Fields, S., Proteomics in genomeland. *Science*, 291, 5507, 1221–1224, 2001.
67. Patterson, S.D. and Aebersold, R.H., Proteomics: The first decade and beyond. *Nat. Genet.*, 33, 3, 311–323, 2003.
68. Wishart, D.S., Applications of metabolomics in drug discovery and development. *Drugs R D.*, 9, 5, 307–322, 2008.
69. Putri, S.P., Nakayama, Y., Matsuda, F. *et al.*, Current metabolomics: Practical applications. *J. Biosci. Bioeng.*, 115, 6, 579–589, 2013.
70. Hayashi, S., Akiyama, S., Tamaru, Y. *et al.*, A novel application of metabolomics in vertebrate development. *Biochem. Biophys. Res. Commun.*, 386, 1, 268–272, 2009.
71. Rochfort, S., Metabolomics reviewed: A new "omics" platform technology for systems biology and implications for natural products research. *J. Nat. Prod.*, 68, 12, 1813–1820, 2005.
72. Wishart, D.S., Emerging applications of metabolomics in drug discovery and precision medicine. *Nat. Rev. Drug Discovery*, 15, 7, 473–484, 2016.
73. Baker, M., Metabolomics: From small molecules to big ideas. *Nat. Methods*, 8, 2, 117–121, 2011.
74. Watkins, S.M., Lipomic profiling in drug discovery, development and clinical trial evaluation. *Curr. Opin. Drug Discovery Dev.*, 7, 1, 112–117, 2004.
75. Liebisch, G., Ahrends, R., Makoto, A. *et al.*, Lipidomics needs more standardization. *Nat. Metab.*, 1, 745–747, 2019.

76. Züllig, T., Trötzmüller, M., Köfeler, H.C., Lipidomics from sample preparation to data analysis: A primer. *Anal. Bioanal. Chem.*, 412, 10, 2191–2209, 2020.
77. Sharma, R. and Prajapati, P.K., Predictive, preventive and personalized medicine: Leads from ayurvedic concept of prakriti (human constitution). *Curr. Pharmacol. Rep.*, 6, 6, 441–450, 2020.
78. Wallace, R.K., Ayurgenomics and modern medicine. *Medicina*, 56, 12, 661, 2020.
79. Kulkarni, A.B., Ayurveda, research, and my experience. *Deerghayu Int.*, 32, 125, 90–96, 2016.
80. Sethi, T.P., Prasher, B., Mukerji, M., Ayurgenomics: A new way of threading molecular variability for stratified medicine. *ACS Chem. Biol.*, 6, 9, 875–880, 2011.
81. Singh, S., Gehlot, S., Agrawal, N.K., Basis of disease manifestation: A molecular and ayurvedic approach with an integrated concept of ayurgenomics. *J. Nat. Remedies*, 19, 3, 99–113, 2019.
82. Huang, Z., Chavda, V.P., Bezbaruah, R. *et al.*, An ayurgenomics approach: Prakriti-based drug discovery and development for personalized care. *Front. Pharmacol.*, 13, 1–9, 2022. [Internet] Available from: https://www.frontiersin.org/article/10.3389/fphar.2022.866827.
83. Milos, P.M. and Seymour, A.B., Emerging strategies and applications of pharmacogenomics. *Hum. Genomics*, 1, 6, 1–12, 2004.
84. Ingelman-Sundberg, M., Pharmacogenetics: An opportunity for a safer and more efficient pharmacotherapy. *J. Intern. Med.*, 250, 3, 186–200, 2001.
85. Roses, A.D., Genome-based pharmacogenetics and the pharmaceutical industry. *Nat. Rev. Drug Discovery*, 1, 7, 541–549, 2002.
86. Zang, R., Li, D., Tang, I.-C., Wang, J., Yang, S.-T., Cell-based assays in high-throughput screening for drug discovery. *Int. J. Biotech. Well. Ind.*, 1, 1, 31–51, 2012.
87. North, M. and Vulpe, C.D., Functional toxicogenomics: Mechanism-centered toxicology. *Int. J. Mol. Sci.*, 11, 12, 4796–4813, 2010.
88. Andersen, M.E. and Krewski, D., Toxicity testing in the 21st century: Bringing the vision to life. *Toxicol. Sci.*, 107, 2, 324–330, 2009.
89. Hamadeh, H.K., Amin, R.P., Paules, R.S., Afshari, C.A., An overview of toxicogenomics. *Curr. Issues Mol. Biol.*, 4, 2, 45–56, 2002.
90. Hayes, K.R., Advances in toxicogenomics. *Chem. Res. Toxicol.*, 18, 403–414, 2005.
91. David, R., The promise of toxicogenomics for genetic toxicology: Past, present and future. *Mutagenesis*, 35, 2, 153–159, 2020.
92. Liu, Z., Huang, R., Roberts, R., Tong, W., Toxicogenomics: A 2020 vision. *Trends Pharmacol. Sci.*, 40, 2, 92–103, 2019.
93. Jayapal, M., Bhattacharjee, R.N., Melendez, A.J., Hande, M.P., Environmental toxicogenomics: A post-genomic approach to analysing biological responses to environmental toxins. *Int. J. Biochem.*, 42, 2, 230–240, 2009.

94. Aardema, M.J. and MacGregor, J.T., Toxicology and genetic toxicology in the new era of "toxicogenomics": Impact of "-omics" technologies. *Mutat. Res.*, 499, 13–25, 2002.
95. Uehara, T., Ono, A., Maruyama, T. *et al.*, The Japanese toxicogenomics project: Application of toxicogenomics. *Mol. Nutr. Food Res.*, 54, 2, 218–227, 2010.
96. Mulrane, L., Rexhepaj, E., Smart, V. *et al.*, Creation of a digital slide and tissue microarray resource from a multi-institutional predictive toxicology study in the rat: An initial report from the PredTox group. *Exp. Toxicol. Pathol.*, 60, 4–5, 235–245, 2008.
97. Vlaanderen, J., Moore, L.E., Smith, M.T. *et al.*, Application of OMICS technologies in occupational and environmental health research; Current status and projections. *Occup. Environ. Med.*, 67, 2, 136–143, 2010.
98. Gatzidou, E.T., Zira, A.N., Theocharis, S.E., Toxicogenomics: A pivotal piece in the puzzle of toxicological research. *J. Appl. Toxicol.*, 27, 4, 302–309, 2007.
99. Paules, R., Phenotypic anchoring: Linking cause and effect. *Environ. Health Perspect.*, 111, 6, A338–A339, 2003.
100. Hieter, P. and Boguski, M., Functional genomics: It's all how you read it. *Science*, 278, 5338, 601–602, 1997.
101. Waters, M.D. and Fostel, J.M., Toxicogenomics and systems toxicology: Aims and prospects. *Nat. Rev. Genet.*, 5, 12, 936–948, 2004.
102. Hamadeh, H.K., Amin, R.P., Paules, R.S., Afshari, C.A., An overview of toxicogenomics. *Curr. Issues Mol. Biol.*, 4, 2, 45–56, 2002.

Part II

BIOINFORMATICS TOOLS FOR PHARMACEUTICAL SECTOR

8

Bioinformatics and Cheminformatics Tools in Early Drug Discovery

Palak K. Parikh[1], Jignasa K. Savjani[2], Anuradha K. Gajjar[1] and Mahesh T. Chhabria[3]*

[1]Department of Pharmaceutical Chemistry and Quality Assurance, L. M. College of Pharmacy, Navrangpura, Ahmedabad, Gujarat, India
[2]Department of Pharmaceutical Chemistry, Institute of Pharmacy, Nirma University, Ahmedabad, Gujarat, India
[3]L. M. College of Pharmacy, Navrangpura, Ahmedabad, Gujarat, India

Abstract
Drug discovery is an important domain of research for chemical scientists and pharmaceutical industries. However, this process encompasses several challenges of increasing cost, high time consumption, off-target delivery and a high risk of failure. The advances in bioinformatics and cheminformatics have modernized this process by integrating computational tools and contributed significantly to overcoming challenges and complexity observed at different stages of the drug discovery and development pipeline. Different computer aided drug design (CADD) approaches are employed at almost every stage of the early discovery process to identify molecules that have desirable characteristics to make acceptable drugs. The present chapter discusses various CADD approaches along with major available tools and software used in the rational designing of drugs. Thus, the main aim of present compilation is to provide an outline of different computational approaches along with their effective applications in the early drug discovery.

Keywords: Bioinformatics, cheminformatics, drug discovery, computer aided drug design, docking, QSAR, pharmacophore modeling, ADMET

**Corresponding author*: mahesh.chhabria@rediffmail.com

Vivek Chavda, Krishnan Anand and Vasso Apostolopoulos (eds.) Bioinformatics Tools for Pharmaceutical Drug Product Development, (149–182) © 2023 Scrivener Publishing LLC

Abbreviations

ADMET	Absorption, distribution, metabolism, excretion and toxicity
ANNs	Artificial neural networks
CADD	Computer aided drug design
CoMFA	Comparative molecular field analysis
CoMSIA	Comparative molecular similarity indices
DNA	Deoxyribonucleic acid
FDA	Food and Drug Administration
GFA	Genetic function approximation
GH score	Güner-Henry score
GPCR	G-protein-coupled receptor
GQSAR	Group based QSAR
GWAS	Genome-wide association study
hERG	human Ether-à-go-go Related Gene
HQSAR	Hologram QSAR
HTS	High-throughput screening
*k*NN	*k*-nearest neighbor
LBDD	Ligand based drug design
LDA	Linear discriminant analysis
MD	Molecular dynamics
MFA	Molecular field analysis
MIA-QSAR	Multi-variate image analysis-QSAR
MLR	Multiple linear regression
MOE	Molecular Operating Environment
NCE	New chemical entity
PBPK	Physiologically based pharmacokinetic
PCA	Principal component analysis
PCR	Principal component regression
PDB	Protein data bank
PLS	Partial least square analysis
QSAR	Quantitative structure activity relationship
RMSD	Root mean square deviation
RMSF	Root mean square fluctuation
ROC curve	Receiver operating characteristic curve
RoG	Radius of gyration
SBDD	Structure based drug design
SLR	Simple linear regression
SVM	Support vector machine

8.1 Introduction

Drug discovery is a knowledge-intensive complex process of identifying a small molecule or a large biological molecule with the potential to become a drug candidate. A new medicine takes an average of 10-15 years from discovery to approval and costs more than US$ 2 billion to launch a new molecule [1–3]. The drug discovery process encompasses the early stage of research starting with the identification of the disease condition and its unmet need, target discovery and validation, assay development, identification of hit using numerous screening approaches, hit optimization and lead discovery, medicinal chemistry and lead optimization and preclinical candidate development. The process of drug discovery has been accelerated because of the development of various computational tools/methods by eliminating unsuitable drug candidates in the early stage of drug discovery process. Furthermore, the use of informatics with complementary experimental techniques increases the probabilities of success in several stages of the discovery process. Figure 8.1 describes an overview of drug discovery process with role of multiple computational approaches that can be applied in various stages of the drug discovery [4–8]. The use of computational tools saves up to 30% of the time and money for the drug discovery and development process and are employed regularly for the research and development in academia and pharmaceutical industries [9]. Computer aided drug design (CADD) has contributed significantly in the discovery process of greater than 70 pharmaceutical drugs that have been approved by the Food and Drug Administration (FDA) and reached the clinic [10]. Moreover, the evolution of drug discovery relies on numerous factors such as the identification of an increasing number of novel drug targets, accumulated data revealing the 3D protein structures, recent developments in

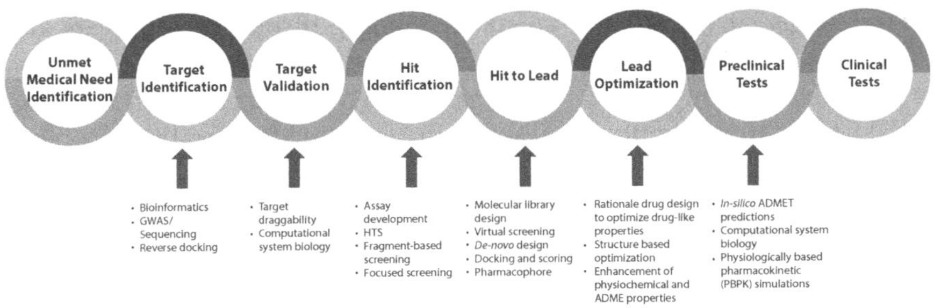

Figure 8.1 Overview of drug discovery process.

computing power of informatics and availability of numerous CADD software and tools [11].

8.2 Informatics and Drug Discovery

Being a multistep process, drug design and discovery involve genomics, proteomics, bioinformatics and cheminformatics studies to find a new chemical entity (NCE) or a biological therapeutic with a novel mechanism of action. Bioinformatics techniques have revealed information about various diseases for medication development; thanks to the advances in current structural biology. Proteins, enzymes, and deoxyribonucleic acid (DNA) have all been related to the disease condition. The Protein Data Bank (PDB) is an open-source database containing 3D protein structures, enzymes, and DNA as therapeutic targets for any research purpose [12–15]. Cheminformatics is a tool that primarily focuses on the processing of chemical information extracted from the structure of the molecule using computer technologies, which is then investigated to establish a meaningful relationship between the structural features of a chemical compound and its function [16, 17]. Being interdisciplinary fields, bioinformatics and cheminformatics complement each other for exploring the physiological processes in living systems. Furthermore, computational approaches involving bioinformatics and cheminformatics are increasingly used in the research [16]. Several computational approaches, also called as CADD techniques are available to discover new drug like candidates and can be divided into two general categories (i) Structure based drug design (SBDD) (ii) Ligand based drug design (LBDD) (Figure 8.2) [6]. SBDD relies on the knowledge of 3D macromolecular biological target or homology model of an unavailable target structure compared to a similar homologous protein structure (template). It is one of the most useful strategies in CADD to screen promising molecules from the chemical library for a selected biological target. It necessitates an understanding of biological targets and their 3D characteristics extracted via NMR spectroscopy or X-ray crystallography. Docking and *de novo* ligand design are the main strategies of SBDD. High-throughput virtual screening enables identification of potential drug like candidates, which may be validated further by using molecular dynamics (MD) simulation and visualization approaches [18–20]. LBDD depends on the knowledge of known ligands/small molecules in the absence of structural data of known proteins. Commonly used LBDD techniques include quantitative structure activity relationship (QSAR) studies, pharmacophore modeling and molecular similarity searches. It is

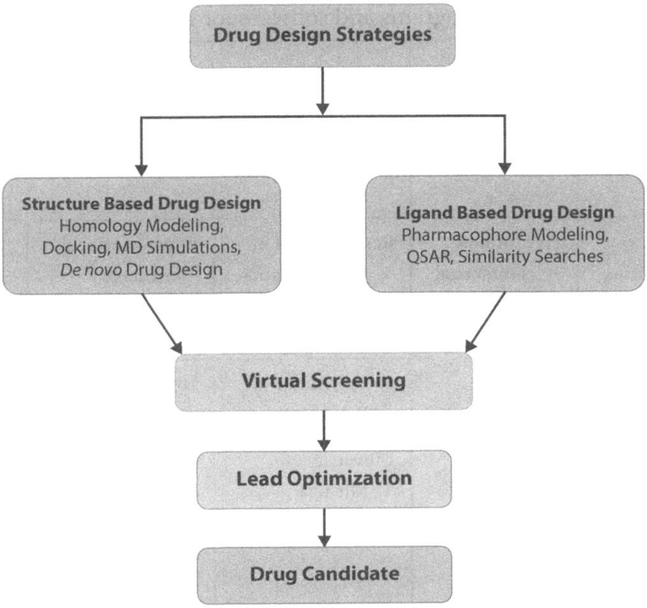

Figure 8.2 Schematic representation of CADD strategies.

an alternative to SBDD or in the case where the prediction of target structure using homology modeling is challenging [18, 21].

8.3 Computational Methods in Drug Discovery

8.3.1 Homology Modeling

Homology modeling is an *in-silico* structure prediction tool for creating reliable 3D coordinates of the target protein from its amino acid sequence, and it is employed in a broad range of biological applications [22]. 3D structure of a query protein can be predicted using template protein sequence alignment using homology modeling. The basic workflow of homology modeling is generally comprised of several systematic tasks including (i) selection of the suitable template for a given target sequence using the BLAST search; (ii) global sequence alignment; (iii) model creation for the target using 3D structural information from the template; (iv) model refinement, analysis of alignments, gap additions, deletions, and substitutions and lastly (v) model validation [23, 24]. Different software and server based tools that are widely used for protein modeling are listed in Table 8.1. The reliability of the

Table 8.1 List of selected programs and software for protein modeling.

Program/ software	Availability	Organization	URL	Reference
MODELLER	Free for academic use	Sali Lab, University of California at San Francisco	https://salilab.org/modeller/	[28]
PRIMO	Free for non-commercial use	Research Unit in Bioinformatics (RUBi), Rhodes University	https://primo.rubi.ru.ac.za/	[29]
SWISS-MODEL	Free	Swiss Institute of Bioinformatics	https://swissmodel.expasy.org/	[30]
I-TASSER	Free for academic and non-profit research	University of Michigan	https://zhanggroup.org/I-TASSER/	[31]
Robetta	Free for academic use	University of Washington	https://robetta.bakerlab.org/	[32]
Phyre2	Free	Structural Bioinformatics Group, Imperial College London	http://www.sbg.bio.ic.ac.uk/phyre2	[33]
HH-suite3	Free	Söding Lab, Quantitative and Computational Biology Group, Max-Planck Institute for Biophysical Chemistry	https://github.com/soedinglab/hh-suite	[34]
PyMod3	Free	Department of Biochemical Sciences, Sapienza University of Rome	https://github.com/pymodproject/pymod	[35]

(*Continued*)

Table 8.1 List of selected programs and software for protein modeling. (*Continued*)

Program/ software	Availability	Organization	URL	Reference
ProModel	Commercial	VLife Technologies	https://www.vlifesciences.com/products/VLifeMDS/Protein_Modeller.php	[36]
Prime	Commercial	Schrödinger	https://www.schrodinger.com/products/prime	[37, 38]
Molecular Operating Environment (MOE)	Commercial	Chemical Computing Group	https://www.chemcomp.com/Products.htm	[39]
ICM-Pro	Commercial	Molsoft LLC	https://www.molsoft.com/homology.html	[40]

homology modeling depends on the sequence homology between the target protein and its template. Hence, when a template is selected for homology modeling one should consider the consistency of the target protein's activation state. High quality homology models should be considered for molecular docking based virtual screening [25]. Ramachandran plot and favorable energies are evaluated to validate the accuracy of the predicted target protein structure [26]. MolProbity, RAMPAGE, PDBsum, ZLab, STAN and others are a few tools and/or servers used to create the Ramachandran plot. Various types of stereochemical aspects of the protein structure can be predicted using popular tools and a comprehensive toolkit like SAVESv6.0 (https://saves.mbi.ucla.edu/) (a toolkit with five tools such as ERRAT, VERIFY3D, PROVE, PROCHECK, and WHAT_CHECK) [27].

8.3.2 Docking Studies

Molecular docking is one of the most popular computational techniques used for the prediction of target protein-ligand binding interactions. It is also one of the most critical methods in virtual screening, which involves docking compound libraries against a single pharmacological target to retrieve the best hit. According to the type of ligand, docking can be divided into the following classes (i) protein-small molecule (ligand) docking; (ii) protein-protein docking and (iii) protein-nucleic acid docking [41, 42]. The first and most crucial step before docking is identifying the active site amino acids of the protein involved in the binding. If the crystal structure of a protein is available in PDB, the co-crystalized ligand can be extracted to get knowledge about the active site; otherwise, blind docking can be performed without predicting the active site of the selected protein structure. Programs like LigA Site, Q-SiteFinder, Meta Pocket and CASTp are helpful for active site identification in either case [43]. Table 8.2 describes the molecular docking software tools and their features.

According to the degree of simplification, docking protocols can be divided into different classes *i.e.* rigid docking, semi-flexible docking,

Table 8.2 List of selected programs and software for docking.

Program/ software	Availability	Organization	URL	Reference
AutoDock	Free	The Scripps Research Institute	https://autodock.scripps.edu/	[51]
AutoDock Vina	Free	The Scripps Research Institute	https://vina.scripps.edu/	[52]
Swiss Dock	Free	Swiss Institute of Bioinformatics	http://www.swissdock.ch/	[53]
ZDOCK	Free for academic and non-profit use	Zhiping Weng's lab (ZLAB), University of Massachusetts Medical School	https://zdock.umassmed.edu/	[54]
pyDOCK	Free for academic use	Barcelona Supercomputing Centre	https://life.bsc.es/pid/pydock/	[55]
iGEMDOCK	Free for non-commercial research	Department of Biological Science and Technology & Institute of Bioinformatics, National Chiao Tung University	http://gemdock.life.nctu.edu.tw/dock/igemdock.php	[56]

(*Continued*)

Table 8.2 List of selected programs and software for docking. (*Continued*)

Program/ software	Availability	Organization	URL	Reference
rDOCK	Free	University of Barcelona and University of York	http://rdock.sourceforge.net/	
FlexX	Commercial	BioSolveIT GmbH	https://www.biosolveit.de/products/#FlexX	[57]
GOLD	Commercial	Cambridge Crystallographic Data Centre (CCDC)	https://www.ccdc.cam.ac.uk/solutions/csd-discovery/components/gold/	[58]
Glide	Commercial	Schrödinger	https://www.schrodinger.com/products/glide	[59]
BIOVIA Discovery Studio	Commercial	Dassault Systèmes	https://www.3ds.com/products-services/biovia/products/molecular-modeling-simulation/biovia-discovery-studio/	[60]
VLifeDock	Commercial	VLife Technologies	https://www.vlifesciences.com/products/Functional_products/VLifeDock.php	[36]
Molecular Operating Environment (MOE)	Commercial	Chemical Computing Group	https://www.chemcomp.com/Products.htm	[39]

and flexible docking [44]. During rigid docking, the structure of molecules does not change. Rigid docking is better for studying macromolecular interactions like protein-protein and protein-nucleic acid as it is simple and focuses on the conformation of macromolecules. Semi-flexible docking is suitable for protein-ligand interactions because the shape of the ligand can be changed within a narrow range. The structures of small molecules can be manipulated, whereas the structure of macromolecules remains rigid or may contain a few rotatable amino acid residues to reduce the computational power. In flexible docking, the docking procedure allows the docking system (protein and ligand) conformations to be readily modified [45–47].

A strategy for predicting if and how a ligand and a protein will interact is known as molecular docking. This is usually performed in two steps, namely (i) identifying potential structural matches and (ii) assigning a score to those matches. Protein preparation is a crucial step and involves the knowledge of induced fit effects and water molecules to be retained for protein geometry. This can be achieved through a comparison of the active sites for multiple PDB structures for the same target. The validation of a docking protocol would involve (i) recreating the empirically proven binding mechanism for known ligands and (ii) extracting known active compounds from a decoy collection. The scoring function in the docking evaluates how strong the binding is between a protein and a ligand by predicting the binding affinity of the pose. Scoring functions used in docking algorithms are divided into three groups (i) force-field based; (ii) knowledge-based and (iii) empirical scoring functions [47–49].

Prediction of the complex interactions can be done utilizing protein-protein docking instead of studying individual protein structures. However, protein-protein docking is one of the most challenging areas in CADD because the determination of the 3D protein-protein complex is more difficult than a single protein structure. Docking provides the structural information for drug design and gives tools for fundamental research of protein interactions. The steric and electrostatic interactions between the protein structures can be analyzed using the docking approach. In HTS, conformational changes between bound and unbound structures can be analyzed through docking techniques, which is required for modeling extensive networks of protein interactions [50].

8.3.3 Molecular Dynamics Simulations

MD simulations have evolved into an important computational technique that is performed to evaluate the stability of a protein-ligand complex.

It follows Newton's second law equation for the simulation of molecular systems. It involves simulation of time-dependent atomic motions of a molecular system (treating all the entities-ligand, protein, as well as water molecules in the simulation box as flexible) and thus provides insights into conformational rearrangements or flexibility of a molecular system. The trajectories produced by the molecular system simulation contain all the molecular properties of the protein and cocrystal structure.

MD simulation is performed on the docked protein-ligand complex with the best score [47, 61–63]. The common workflow involves the following steps for MD simulation: (i) system preparation involving 3D structure preparation; (ii) minimization; (iii) heating and equilibrium; (iv) MD simulation and (v) post trajectory analysis. The protein topology is first determined using standard parameters such as GROMACS or the LEap software. The PRODRG online server application generates the ligand topology. The commonly used force fields in MD simulations include AMBER, OPLS, CHARMM and GROMOS. The protein and ligand complexes are solvated with water and placed in the cubic box with some space. Proteins being charged molecules, counter ions such as Na^+ or Cl^- are used to neutralize the system. The systems' energy is minimized for 1000 steps using the steepest descent algorithm. MD simulations are typically performed under normal volume and temperature dynamics (NVT) at 300 K, followed by production simulations under normal pressure and temperature dynamics (NPT). Finally, the complex is subjected to MD simulation. The root mean square deviation (RMSD), root mean square fluctuation (RMSF), radius of gyration (RoG) and intermolecular hydrogen bonds are common analyses computed after simulation for the assessment of the stability of the complex [9, 64–66]. AMBER (https://ambermd.org), GROMACS (http://www.gromacs.org), NAMD (https://www.ks.uiuc.edu/Research/namd/), LAMMPS (https://lammps.sandia.gov), Desmond (https://www.deshawresearch.com/resources_desmond.html) and CHARMM (https://www.charmm.org/) are among the software utilized for MD simulations [62, 67–72].

8.3.4 *De Novo* Drug Design

It is a method aiming to fill the binding sites of a macromolecular target by using small molecular fragments. In the *de novo* ligand design process, the stepwise growing of components with the required properties is utilized to generate ligands. The process is repeated until one or more ligands possess the required properties. The selection of fragment sets that have the potential to be a part of new ligand compounds with ideal physicochemical and pharmacological properties is one of the most critical challenges of this technique [6, 73, 74].

Two main types of *de novo* design methods are available namely, structure-based and ligand-based. In structure-based methods, different molecular fragments or building blocks with desirable predicted interactions are grown within the constraints of a binding pocket of a macromolecular target to generate novel molecular structures. In the absence of the 3D structure of a macromolecular target, ligand-based *de novo* design methods can suggest a new molecule based structure analogous to the known ligand molecule [75, 76]. Examples of structure-based *de novo* design are LUDI, LigBuilder V3, and PRO_LIGAND [77–79]. DOGS, SYNOPSIS and TOPAS are some examples of ligand-based *de novo* drug design tools [80–82].

8.3.5 Quantitative Structure Activity Relationships

The goal of QSAR modeling is to reveal a mathematical relationship between molecular properties (considered as molecular descriptors) of chemical compounds to their biological function in order to accurately predict the biological function of closely related target compounds [83, 84]. Since the seminal work reported by Hansch and Fujita in the 1960s, QSAR modeling remains the most popular ligand-based designing method for drug discovery and lead optimization [85, 86]. During past 60 years, QSAR modeling has witnessed several transformations in terms of different dimensions of descriptors ranging from 1D to 7D and several statistical methods used to determine the correlation between the molecular properties of chemical structures with their biological function or response variable [87, 88]. Molecular descriptors represent different dimensions of a chemical structure and fall into different categories *viz.* global molecular properties (1D), structural patterns concerning two-dimensional molecular representations (2D), single state three-dimensional structure representations (3D), ensemble of ligand representations (4D), explicit induced fit ligand-based virtual or pseudo receptor models (5D), different solvation scenarios (6D) and target-based receptor model data (7D) [89, 90].

The process of QSAR modeling is generally comprised of several systematic tasks including (i) collection and curation of data; (ii) calculation of molecular descriptors; (iii) transformation of data (scaling of biological function with a logarithmic function) and division of dataset (partitioning data into training, test and/or external validation sets); (iv) selection of appropriate features and construction of a QSAR model by application of suitable modeling algorithm; (v) selection of models with high internal and external accuracy; (vi) validation assessment of applicability domain and (vii) use of a derived model for prediction of novel components [91–93]. Furthermore, following are the most important key points having a considerable influence in the construction of a predictive QSAR model: (i) the chemical diversity with known activities must be covered fully during splitting the dataset into training and test sets; (ii) defining suitable molecular descriptors; (iii) reliable model construction and validation and (iv) predictive reliability of the model to predict the target property of new untested compounds [91, 94, 95].

Statistical methods or machine learning techniques are used to build QSAR models which include linear regression analysis (simple linear regression [SLR], multiple linear regression [MLR], linear discriminant analysis [LDA], stepwise MLR, *etc.*), multivariate data analysis (principal component analysis [PCA], partial least square analysis [PLS], principal component regression [PCR], genetic function approximation [GFA], *etc.*), pattern recognition (artificial neural networks [ANNs], cluster analysis, *k*-nearest neighbor [*k*NN], *etc.*), support vector machine [SVM], decision tree, random forest and so on [96, 97]. Qualified validation is highly important for developed QSAR models and therefore, different validation approaches must be applied to check the reliability of a QSAR model using leave-one-out (LOO) cross-validation (q^2), square of the correlation coefficient (r^2), bootstrap resampling, Y-randomization (randomization of biological function or activity) and predication for test sets (external validation) [98]. After qualified external validation, the QSAR model can be used for virtual screening of available databases of chemical compounds and new untested compounds. Therefore, it is crucial to establish the applicability domain of a developed model prior to its application for improvement of the predictive performance [99, 100]. There are different types of QSAR techniques that evolved with time, from Hansch and Free-Wilson's 1D or 2D linear free-energy relationships to multidimensional QSAR modeling including real receptor or target-based 7D QSAR [88, 96, 101]. Among them, Group based QSAR (GQSAR), Hologram QSAR (HQSAR), comparative molecular field analysis (CoMFA), topomer CoMFA, comparative molecular similarity indices (CoMSIA), molecular field analysis (MFA) and multi-variate image analysis-QSAR (MIA-QSAR) are popularly used QSAR modeling techniques [93, 102, 103]. Several free and commercial tools/software available for QSAR modeling are listed in Table 8.3.

8.3.6 Pharmacophore Modeling

A pharmacophore is known as a set of molecular frameworks that represent an optimal supramolecular binding pattern between a specific macromolecular target and ligands. The term "pharmacophore" was initially presented

Table 8.3 List of selected programs and software for QSAR modeling.

Program/ software	Availability	Organization	URL	Reference
Open3DQSAR	Free	University of Turin (Paolo Tosco), University of Sydney (Thomas Balleb)	http://open3dqsar.sourceforge.net/	[104]
QSAR-Co-X	Free	University of Porto	https://github.com/ncordeirfcup/QSAR-Co-X	[105]
StarDrop™	Commercial	Optibrium	http://www.optibrium.com	[106]
QSARpro®	Commercial	Vlife Technologies	https://www.vlifesciences.com/products/QSARPro/Product_QSARpro.php	[36]
BIOVIA Discovery Studio	Commercial	Dassault Systèmes	https://www.3ds.com/products-services/biovia/products/molecular-modeling-simulation/biovia-discovery-studio/	[60]
Flare™	Commercial	Cresset Software	https://www.cresset-group.com/software/flare/	[107]
AutoQSAR	Commercial	Schrödinger	https://www.schrodinger.com/products/autoqsar	[108]

(*Continued*)

Table 8.3 List of selected programs and software for QSAR modeling. (*Continued*)

Program/ software	Availability	Organization	URL	Reference
Field-Based QSAR	Commercial	Schrödinger	https://www.schrodinger.com/products/field-based-qsar	[109]
FLAP and Pentacle	Commercial	Molecular Discovery	https://www.moldiscovery.com/software/	[110]
GUSAR	Commercial	geneXplain GmbH	https://genexplain.com/gusar/	
Molecular Operating Environment (MOE)	Commercial	Chemical Computing Group	https://www.chemcomp.com/Products.htm	[39]

by Paul Ehrlich in the early 1900s [111, 112]. The most common pharmacophoric features that represent molecular functionalities include "Hydrogen-bond acceptor", "Hydrogen-bond donor", "Aromatic", "Hydrophobic", "Positive ionizable" or "Negative ionizable" and any logical combinations of these [113, 114]. A derived pharmacophore model encompasses a distinct spatial arrangement of features that represent the chemical functionalities of active chemical entities [115].

The pharmacophore modeling can be done by two different approaches. In ligand-based modeling, a set of ligands is superimposed to identify common interaction features that are essential for biological response. In another way, the pharmacophore model can be derived by probing probable interaction points between a 3D structure of a macromolecular target and ligands. Such pharmacophore modeling is known as structure-based pharmacophore [116, 117]. A general protocol used to derive a ligand-based pharmacophore model comprises the following steps: (i) collection of compounds with definite biological activity against a macromolecular target and picking up the right set of compounds (active and inactive compounds); (ii) preparation of training and test sets; (iii) exhaustive conformational search; (iv) extraction of features and representation; (v) identification of the pattern and scoring and (vi) external validation [115, 118, 119]. The modeling of a structure-based pharmacophore requires 3D structure of a macromolecular target or a macromolecule-ligand complex. A common framework for structure-based pharmacophore modeling involves the following steps: (i) identification of the active site; (ii) analysis of the complementary chemical features for the active site and their spatial relationships and (iii) assembling of selected chemical features to derive the model and hit analysis [115, 120]. There are several pharmacophore generating programs such as PHASE, CATALYST, MOE, LigandScout and other free academic software/tools (Table 8.4).

The validation of a derived pharmacophore model is significantly important to ascertain its quality and reliability. The derived pharmacophore model should be statistically significant for successive applications in various molecular modeling tasks. Based on the acceptable correlation

Table 8.4 List of selected programs and software for pharmacophore modeling.

Program/ software	Availability	Organization	URL	Reference
Pharmmaker	Free	University of Pittsburgh	http://prody.csb.pitt.edu/pharmmaker/	[126]
PharmMapper	Free	East China University of Science and Technology, Peking University	http://www.lilab-ecust.cn/pharmmapper/	[127]
PharmaGist	Free	Tel Aviv University	https://bioinfo3d.cs.tau.ac.il/PharmaGist/php.php	[128]
ZINCPharmer	Free	University of Pittsburgh	http://zincpharmer.csb.pitt.edu/	[129]
LigandScout	Commercial	Inte:Ligand Software-Entwicklungs und Consulting GmbH	http://www.inteligand.com/ligandscout/	[130]
Flare™	Commercial	Cresset Software	https://www.cresset-group.com/software/flare/	[107]
PHASE	Commercial	Schrödinger	https://www.schrodinger.com/products/phase	[131]
FLAP	Commercial	Molecular Discovery	https://www.moldiscovery.com/software/flap/	[132]

(*Continued*)

Table 8.4 List of selected programs and software for pharmacophore modeling. (*Continued*)

Program/ software	Availability	Organization	URL	Reference
CATALYST	Commercial	BIOVIA Discovery Studio	https://www.3ds.com/products-services/biovia/products/molecular-modeling-simulation/biovia-discovery-studio/pharmacophore/	[133]
Molecular Operating Environment (MOE)	Commercial	Chemical Computing Group	https://www.chemcomp.com/Products.htm	[39]
MolSign	Commercial	Vlife Technologies	https://www.vlifesciences.com/products/Functional_products/Molsign.php	[36]

coefficient and cost analysis, the derived model should be validated using commonly used validation methods *viz.*, test set prediction, Fischer's randomization test, Güner-Henry (GH) score calculation, receiver operating characteristic (ROC) curve, enrichment factor, *etc.* [42, 121, 122]. A derived pharmacophore model can be used for virtual screening to identify potential ligands that possess essential structural features in correct 3D conformation. This technique is also useful to design the library for hit discovery and to optimize the leads to final drug candidates. Furthermore, it can be used for absorption, distribution, metabolism, excretion and toxicity (ADMET) predictions, off-target predictions and target identification [123–125].

8.3.7 Absorption, Distribution, Metabolism, Excretion and Toxicity Profiling

Undesirable pharmacokinetics including ADMET and pharmacodynamics are the common reasons for high attrition rates in pharmaceutical R&D.

It has been frequently recognized that early ADMET profiling can save time and money as well as help to avoid drug failure at late stages in the drug development process and drug recalls [4, 134]. Despite the availability of numerous high-throughput *in-vitro* ADMET screening models, the use of *in-silico* tools in the comprehensive profiling of ADMET parameters is one of the most popular CADD strategies due to their relatively lower cost and faster prediction ability [135].

In-silico ADMET predictions assist medicinal chemists to exclude undesirable NCEs at the initial stage of drug design and provide timely feedback on ADMET profile for lead optimization as well as reduce animal testing in the laboratory [136, 137]. Over the past two decades, a wide range of ADMET tools have been developed and are widely used across various organizations for *in-silico* ADMET predictions [138–140]. *In-silico* approaches used for ADMET predictions are categorized into two categories *viz.* data modeling and molecular modeling. The data modeling method is based on database approaches such as physiologically based pharmacokinetic (PBPK) and QSAR modeling. Molecular modeling includes different methods like docking, MD simulations and quantum mechanics calculations and is based on the 3D structure of the protein [4, 141–143]. Furthermore, these methods comprise machine learning, regression, network analysis tools, data mining, data visualization and data analysis tools using computers [137, 144]. A series of *in-silico* ADMET tools are currently available that are capable of predicting comprehensive properties just from the chemical structure of NCEs. They are implemented to model physicochemical properties including drug-likeness, acute toxicity, human intestinal absorption, metabolism, membrane transporters, human ether-à-go-go-related gene (hERG) toxicity, genotoxicity, broad scale pharmacology profiling, *etc.* [135, 145]. A wide range of computational tools for predicting different aspects of pharmacokinetics and safety evaluations of drug-like molecules are listed in Table 8.5.

Table 8.5 List of selected programs and software for ADMET prediction.

Program/software	Availability	Organization	URL	Reference
ADMETlab 2.0	Free	Xiangya School of Pharmaceutical Sciences, Central South University	https://admetmesh.scbdd.com/	[136]
admetSAR 2.0	Free	East China University of Science and Technology	http://lmmd.ecust.edu.cn/admetsar2/	[146]

(*Continued*)

Table 8.5 List of selected programs and software for ADMET prediction. (*Continued*)

Program/software	Availability	Organization	URL	Reference
CypReact	Free	University of Alberta	https://bitbucket.org/Leon_Ti/cypreact	[147]
CypRules	Free	National Taiwan University	https://cyprules.cmdm.tw/	[148]
DrugMint	Free	Institute of Microbial Technology	http://crdd.osdd.net/oscadd/drugmint/	[149]
*e*ToxPred	Free	Louisiana State University	https://github.com/pulimeng/etoxpred	[150]
FP-ADMET	Free	Norwegian University of Science and Technology	https://gitlab.com/vishsoft/fpadmet	[151]
NERDD (CYPstrate, CYPlebrity, FAMe 3, GLORY, GLORYx, NP-Scout, Skin Doctor CP)	Free	Universität Hamburg	https://nerdd.univie.ac.at/	[152]
OSIRIS property explorer	Free	Idorsia Pharmaceuticals Ltd,	https://www.organic-chemistry.org/prog/peo/	[153]
SwissADME	Free	Swiss Institute of Bioinformatics	http://www.swissadme.ch/	[154]
vNN-ADMET	Free	Biotechnology High Performance Computing Software Applications Institute	https://vnnadmet.bhsai.org/vnnadmet/login.xhtml	[155]
pkCSM	Free	University of Melbourne/University of Cambridge	http://biosig.unimelb.edu.au/pkcsm/prediction	[156]

(*Continued*)

Table 8.5 List of selected programs and software for ADMET prediction. (*Continued*)

Program/software	Availability	Organization	URL	Reference
Pred-hERG	Free	LabMol (Laboratory for Molecular modeling and Drug Design)	http://predherg.labmol.com.br/	[157]
PASS	Commercial	geneXplain	https://genexplain.com/pass/	[158]
ADMET Predictor®	Commercial	Simulations Plus	https://www.simulations-plus.com/software/admetpredictor/	[159]
QikProp	Commercial	Schrodinger	https://www.schrodinger.com/products/qikprop	[160]

8.4 Conclusion

The advances in bioinformatics and cheminformatics have contributed significantly at various stages of the drug discovery and development pipeline in academia and pharmaceutical industries by integrating computational tools. Different CADD approaches have effectively accelerated and economized the process of drug discovery. Various computational strategies discussed in this chapter are used extensively at the early stages of discovery processes from initial target discovery and validation, hit identification and optimization, medicinal chemistry and lead optimization and preclinical development. This chapter summarized different CADD software and tools, which are commonly employed in academia and pharmaceutical industries for early drug discovery. Despite several advances and successes, bioinformatics, cheminformatics and related fields need to be explored further for more efficient algorithms and software tools to mimic the underlying principles and functions of the physiological system.

References

1. Davenport, T.H. and Peitsch, M.C., Human aspects of the management of drug discovery knowledge. *Drug Discov. Today Technol.*, 2, 3, 205–209, 2005.
2. Hughes, J.P., Rees, S.S., Kalindjian, S.B., Philpott, K.L., Principles of early drug discovery. *Br. J. Pharmacol.*, 162, 6, 1239–1249, 2011. [Internet] Available from: /pmc/articles/PMC3058157/.
3. Berdigaliyev, N. and Aljofan, M., An overview of drug discovery and development. *Future Med. Chem.*, 12, 10, 939–947, 2020.
4. Wu, F., Zhou, Y., Li, L. *et al.*, Computational approaches in preclinical studies on drug discovery and development. *Front. Chem.*, 8, 726, 2020.
5. Sinha, S. and Vohora, D., Drug discovery and development: An overview, in: *Pharmaceutical Medicine and Translational Clinical Research*, pp. 19–32, Academic Press, London, United Kingdom, 2018, [Internet] Available from: http://dx.doi.org/10.1016/B978-0-12-802103-3.00002-X.
6. Ou-Yang, S.S., Lu, J.Y., Kong, X.Q., Liang, Z.J., Luo, C., Jiang, H., Computational drug discovery. *Acta Pharmacol. Sin.*, 33, 9, 1131–1140, 2012. [Internet] Available from: https://www.nature.com/articles/aps2012109.
7. Tang, Y., Zhu, W., Chen, K., Jiang, H., New technologies in computer-aided drug design: Toward target identification and new chemical entity discovery. *Drug Discov. Today Technol.*, 3, 3, 307–313, 2006.
8. Bajorath, J., Rational drug discovery revisited: Interfacing experimental programs with bio- and chemo-informatics. *Drug Discov. Today*, 6, 19, 989–995, 2001.
9. Sharma, V., Wakode, S., Kumar, H., Structure- and ligand-based drug design: Concepts, approaches, and challenges, in: *Chemoinformatics and Bioinformatics in the Pharmaceutical Sciences*, pp. 27–53, Academic Press, London, United Kingdom, 2021.
10. Sabe, V.T., Ntombela, T., Jhamba, L.A. *et al.*, Current trends in computer aided drug design and a highlight of drugs discovered via computational techniques: A review. *Eur. J. Med. Chem.*, 224, 113705, 2021. [Internet] Available from: https://doi.org/10.1016/j.ejmech.2021.113705.
11. Ataya, F.S., Bioinformatics, genomics, and proteomics tools in drug design. *J. Drug Res. Dev.*, 5, 1, 1–6, 2019.
12. Lage, O.M., Ramos, M.C., Calisto, R., Almeida, E., Vasconcelos, V., Vicente, F., Current screening methodologies in drug discovery for selected human diseases. *Mar. Drugs*, 16, 8, 279, 2018.
13. Macalino, S.J.Y., Gosu, V., Hong, S., Choi, S., Role of computer-aided drug design in modern drug discovery. *Arch. Pharm. Res.*, 38, 9, 1686–1701, 2015.
14. Patel, C.N., Kumar, S.P., Rawal, R.M., Patel, D.P., Gonzalez, F.J., Pandya, H.A., A multiparametric organ toxicity predictor for drug discovery. *Toxicol. Mech. Methods*, 30, 3, 159–166, 2020.

15. Xia, X., Bioinformatics and drug discovery. *Curr. Top. Med. Chem.*, 17, 15, 1709–1726, 2017.
16. López-López, E., Bajorath, J., Medina-Franco, J.L., Informatics for chemistry, biology, and biomedical sciences. *J. Chem. Inf. Model.*, 61, 1, 26–35, 2021.
17. Xu, J. and Hagler, A., Chemoinformatics and drug discovery. *Molecules*, 7, 8, 566–600, 2002. [Internet] Available from: /pmc/articles/PMC6146447/.
18. Macalino, S.J.Y., Gosu, V., Hong, S., Choi, S., Role of computer-aided drug design in modern drug discovery. *Arch. Pharm. Res.*, 38, 9, 1686–1701, 2015.
19. Huang, H.J., Yu, H.W., Chen, C.Y. *et al.*, Current developments of computer-aided drug design. *J. Taiwan Inst. Chem. Eng.*, 41, 6, 623–635, 2010. [Internet] Available from: http://dx.doi.org/10.1016/j.jtice.2010.03.017.
20. Schaduangrat, N., Lampa, S., Simeon, S., Gleeson, M.P., Spjuth, O., Nantasenamat, C., Towards reproducible computational drug discovery. *J. Cheminform.*, 12, 1, 1–30, 2020. [Internet] Available from: https://doi.org/10.1186/s13321-020-0408-x.
21. Leelananda, S.P. and Lindert, S., Computational methods in drug discovery. *Beilstein J. Org. Chem.*, 12, 1, 2694–2718, 2016.
22. Muhammed, M.T. and Aki-Yalcin, E., Homology modeling in drug discovery: Overview, current applications, and future perspectives. *Chem. Biol. Drug Des.*, 93, 1, 12–20, 2019. [Internet] Available from: https://onlinelibrary.wiley.com/doi/full/10.1111/cbdd.13388.
23. Vyas, V.K., Ukawala, R.D., Ghate, M., Chintha, C., Homology modeling a fast tool for drug discovery: Current perspectives. *Indian J. Pharm. Sci.*, 74, 1, 1–17, 2012. [Internet] Available from: /pmc/articles/PMC3507339/.
24. Gromiha, M.M., Nagarajan, R., Selvaraj, S., Protein structural bioinformatics: An overview, in: *Encyclopedia of Bioinformatics and Computational Biology: ABC of Bioinformatics*, pp. 445–459, Elsevier Inc., Amsterdam, Netherlands, 2019.
25. Hongmao, S., Homology modeling and ligand-based molecule design, in: *A Practical Guide to Rational Drug Design*, pp. 109–160, Woodhead Publishing, Cambridge, United Kingdom, 2016.
26. Ramachandran, G.N. and Sasisekharan, V., Conformation of polypeptides and proteins. *Adv. Protein Chem.*, 23, 283–437, 1968. [Internet] Available from: https://pubmed.ncbi.nlm.nih.gov/4882249/.
27. Agnihotry, S., Pathak, R.K., Singh, D.B., Tiwari, A., Hussain, I., Protein structure prediction, in: *Bioinformatics*, pp. 177–188, Academic Press, London, United Kingdom, 2022.
28. Webb, B. and Sali, A., Comparative protein structure modeling using MODELLER. *Curr. Protoc. Bioinf.*, 54, 5.6.1–5.6.37, 2016. [Internet] Available from: https://pubmed.ncbi.nlm.nih.gov/27322406/.
29. Hatherley, R., Brown, D.K., Glenister, M., Bishop, Ö.T., PRIMO: An interactive homology modeling pipeline. *PloS One*, 11, 11, e0166698, 2016. [Internet] Available from: https://journals.plos.org/plosone/article?id=10.1371/journal.pone.0166698.

30. Waterhouse, A., Bertoni, M., Bienert, S. *et al.*, SWISS-MODEL: Homology modelling of protein structures and complexes. *Nucleic Acids Res.*, 46, W1, W296–W303, 2018. [Internet] Available from: https://academic.oup.com/nar/article/46/W1/W296/5000024.
31. Yang, J. and Zhang, Y., Protein structure and function prediction using I-TASSER. *Curr. Protoc. Bioinf.*, 52, 1, 5.8.1–5.8.15, 2015. [Internet] Available from: /pmc/articles/PMC4871818/.
32. Kim, D.E., Chivian, D., Baker, D., Protein structure prediction and analysis using the Robetta server. *Nucleic Acids Res.*, 32, suppl_2, W526–W531, 2004. [Internet] Available from: https://pubmed.ncbi.nlm.nih.gov/15215442/.
33. Kelley, L.A., Mezulis, S., Yates, C.M., Wass, M.N., Sternberg, M.J.E., The phyre2 web portal for protein modeling, prediction and analysis. *Nat. Protoc.*, 10, 6, 845–858, 2015. [Internet] Available from: https://www.nature.com/articles/nprot.2015.053.
34. Steinegger, M., Meier, M., Mirdita, M., Vöhringer, H., Haunsberger, S.J., Söding, J., HH-suite3 for fast remote homology detection and deep protein annotation. *BMC Bioinf.*, 20, 1, 1–15, 2019. [Internet] Available from: https://bmcbioinformatics.biomedcentral.com/articles/10.1186/s12859-019-3019-7.
35. Janson, G. and Paiardini, A., PyMod 3: A complete suite for structural bioinformatics in PyMOL. *Bioinformatics*, 37, 10, 1471–1472, 2021. [Internet]. Available from: https://academic.oup.com/bioinformatics/article/37/10/1471/5917627.
36. VLife products protein modeling and docking, protein ligand docking, QSAR. *Cheminformatics*. [Internet]. Available from: https://www.vlifesciences.com/products/Products.php (Accessed on 27th February 2022).
37. Jacobson, M.P., Pincus, D.L., Rapp, C.S. *et al.*, A hierarchical approach to all-atom protein loop prediction. *Proteins Struct. Funct. Genet.*, 55, 2, 351–367, 2004. [Internet] Available from: https://onlinelibrary.wiley.com/doi/full/10.1002/prot.10613.
38. Jacobson, M.P., Friesner, R.A., Xiang, Z., Honig, B., On the role of the crystal environment in determining protein side-chain conformations. *J. Mol. Biol.*, 320, 3, 597–608, 2002.
39. Molecular operating environment (MOE) | MOEsaic | PSILO. [Internet]. Available from: https://www.chemcomp.com/Products.htm (Accessed on 27th February 2022).
40. Cardozo, T., Totrov, M., Abagyan, R., Homology modeling by the ICM method. *Proteins Struct. Funct. Bioinf.*, 23, 3, 403–414, 1995. [Internet] Available from: https://onlinelibrary.wiley.com/doi/full/10.1002/prot.340230314.
41. Meng, X.-Y., Zhang, H.-X., Mezei, M., Cui, M., Molecular docking: A powerful approach for structure-based drug discovery. *Curr. Comput. Aided-Drug Des.*, 7, 2, 146–157, 2011.
42. Roy, K., Kar, S., Das, R.N., Other related techniques, in: *Understanding the Basics of QSAR for Applications in Pharmaceutical Sciences and Risk Assessment*, pp. 357–425, Academic Press, London, United Kingdom, 2015.

43. Laurie, A.T.R. and Jackson, R.M., Q-SiteFinder: An energy-based method for the prediction of protein-ligand binding sites. *Bioinformatics*, 21, 9, 1908–1916, 2005.
44. Tao, X., Huang, Y., Wang, C. *et al.*, Recent developments in molecular docking technology applied in food science: A review. *Int. J. Food Sci. Technol.*, 55, 1, 33–45, 2020. [Internet] Available from: https://onlinelibrary.wiley.com/doi/full/10.1111/ijfs.14325.
45. de Ruyck, J., Brysbaert, G., Blossey, R., Lensink, M.F., Molecular docking as a popular tool in drug design, an *in silico* travel. *Adv. Appl. Bioinform. Chem.*, 9, 1–11, 2016.
46. Ferreira, L.G., Dos Santos, R.N., Oliva, G., Andricopulo, A.D., Molecular docking and structure-based drug design strategies. *Molecules*, 20, 7, 13384–13421, 2015.
47. Salmaso, V. and Moro, S., Bridging molecular docking to molecular dynamics in exploring ligand-protein recognition process: An overview. *Front. Pharmacol.*, 9, 923, 2018.
48. Lu, Y., Wang, R., Yang, C.Y., Wang, S., Analysis of ligand-bound water molecules in high-resolution crystal structures of protein-ligand complexes. *J. Chem. Inf. Model.*, 47, 2, 668–675, 2007. [Internet] Available from: https://pubs.acs.org/doi/abs/10.1021/ci6003527.
49. Guedes, I.A., Pereira, F.S.S., Dardenne, L.E., Empirical scoring functions for structure-based virtual screening: Applications, critical aspects, and challenges. *Front. Pharmacol.*, 9, 1089, 2018.
50. Vakser, I.A., Protein-protein docking: From interaction to interactome. *Biophys. J.*, 107, 8, 1785–1793, 2014.
51. Österberg, F., Morris, G.M., Sanner, M.F., Olson, A.J., Goodsell, D.S., Automated docking to multiple target structures: Incorporation of protein mobility and structural water heterogeneity in autodock. *Proteins*, 46, 1, 34–40, 2002. [Internet] Available from: https://pubmed.ncbi.nlm.nih.gov/11746701/.
52. Trott, O. and Olson, A.J., Autodock vina: Improving the speed and accuracy of docking with a new scoring function, efficient optimization, and multithreading. *J. Comput. Chem.*, 31, 2, 455–461, 2010. [Internet] Available from: https://onlinelibrary.wiley.com/doi/full/10.1002/jcc.21334.
53. Grosdidier, A., Zoete, V., Michielin, O., Swissdock, a protein-small molecule docking web service based on EADock DSS. *Nucleic Acids Res.*, 39, suppl_2, W270–W277, 2011. [Internet] Available from: /pmc/articles/PMC3125772/.
54. Pierce, B.G., Wiehe, K., Hwang, H., Kim, B.H., Vreven, T., Weng, Z., ZDOCK server: Interactive docking prediction of protein–protein complexes and symmetric multimers. *Bioinformatics*, 30, 12, 1771–1773, 2014. [Internet] Available from: /pmc/articles/PMC4058926/.
55. Cheng, T.M.K., Blundell, T.L., Fernandez-Recio, J., pyDock: Electrostatics and desolvation for effective scoring of rigid-body protein–protein docking. *Proteins Struct. Funct. Bioinf.*, 68, 2, 503–515, 2007. [Internet] Available from: https://onlinelibrary.wiley.com/doi/full/10.1002/prot.21419.

56. Hsu, K.C., Chen, Y.F., Lin, S.R., Yang, J.M., iGEMDOCK: A graphical environment of enhancing gemdock using pharmacological interactions and post-screening analysis. *BMC Bioinf.*, 12, 1, 1–11, 2011. [Internet] Available from: https://bmc-bioinformatics.biomedcentral.com/articles/10.1186/1471-2105-12-S1-S33.
57. Rarey, M., Kramer, B., Lengauer, T., Klebe, G., A fast flexible docking method using an incremental construction algorithm. *J. Mol. Biol.*, 261, 3, 470–489, 1996. [Internet] Available from: https://pubmed.ncbi.nlm.nih.gov/8780787/.
58. Jones, G., Willett, P., Glen, R.C., Leach, A.R., Taylor, R., Development and validation of a genetic algorithm for flexible docking. *J. Mol. Biol.*, 267, 3, 727–748, 1997.
59. Friesner, R.A., Banks, J.L., Murphy, R.B. *et al.*, Glide: A new approach for rapid, accurate docking and scoring. 1. Method and assessment of docking accuracy. *J. Med. Chem.*, 47, 7, 1739–1749, 2004. [Internet] Available from: https://pubs.acs.org/doi/abs/10.1021/jm0306430.
60. BIOVIA-Dassault Systèmes®, BIOVIA Discovery studio. [Internet]. Available from: https://www.3ds.com/products-services/biovia/products/molecular-modeling-simulation/biovia-discovery-studio/ (Accessed on 27th February 2022).
61. Durrant, J.D. and Mc Cammon, J.A., Molecular dynamics simulations and drug discovery. *BMC Biol.*, 9, 1, 1–9, 2011. [Internet] Available from: https://bmcbiol.biomedcentral.com/articles/10.1186/1741-7007-9-71.
62. Hollingsworth, S.A. and Dror, R.O., Molecular dynamics simulation for all. *Neuron*, 99, 6, 1129–1143, 2018. [Internet] Available from: /pmc/articles/PMC6209097/.
63. Hospital, A., Goñi, J.R., Orozco, M., Gelpí, J.L., Molecular dynamics simulations: Advances and applications. *Adv. Appl. Bioinform. Chem.*, 8, 1, 37–47, 2015. [Internet] Available from: https://www.dovepress.com/molecular-dynamics-simulations-advances-and-applications-peer-reviewed-fulltext-article-AABC.
64. Lopes, P.E.M., Guvench, O., Mackerell, A.D., Current status of protein force fields for molecular dynamics. *Methods in Molecular Biology*, vol. 1215, pp. 47–71, Humana Press, New York, NY, USA, 2015. https://doi.org/10.1007/978-1-4939-1465-4_3
65. Schüttelkopf, A.W. and Van Aalten, D.M.F., PRODRG: A tool for high-throughput crystallography of protein-ligand complexes. *Acta Crystallogr. Sect. D Biol. Crystallogr.*, 60, 8, 1355–1363, 2004.
66. Browne, R.B., Thomas, S.C., Roy, J.D., Bioinfomatics as a tool in drug designing, in: *Computation in Bioinformatics: Multidisciplinary Applications*, pp. 1–24, Wiley-Scrivener, Hoboken, NJ, USA, 2021.
67. Case, D.A., Cheatham, T.E., Darden, T. *et al.*, The amber biomolecular simulation programs. *J. Comput. Chem.*, 26, 16, 1668–1688, 2005. [Internet] Available from: /pmc/articles/PMC1989667/.
68. Van Der Spoel, D., Lindahl, E., Hess, B., Groenhof, G., Mark, A.E., Berendsen, H.J.C., GROMACS: Fast, flexible, and free. *J. Comput. Chem.*, 26, 16, 1701–1718, 2005.

69. Phillips, J.C., Braun, R., Wang, W. *et al.*, Scalable molecular dynamics with NAMD. *J. Comput. Chem.*, 26, 16, 1781–1802, 2005. [Internet] Available from: /pmc/articles/PMC2486339/.
70. Thompson, A.P., Aktulga, H.M., Berger, R. *et al.*, LAMMPS-a flexible simulation tool for particle-based materials modeling at the atomic, meso, and continuum scales. *Comput. Phys. Commun.*, 271, 108171, 2022.
71. Plimpton, S., Fast parallel algorithms for short-range molecular dynamics. *J. Comput. Phys.*, 117, 1, 1–19, 1995.
72. Brooks, B.R., Brooks, C.L., Mackerell, A.D. *et al.*, CHARMM: The biomolecular simulation program. *J. Comput. Chem.*, 30, 10, 1545–1614, 2009. [Internet] Available from: /pmc/articles/PMC2810661/.
73. Nicolaou, C., Kannas, C., Loizidou, E., Multi-objective optimization methods in *de novo* drug design. *Mini Rev. Med. Chem.*, 12, 10, 979–987, 2012.
74. Kutchukian, P.S. and Shakhnovich, E.I., *De novo* design: Balancing novelty and confined chemical space. *Expert Opin. Drug Discov.*, 5, 8, 789–812, 2010. [Internet] Available from: https://www.tandfonline.com/doi/abs/10.1517/17460441.2010.497534.
75. Lin, X., Li, X., Lin, X., A review on applications of computational methods in drug screening and design. *Molecules*, 25, 6, 1375, 2020.
76. Mouchlis, V.D., Afantitis, A., Serra, A. *et al.*, Advances in *de novo* drug design: From conventional to machine learning methods. *Int. J. Mol. Sci.*, 22, 4, 1676, 2021. [Internet] Available from: https://www.mdpi.com/1422-0067/22/4/1676/htm.
77. Böhm, H.J., LUDI: Rule-based automatic design of new substituents for enzyme inhibitor leads. *J. Comput. Mol. Des.*, 6, 6, 593–606, 1992. [Internet] Available from: https://link.springer.com/article/10.1007/BF00126217.
78. Yuan, Y., Pei, J., Lai, L., LigBuilder V3: A multi-target *de novo* drug design approach. *Front. Chem.*, 8, 142, 2020.
79. Clark, D.E., Frenkel, D., Levy, S.A. *et al.*, PRO_LIGAND: An approach to *de novo* molecular design. 1. Application to the design of organic molecules. *J. Comput. Mol. Des.*, 9, 1, 13–32, 1995. [Internet] Available from: https://link.springer.com/article/10.1007/BF00117275.
80. Hartenfeller, M., Zettl, H., Walter, M. *et al.*, DOGS: Reaction-driven *de novo* design of bioactive compounds. *Plos Comput. Biol.*, 8, 2, e1002380, 2012. [Internet] Available from: https://journals.plos.org/ploscompbiol/article?id=10.1371/journal.pcbi.1002380.
81. Vinkers, H.M., De Jonge, M.R., Daeyaert, F.F.D. *et al.*, SYNOPSIS: Synthesize and optimize system *in silico*. *J. Med. Chem.*, 46, 13, 2765–2773, 2003. [Internet] Available from: https://pubs.acs.org/doi/abs/10.1021/jm030809x.
82. Schneider, G., Lee, M.L., Stahl, M., Schneider, P., *De novo* design of molecular architectures by evolutionary assembly of drug-derived building blocks. *J. Comput. Aided Mol. Des.*, 14, 5, 487–494, 2000. [Internet] Available from: https://link.springer.com/article/10.1023/A:1008184403558.
83. Kwon, S., Bae, H., Jo, J., Yoon, S., Comprehensive ensemble in QSAR prediction for drug discovery. *BMC Bioinf.*, 20, 1, 1–12, 2019. [Internet] Available

from: https://bmcbioinformatics.biomedcentral.com/articles/10.1186/s12859-019-3135-4.
84. Vilar, S. and Costanzi, S., Predicting the biological activities through QSAR analysis and docking-based scoring. *Methods in Molecular Biology*, vol. 914, pp. 271–284, Humana Press, Totowa, NJ, USA, 2012. https://doi.org/10.1007/978-1-62703-023-6_16
85. Hansch, C., Maloney, P.P., Fujita, T., Muir, R.M., Correlation of biological activity of phenoxyacetic acids with Hammett substituent constants and partition coefficients. *Nature*, 194, 4824, 178–180, 1962.
86. Hansch, C. and Fujita, T., ρ-σ-π Analysis. A method for the correlation of biological activity and chemical structure. *J. Am. Chem. Soc.*, 86, 8, 1616–1626, 1964. [Internet] Available from: https://pubs.acs.org/doi/abs/10.1021/ja01062a035.
87. Neves, B.J., Braga, R.C., Melo-Filho, C.C., Moreira-Filho, J.T., Muratov, E.N., Andrade, C.H., QSAR-based virtual screening: Advances and applications in drug discovery. *Front. Pharmacol.*, 9, 1275, 2018.
88. Polanski, J., Receptor dependent multidimensional QSAR for modeling drug-receptor interactions. *Curr. Med. Chem.*, 16, 25, 3243–3257, 2009.
89. Lill, M.A., Multi-dimensional QSAR in drug discovery. *Drug Discov. Today*, 12, 23–24, 1013–1017, 2007.
90. Roy, K., Kar, S., Das, R.N., Newer directions in QSAR/QSPR, in: *A Primer on QSAR/QSPR Modeling Fundamental Concepts. SpringerBriefs in Molecular Science*, pp. 105–121, Springer, Cham, Switzerland, 2015.
91. Wang, T., Wu, M.B., Lin, J.P., Yang, L.R., Quantitative structure-activity relationship: Promising advances in drug discovery platforms. *Expert Opin. Drug Discov.*, 10, 12, 1283–1300, 2015.
92. Kausar, S. and Falcao, A.O., An automated framework for QSAR model building. *J. Cheminformatics*, 10, 1, 1–23, 2018. [Internet] Available from: https://jcheminf.biomedcentral.com/articles/10.1186/s13321-017-0256-5.
93. Cherkasov, A., Muratov, E.N., Fourches, D. *et al.*, QSAR modeling: Where have you been? Where are you going to? *J. Med. Chem.*, 57, 12, 4977–5010, 2014. [Internet] Available from: /pmc/articles/PMC4074254/.
94. Kaushik, A.C., Kumar, A., Bharadwaj, S., Chaudhary, R., Sahi, S., Ligand-based approach for *in-silico* drug designing, in: *Bioinformatics Techniques for Drug Discovery. Springer Briefs in Computer Science*, pp. 11–19, Springer, Cham, Switzerland, 2018.
95. Gramatica, P., On the development and validation of QSAR models, in: *Computational Toxicology. Methods in Molecular Biology (Methods and Protocols)*, pp. 499–526, Humana Press, Totowa, NJ, USA, 2013.
96. Verma, J., Khedkar, V., Coutinho, E., 3D-QSAR in drug design-a review. *Curr. Top. Med. Chem.*, 10, 1, 95–115, 2010. [Internet]. Available from: http://www.eurekaselect.com/openurl/content.php?genre=article&issn=1568-0266&volume=10&issue=1&spage=95.
97. Keyvanpour, M.R. and Shirzad, M.B., An analysis of QSAR research based on machine learning concepts. *Curr. Drug Discov. Technol.*, 18, 1, 17–30, 2021.

98. Tropsha, A. and Golbraikh, A., Predictive quantitative structure-activity relationships modeling: Development and validation of QSAR models, in: *Handbook of Chemoinformatics Algorithms*, pp. 211–232, Chapman and Hall/CRC, Boca Raton, FL, USA, 2010.
99. Tropsha, A. and Golbraikh, A., Predictive quantitative structure-activity relationships modeling: Data preparation and the general modeling workflow, in: *Handbook of Chemoinformatics Algorithms*, pp. 173–210, Chapman and Hall/CRC, Boca Raton, FL, USA, 2010.
100. Weaver, S. and Gleeson, M.P., The importance of the domain of applicability in QSAR modeling. *J. Mol. Graph. Model.*, 26, 8, 1315–1326, 2008.
101. Roy, K., Kar, S., Das, R.N., Background of QSAR and historical developments, in: *Understanding the Basics of QSAR for Applications in Pharmaceutical Sciences and Risk Assessment*, pp. 1–46, Academic Press, London, United Kingdom, 2015.
102. Kar, S., Roy, K., Leszczynski, J., On applications of QSARs in food and agricultural sciences: History and critical review of recent developments, in: *Advances in QSAR Modeling. Challenges and Advances in Computational Chemistry and Physics*, K. Roy, (Ed.), pp. 203–302, Springer, Cham, Switzerland, 2017.
103. Wang, T., Yuan, X.S., Wu, M.B., Lin, J.P., Yang, L.R., The advancement of multidimensional QSAR for novel drug discovery-where are we headed? *Expert Opin. Drug Discov.*, 12, 8, 769–784, 2017. [Internet] Available from: https://doi.org/10.1080/17460441.2017.1336157.
104. Tosco, P. and Balle, T., Open3DQSAR: A new open-source software aimed at high-throughput chemometric analysis of molecular interaction fields. *J. Mol. Model.*, 17, 1, 201–208, 2011. [Internet] Available from: https://pubmed.ncbi.nlm.nih.gov/20383726/.
105. Halder, A.K. and Cordeiro, M.N.D.S., QSAR-Co-X: An open source toolkit for multitarget QSAR modelling. *J. Cheminformatics*, 13, 1, 1–18, 2021. [Internet] Available from: https://jcheminf.biomedcentral.com/articles/10.1186/s13321-021-00508-0.
106. Lagunin, A.A., Goel, R.K., Gawande, D.Y. *et al.*, Chemo-and bioinformatics resources for *in silico* drug discovery from medicinal plants beyond their traditional use: A critical review. *Nat. Prod. Rep.*, 31, 11, 1585–1611, 2014. [Internet] Available from: http://dx.doi.org/10.1039/C4NP00068D.
107. Cressset Group, Outstanding software for molecule design. [Internet] Available from: https://www.cresset-group.com/software/ (Accessed on 27th February 2022).
108. Dixon, S.L., Duan, J., Smith, E., Von Bargen, C.D., Sherman, W., Repasky, M.P., AutoQSAR: An automated machine learning tool for best-practice quantitative structure-activity relationship modeling. *Future Med. Chem.*, 8, 15, 1825–1839, 2016. [Internet] Available from: https://pubmed.ncbi.nlm.nih.gov/27643715/.
109. Cappel, D., Dixon, S.L., Sherman, W., Duan, J., Exploring conformational search protocols for ligand-based virtual screening and 3-D QSAR modeling.

J. Comput. Mol. Des., 29, 2, 165–182, 2015. [Internet] Available from: https://link.springer.com/article/10.1007/s10822-014-9813-4.
110. Molecular Discovery, Software. [Internet] Available from: https://www.moldiscovery.com/software/ (Accessed on 27th February 2022).
111. Güner, O.F. and Bowen, J.P., Setting the record straight: The origin of the pharmacophore concept. *J. Chem. Inf. Model.*, 54, 5, 1269–1283, 2014.
112. Ehrlich, P., Über den jetzigen Stand der chemotherapie. *Ber. Dtsch. Chem. Ges.*, 42, 1, 17–47, 1909. [Internet] Available from: https://onlinelibrary.wiley.com/doi/full/10.1002/cber.19090420105.
113. Voet, A. and Zhang, K.Y.J., Pharmacophore modelling as a virtual screening tool for the discovery of small molecule protein-protein interaction inhibitors. *Curr. Pharm. Des.*, 18, 30, 4586–4598, 2012.
114. Seidel, T., Wieder, O., Garon, A., Langer, T., Applications of the pharmacophore concept in natural product inspired drug design. *Mol. Inform.*, 39, 11, 2000059, 2020.
115. Choudhury, C. and Sastry, G.N., Pharmacophore modelling and screening: Concepts, recent developments and applications in rational drug design, in: *Structural Bioinformatics: Applications in Preclinical Drug Discovery Process. Challenges and Advances in Computational Chemistry and Physics*, Mohan, C. (ed.), pp. 25–53, Springer, Cham, Switzerland, 2019.
116. Yang, S.Y., Pharmacophore modeling and applications in drug discovery: Challenges and recent advances. *Drug Discov. Today*, 15, 11–12, 444–450, 2010. [Internet] Available from: http://dx.doi.org/10.1016/j.drudis.2010.03.013.
117. Langer, T. and Hoffmann, R.D., Pharmacophore modelling: Applications in drug discovery. *Expert Opin. Drug Discov.*, 1, 3, 261–267, 2006.
118. Noha, S.M. and Schuster, D., Pharmacophore modeling, in: *In Silico Drug Discovery and Design*, pp. 80–93, Future Science Ltd., London, United Kingdom, 2013.
119. Kutlushina, A., Khakimova, A., Madzhidov, T., Polishchuk, P., Ligand-based pharmacophore modeling using novel 3D pharmacophore signatures. *Molecules*, 23, 12, 3094, 2018. [Internet] Available from: /pmc/articles/PMC6321403/.
120. Gaurav, A. and Gautam, V., Structure-based three-dimensional pharmacophores as an alternative to traditional methodologies. *J. Recept. Ligand Channel Res.*, 7, 27–38, 2014. [Internet] Available from: https://www.dovepress.com/structure-based-three-dimensional-pharmacophores-as-an-alternative-to–peer-reviewed-fulltext-article-JRLCR.
121. Chandrasekaran, B., Agrawal, N., Kaushik, S., Pharmacophore development, in: *Encyclopedia of Bioinformatics and Computational Biology: ABC of Bioinformatics*, pp. 677–687, Elsevier Inc., Amsterdam, Netherlands, 2019.
122. Schaller, D., Šribar, D., Noonan, T. *et al.*, Next generation 3D pharmacophore modeling. *Wiley Interdiscip. Rev. Comput. Mol. Sci.*, 10, 4, 1–20, 2020.
123. Lu, X., Yang, H., Chen, Y. *et al.*, The development of pharmacophore modeling: Generation and recent applications in drug discovery. *Curr. Pharm. Des.*, 24, 29, 3424–3439, 2018.

124. Khedkar, S., Malde, A., Coutinho, E., Srivastava, S., Pharmacophore modeling in drug discovery and development: An overview. *Med. Chem. (Los. Angeles)*, 3, 2, 187–197, 2007.
125. Tyagi, R., Singh, A., Chaudhary, K.K., Yadav, M.K., Pharmacophore modeling and its applications, in: *Bioinformatics*, pp. 269–289, Academic Press, Elsevier Inc., London, United Kingdom, 2022.
126. Lee, J.Y., Krieger, J.M., Li, H., Bahar, I., Pharmmaker: Pharmacophore modeling and hit identification based on druggability simulations. *Protein Sci.*, 29, 1, 76–86, 2020. [Internet] Available from: https://onlinelibrary.wiley.com/doi/full/10.1002/pro.3732.
127. Wang, X., Shen, Y., Wang, S. *et al.*, PharmMapper 2017 update: A web server for potential drug target identification with a comprehensive target pharmacophore database. *Nucleic Acids Res.*, 45, W1, W356–W360, 2017. Available from: https://pubmed.ncbi.nlm.nih.gov/28472422/.
128. Schneidman-Duhovny, D., Dror, O., Inbar, Y., Nussinov, R., Wolfson, H.J., PharmaGist: A webserver for ligand-based pharmacophore detection. *Nucleic Acids Res.*, 36, suppl_2, W223–W228, 2008. [Internet] Available from: /pmc/articles/PMC2447755/.
129. Koes, D.R. and Camacho, C.J., ZINCPharmer: Pharmacophore search of the ZINC database. *Nucleic Acids Res.*, 40, W1, W409-W414, 2012. [Internet] Available from: /pmc/articles/PMC3394271/.
130. Wolber, G. and Langer, T., LigandScout: 3-D pharmacophores derived from protein-bound ligands and their use as virtual screening filters. *J. Chem. Inf. Model.*, 45, 1, 160–169, 2004. [Internet] Available from: https://pubs.acs.org/doi/abs/10.1021/ci049885e.
131. Dixon, S.L., Smondyrev, A.M., Rao, S.N., PHASE: A novel approach to pharmacophore modeling and 3D database searching. *Chem. Biol. Drug Des.*, 67, 5, 370–372, 2006. [Internet] Available from: https://onlinelibrary.wiley.com/doi/full/10.1111/j.1747-0285.2006.00384.x.
132. Baroni, M., Cruciani, G., Sciabola, S., Perruccio, F., Mason, J.S., A common reference framework for analyzing/comparing proteins and ligands. Fingerprints for Ligands and Proteins (FLAP): Theory and application. *J. Chem. Inf. Model.*, 47, 2, 279–294, 2007. [Internet] Available from: https://pubmed.ncbi.nlm.nih.gov/17381166/.
133. Barnum, D., Greene, J., Smellie, A., Sprague, P., Identification of common functional configurations among molecules. *J. Chem. Inf. Comput. Sci.*, 36, 3, 563–571, 1996. [Internet] Available from: https://pubs.acs.org/doi/abs/10.1021/ci950273r.
134. Bocci, G., Carosati, E., Vayer, P., Arrault, A., Lozano, S., Cruciani, G., ADME-space: A new tool for medicinal chemists to explore ADME properties. *Sci. Rep.*, 7, 1, 1–13, 2017.
135. Daoud, N.E.-H., Borah, P., Deb, P.K. *et al.*, ADMET Profiling in drug discovery and development: Perspectives of *in silico, in vitro* and integrated approaches. *Curr. Drug Metab.*, 22, 7, 503–522, 2021.

136. Xiong, G., Wu, Z., Yi, J. *et al.*, ADMETlab 2.0: An integrated online platform for accurate and comprehensive predictions of ADMET properties. *Nucleic Acids Res.*, 49, W1, W5–W14, 2021.
137. Raunio, H., *In silico* toxicology non-testing methods. *Front. Pharmacol.*, 2, 33, 2011.
138. Madden, J.C., Enoch, S.J., Paini, A., Cronin, M.T.D., A review of *in silico* tools as alternatives to animal testing: Principles, resources and applications. *Altern. Lab. Anim.*, 48, 4, 146–172, 2020. [Internet] Available from: https://journals.sagepub.com/doi/full/10.1177/0261192920965977.
139. Djoumbou-Feunang, Y., Fiamoncini, J., Gil-de-la-Fuente, A., Greiner, R., Manach, C., Wishart, D.S., BioTransformer: A comprehensive computational tool for small molecule metabolism prediction and metabolite identification. *J. Cheminformatics*, 11, 1, 1–25, 2019. [Internet] Available from: https://jcheminf.biomedcentral.com/articles/10.1186/s13321-018-0324-5.
140. Göller, A.H., Kuhnke, L., Montanari, F. *et al.*, Bayer's *in silico* ADMET platform: A journey of machine learning over the past two decades. *Drug Discov. Today*, 25, 9, 1702–1709, 2020. [Internet] Available from: https://doi.org/10.1016/j.drudis.2020.07.001.
141. Idakwo, G., Luttrell, J., Chen, M. *et al.*, A review on machine learning methods for *in silico* toxicity prediction. *J. Environ. Sci. Health, Part C*, 36, 4, 169–191, 2018. https://doi.org/10.1080/10590501.2018.1537118 [Internet] Available from: https://www.tandfonline.com/doi/abs/10.1080/10590501.2018.1537118.
142. Bhhatarai, B., Walters, W.P., Hop, C.E.C.A., Lanza, G., Ekins, S., Opportunities and challenges using artificial intelligence (AI) in ADME/tox. *Nat. Mater.*, 18, 5, 418–422, 2019. [Internet] Available from: /pmc/articles/PMC6594826/.
143. Khan, M.T.H., Predictions of the ADMET properties of candidate drug molecules utilizing different QSAR/QSPR modelling approaches. *Curr. Drug Metab.*, 11, 4, 285–295, 2010.
144. Cáceres, E.L., Tudor, M., Cheng, A.C., Deep learning approaches in predicting ADMET properties. *Future Med. Chem.*, 12, 22, 1995–1999, 2020. https://doi.org/10.4155/fmc-2020-0259 [Internet] Available from: https://www.future-science.com/doi/abs/10.4155/fmc-2020-0259.
145. Wang, Y., Xing, J., Xu, Y. *et al.*, *In silico* ADME/T modelling for rational drug design. *Q. Rev. Biophys.*, 48, 4, 488–515, 2015.
146. Yang, H., Lou, C., Sun, L. *et al.*, AdmetSAR 2.0: Web-service for prediction and optimization of chemical ADMET properties. *Bioinformatics*, 35, 6, 1067–1069, 2019. [Internet] Available from: https://academic.oup.com/bioinformatics/article/35/6/1067/5085368.
147. Tian, S., Djoumbou-Feunang, Y., Greiner, R., Wishart, D.S., CypReact: A software tool for *in silico* reactant prediction for human cytochrome P450

enzymes. *J. Chem. Inf. Model.*, 58, 6, 1282–1291, 2018. [Internet] Available from: https://pubs.acs.org/doi/abs/10.1021/acs.jcim.8b00035.
148. Shao, C.Y., Su, B.H., Tu, Y.S., Lin, C., Lin, O.A., Tseng, Y.J., CypRules: A rule-based P450 inhibition prediction server. *Bioinformatics*, 31, 11, 1869–1871, 2015. [Internet] Available from: https://pubmed.ncbi.nlm.nih.gov/25617412/.
149. Dhanda, S.K., Singla, D., Mondal, A.K., Raghava, G.P.S., DrugMint: A web-server for predicting and designing of drug-like molecules. *Biol. Direct*, 8, 1, 1–12, 2013. [Internet] Available from: https://biologydirect.biomedcentral.com/articles/10.1186/1745-6150-8-28.
150. Pu, L., Naderi, M., Liu, T., Wu, H.C., Mukhopadhyay, S., Brylinski, M., EToxPred: A machine learning-based approach to estimate the toxicity of drug candidates. *BMC Pharmacol. Toxicol.*, 20, 1, 1–15, 2019.
151. Venkatraman, V., FP-ADMET: A compendium of fingerprint-based ADMET prediction models. *J. Cheminformatics*, 13, 1, 1–12, 2021. [Internet] Available from: https://doi.org/10.1186/s13321-021-00557-5.
152. Stork, C., Embruch, G., Šícho, M. *et al.*, NERDD: A web portal providing access to *in silico* tools for drug discovery. *Bioinformatics*, 36, 4, 1291–1292, 2020. [Internet] Available from: https://pubmed.ncbi.nlm.nih.gov/32077475/.
153. Sander, T., Freyss, J., Von Korff, M., Reich, J.R., Rufener, C., OSIRIS, an entirely in-house developed drug discovery informatics system. *J. Chem. Inf. Model.*, 49, 2, 232–246, 2009. [Internet] Available from: https://pubs.acs.org/doi/abs/10.1021/ci800305f.
154. Daina, A., Michielin, O., Zoete, V., SwissADME: A free web tool to evaluate pharmacokinetics, drug-likeness and medicinal chemistry friendliness of small molecules. *Sci. Rep.*, 7, 1, 1–13, 2017. [Internet] Available from: http://dx.doi.org/10.1038/srep42717.
155. Schyman, P., Liu, R., Desai, V., Wallqvist, A., vNN web server for ADMET predictions. *Front. Pharmacol.*, 8, 889, 2017.
156. Pires, D.E.V., Blundell, T.L., Ascher, D.B., pkCSM: Predicting small-molecule pharmacokinetic and toxicity properties using graph-based signatures. *J. Med. Chem.*, 58, 9, 4066–4072, 2015. [Internet] Available from: https://pubs.acs.org/doi/full/10.1021/acs.jmedchem.5b00104.
157. Braga, R.C., Alves, V.M., Silva, M.F.B. *et al.*, Pred-hERG: A novel web-accessible computational tool for predicting cardiac toxicity. *Mol. Inform.*, 34, 10, 698–701, 2015. [Internet] Available from: https://pubmed.ncbi.nlm.nih.gov/27490970/.
158. Lagunin, A., Stepanchikova, A., Filimonov, D., Poroikov, V., PASS: Prediction of activity spectra for biologically active substances. *Bioinformatics*, 16, 8, 747–748, 2000. [Internet] Available from: https://pubmed.ncbi.nlm.nih.gov/11099264/.

159. Software Products-Simulations Plus. [Internet] Available from: https://www.simulations-plus.com/software/overview/ (Accessed on 27th February 2022).
160. Ioakimidis, L., Thoukydidis, L., Mirza, A., Naeem, S., Reynisson, J., Benchmarking the reliability of qikprop. Correlation between experimental and predicted values. *QSAR Comb. Sci.*, 27, 4, 445–456, 2008. [Internet] Available from: https://onlinelibrary.wiley.com/doi/full/10.1002/qsar.200730051.

9

Artificial Intelligence and Machine Learning-Based Formulation and Process Development for Drug Products

Vivek P. Chavda

Department of Pharmaceutics and Pharmaceutical Technology, L M College of Pharmacy, Ahmedabad, Gujarat, India

Abstract

Artificial intelligence (AI) and machine learning (ML) are constantly evolving techniques that may provide intriguing answers to hard scientific problems. There are some promising instances, such as in molecule design; nevertheless, formulation design is a more difficult domain, and this manuscript will look at what AI/ML can and cannot do to optimize formulation design in this multifarious arena. AI has been more popular in the pharmaceutical and biomedical sectors in recent years. Several AI-based solutions are extensively used in these sectors, resulting in more efficient and automated processes that include predictive and data-driven judgments. Although the drug manufacturing process is lengthy and complicated, it is critical to understand the fundamentals of how this business functions. It is a procedure used in the pharmaceutical industry to synthesize medications on a large scale. ML may be used to collect past batch performance for real-time improvement of crucial process parameters, resulting in optimum output quality. This chapter tries to capture AI/ML application for drug product formulation and process development.

Keywords: Artificial intelligence, machine learning, AI/ML, formulation development, process development, validation, scale up

Email: vivek7chavda@gmail.com

Vivek Chavda, Krishnan Anand and Vasso Apostolopoulos (eds.) Bioinformatics Tools for Pharmaceutical Drug Product Development, (183–196) © 2023 Scrivener Publishing LLC

9.1 Introduction

According to McCarthy J [1], "Artificial Intelligence (AI) has been broadly defined as the science and engineering of making intelligent machines, especially intelligent computer programs. Artificial intelligence can use different techniques, including models based on statistical analysis of data, expert systems that primarily rely on if-then statements, and machine learning. While Machine Learning (ML) is an artificial intelligence technique that can be used to design and train software algorithms to learn from and act on data. Software developers can use machine learning to create an algorithm that is 'locked' so that its function does not change, or 'adaptive' so its behavior can change over time based on new data." COVID-19 vaccines, such as the ground-breaking mRNA vaccines, were developed quickly and widely distributed, demonstrating to consumers what the industry is capable of [2–4]. Simultaneously, new technical advancements are allowing the life sciences sector to make more discoveries that will revolutionize patients' health conditions while possibly saving thousands of lives.

AI/ML has emerged as the technology innovation most expected to have a revolutionary impact on drug discovery and development during the last decade. This is fueled in part by breakthrough developments in computer power and the concurrent dissipation of earlier restrictions to large-scale data collecting and processing. Nevertheless, the cost of getting new pharmaceuticals to market and into the hands of patients has risen dramatically. Recognizing these challenges, the pharmaceutical business is interested in AI/ML approaches because of their robotic approach, pattern recognition, and predicted improved performance. Over the last 15-20 years, ML techniques have become more sophisticated in drug development. Clinical study design, conduct, and analysis are the most current areas of drug research where AI/ML is beginning to have a beneficial impact [5]. Due to a growing dependence on digital technologies in clinical trial execution, the COVID-19 outbreak may hasten the adoption of AI/ML in clinical trials. It's vital to get through the jargon and cacophony as we approach closer to a future where AI/ML is more integrated into R&D [6]. When forming judgments regarding data, it's also critical to remember that the scientific process isn't defunct. This will aid in distinguishing hope from hype and lead to more informed decisions on the best use of AI/ML in drug development [7].

9.2 Current Scenario in Pharma Industry and Quality by Design (QbD)

The worldwide pharmaceutical sector is expected to be valued USD 1.57 trillion by 2023, according to study. Various elements such as market drivers, existing and forthcoming trends, current growth pattern, and market obstacles are used to forecast market growth [8]. Soon after the COVID-19 epidemic wreaked havoc on the planet, it became evident that without new cures, especially vaccinations, the world would be trapped in a never-ending cycle of lockdowns and crises. As a consequence, pharmaceutical businesses moved into the public eye, and the demand to provide results grew swiftly. This was notably true for GSK, Pfizer, Merck & Co., and Sanofi, the worldwide vaccine market leaders [9]. Only Pfizer, in collaboration with German biotech firm BioNTech, has been able to produce a widely-used, safe, and effective vaccine thus far. AstraZeneca, which was not previously known for its vaccine development, collaborated with Oxford University to create a vaccine. Their COVID-19 vaccination is used in almost every country on the planet.

According to Prabal Chakraborty [10], "the Indian pharmaceuticals industry is recognized the world over due to the quality and cost-effectiveness of its products. At present, globally it is one of the fastest-growing industries and contributes 2.4 per cent value wise and 10 per cent volume wise globally. India alone accounts for 20 per cent of global exports in generics. In 2016, the Indian pharma industry exported USD16.89 billion and is expected to touch USD40 billion by 2020. The present generics market has immense potentiality for foreign direct investment (FDI) inflows, and worth USD14.53 billion of FDI inflows came in between April 2000 and December 2016. We have witnessed that Indian pharma companies go for joint ventures with multinational companies, make strategic alliances and co-promotions, contract research and manufacturing services, export, acquisitions and mergers, focus on new markets other than the USA and Europe, buy offshore plants and increase stakes in other companies. India is also becoming an attractive investment for the clinical trials market. The objective of this paper is to analyze the Indian pharmaceuticals industry—opportunity and threats, strategies of the Indian companies particularly after trade-related aspects of intellectual property rights (TRIPS)."

The total process is expedited when QbD features are included into a medicinal product research and validation program. Standardizing a risk-based strategy enables for the documented application of existing information, which leads to a better development strategy and the elimination of superfluous tests. Principal amount will be made in constructing small-scale models for all manufacturing steps, and subsequent robustness experiments may be required. The extra robustness assessments seem to have a dual function in terms of design space delineation and specification setting [12]. By undertaking worst-case assessment of edges instead of complete or partial DOEs, it may be feasible to dramatically decrease robustness assessments when a platform design space is revisited for novel drugs (Figure 9.1). A QbD program may give translational assistance in the long run, particularly for a molecular class array, while also enhancing assistance for ranges and specifications for a specific pharma production process. Some components of "process characterization and validation" activities are initiated roughly 9–12 months prior to the production of qualifying batches, according to the roadmap highlighted in this study. However, formulation robustness multivariate studies should be started considerably earlier as part of therapeutic product development [13].

Submissions that are more standardized, where the end-to-end logic is simpler to follow and the supporting material offers increased confidence in the entire process and product control approach may provide regulatory relief. QbD submissions may be lengthier but stronger, and supplementary submissions may be less necessary over a product's lifespan. To minimize

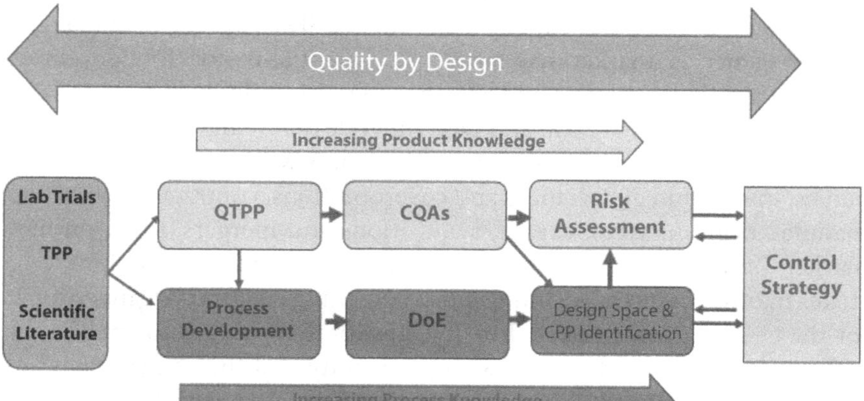

Figure 9.1 QbD roadmap for pharmaceutical product development. (Reprinted with permission from [11]) TPP: target product profile; DOE: design of experiment; QTPP: quality target product profile; CQA: critical quality attributes.

the quantity or kind of submissions, QbD might be used in conjunction with broader change procedures or comparability protocols. A technological transfer of a pharma product process from one location to another may be an example. For the company's assessment, the same work and testing would be done, but instead of a PAS, a yearly update may do [14].

A QbD strategy also allows for the proactive definition of allowed deviations and excursions, as well as some compliance relief. If a temperature excursion occurs at a point in the process that has been caught in the permissible design space, for example, it may become minimal in nature since the lack of influence on product quality has been investigated during design space definition [15].

Finally, a more rigorous and consistent procedure might lead to more predictable approval deadlines and inspection success, as well as more flexibility and post approval process improvement potential. Overall, we think this will improve medicinal product quality for patients while also lowering costs for corporations and regulatory authorities [12–15].

9.3 AI- and ML-Based Formulation Development

Formulation design is presently mostly guided by prior knowledge and experience, with thorough analytical characterization assisting the process. The majority of the research that has been published look at the impact of specific excipients on a range of biophysical parameters. Various excipients, on the other hand, may have a synergistic impact, and their interaction might result in dramatic gains in molecular performance, especially when several attributes must be improved at the same time [16]. Antibody formulation is a dynamic optimization approach that uses specialized pharmaceutical additives to suit the various storage, freeze–thaw, and delivery route criteria for clinical applications [17]. Formulations are traditionally generated *via* substantial trial and error after the discovery and optimization of molecules. Molecules, on the other hand, often suffer in late development due to their incapacity to create a combination with the appropriate characteristics [18]. A machine learning-based paradigm that allows formulation to be addressed during the molecule discovery and optimization stages, allowing for the selection of compounds that can be formed early on [19]. Early selection of the optimal desired formulation options will be aided by machine learning models of local antibody-excipient interactions [20]. Antibody formulation design may be used successfully throughout the molecule optimization phase as a consequence of this technique, cutting the cost of follow-up formulation work and lowering the probability of molecule failure owing to formulation issues.

A research study conducted by Theresa Kruse [21], "The behaviors of three antibodies were simulated in the presence of six excipients: sorbitol, sucrose, trehalose, proline, arginine.HCl, and NaCl. Carbohydrates tended to reduce aggregation propensity due to their preferential interactions with exposed aromatic residues. However, their impact on viscosity was highly dependent on the surface characteristics of the antibody, especially on whether charge effects significantly contributed to the antibody viscosity. Proline tended to interact with aromatic residues, reducing the aggregation of antibodies whose aggregation rate was association-limited. Arginine.HCl could interact via charge effects as well as with hydrophobic residues, while NaCl only interacted via charge effects. The overall impact of these excipients in terms of aggregation and viscosity was highly dependent on the surface charge distribution on the variable region. Finally, these local antibody-excipient interactions were modeled using machine learning techniques." Similarly, Theresa K Cloutier and colleagues have demonstrated ML based algorithm with preferential interactions of formulation excipients that can be used as a platform approach for formulation development [20]. Figure 9.2 summarizes a graphical visualization of deep learning algorithms used for the protein stability. "Bayesian versions of DL models, which are able to provide such uncertainty estimates, are available to researchers via established frameworks such as TensorFlow and PyTorch. Furthermore, new model architectures that are particularly suitable to handle chemistry problems have been developed."

The optimization of "black-box" models, where the fundamental connection between the input and output is unknown and locations in the input–output region can only be found empirically, has become prominent [24]. In a nutshell, Bayesian optimization advises doing trials in a sequential order using a proxy model that replicates the system under investigation based on prior results. The method is capable of attaining optimum conditions quicker and with a lower number of total studies can be done to its characteristic of dynamically evaluating sites [25]. Furthermore, the possibility provided by ML incorporation in drug dosage forms, and more generally in medical sciences, must be seen not just as a way to expedite efforts, but also as a way to discover new materials, unique formulations, and knowledge gained. As a result, we think that machine learning is well positioned to change the way medications are created.

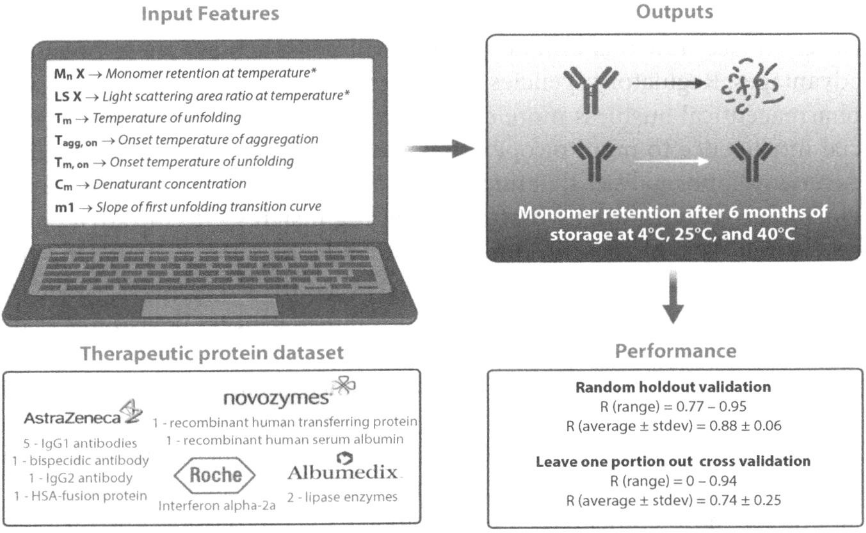

Figure 9.2 Illustration of the study conducted by Gentiluomo *et al.* [22]. The authors investigated various DL model architectures and the authors investigated various DL model architectures and data splitting strategies to predict protein stability (i.e., monomer retention) after six months storage at various temperatures (i.e., 4°C, 25°C and 40°C). Four pharmaceutical companies donated the dataset of therapeutic proteins used in this study, and the authors used experimentally determined metrics as well as preliminary stability data (i.e., up to two weeks) to conduct predictions of long-term stability. The leave-one-protein-out cross-validation approach provided a better means of testing the robustness of the DL model and would likely perform better at predicting the stability of new proteins never seen by the model. (Reprint with permission from [23].)

9.4 AI- and ML-Based Process Development and Process Characterization

Pharma businesses have been able to get a better knowledge of their medicines and related production processes because to QbD. This method may give a greater degree of assurance for customer satisfaction while also potentially improving company and legislative clearance effectiveness. Great strides have been made in establishing the industry methodology and methodology for implementing QbD ideas to pharmaceutical research and development during the last many years. The major tools and tactics for assessing the core parts of QbD, such as CQAs, CPPs, and the control plan, are designed and executed. Some of these critical QbD features have been effectively integrated in current regulatory filings for complicated pharmaceutical medicines, and pharmaceuticals will almost certainly be required in the future [26]. Industry and authorities will be watching closely to see how this unique method will assist achieve these potential advantages. Regulatory agencies and the general public are scrutinizing the pharmaceutical business more closely. Pharma companies may use artificial intelligence to monitor operations on a company-wide scale and discover any abnormalities that might lead to quality concerns or compliance violations. AI is especially useful for offering insights into industrial processes that have historically entailed human labor, such as managing the quality of raw materials and how it affects the finished product. Artificial intelligence-assisted quality assurance promotes process development by detecting flaws in raw materials before they reach the manufacturing line [27]. For example, AI-assisted quality assurance enhances pharmaceutical production by detecting problems in raw materials before they reach the manufacturing process. This technology may assist medicine makers in meeting more strict regulatory criteria as well as meeting customer expectations for more consistency in their goods. Furthermore, some medication manufacturers are also integrating Internet of Things solutions (IoT) technology on manufacturing lines in conjunction with AI-based computer vision to detect defective items or packaging in real time, providing

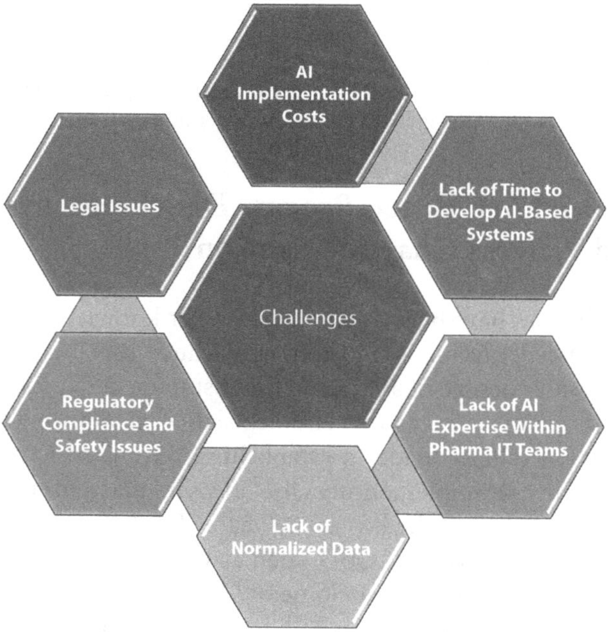

Figure 9.3 Challenges to implementing AI into pharma manufacturing processes.

them an advantage over rivals and helping to boost consumer satisfaction [28]. Figure 9.3 summarizes the current challenges for the implementation of AI in the pharmaceutical industry.

According to Arden NS and Colleagues [29], "Pharmaceutical manufacturing technologies are evolving as the internet of things, artificial intelligence, robots, and advanced computers begin to challenge established pharmaceutical production methodologies, practices, and business models. The adoption of these technologies has the potential to drastically improve the industrial manufacturing of medicines' agility, efficiency, flexibility, and quality. The next generation of pharmaceutical production will be defined by how these technologies are used along the path from data collecting to the signature digital maturity of Industry 4.0 (Figure 9.4)." Comprehensive lean and automatic manufacturing entails capturing all workflow performance metrics via cloud-connected PAT technology, analyzing that data into organized information, applying AI-based algorithms to transform that data into intelligence, and finally applying that expertise to gain overview of the process and improve process control [30]. Because of its capacity to learn, anticipate, and predict process conditions depending on historical information, ANN models may be used for adaptive process control. These principles will allow for real-time data capturing of process performance characteristics and trends, which can then be used to anticipate product quality features further along the manufacturing chain [31].

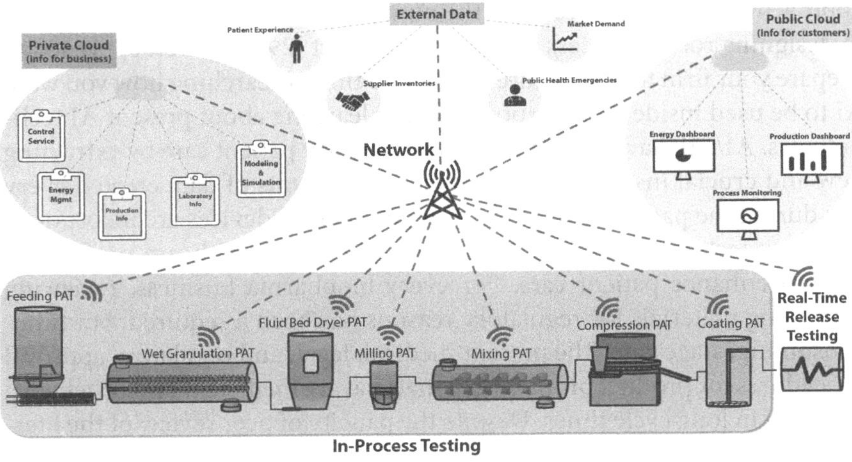

Figure 9.4 AI/ML based modern pharmaceutical manufacturing process. (Adopted under CC BY 4.0 from [29].)

Regulatory authorities regard pharmaceutical continuous production to be an emerging technology, and have established a framework based on good quality risk management. Pharmaceutical continuous manufacturing may address the Quality-by-Design paradigm, which opens the way for the future smart manufacturing outlined by Quality-by-Control, by understanding process dynamics and implementing the right control strategy [32]. Soft sensors seem to be a useful tool in the quest for smart manufacturing. Soft sensors, in fact, have the capacity to preserve the quality characteristics of the final medication product as near to their regulatory agency-set standards as feasible, as well as to avoid unwanted occurrences by possibly discarding out-of-spec goods.

9.5 Concluding Remarks and Future Prospects

Pharmaceuticals manufacturing is a difficult undertaking that needs meticulous planning to guarantee that all operations are monitored for efficiency. Pharma businesses are debating whether or not to improve their systems by incorporating AI into the manufacturing process. There are numerous obstacles to overcome before incorporating AI into drug manufacturing processes. AI is still a fairly new phenomenon in the health industry. The application of AI in manufacturing processes, on the other hand, might be a game-changer for pharmaceutical companies and their manufacturing processes. For pharmaceutical companies, AI Deployment offers better productivity, quality control, cost savings, and more. AI/ML based approaches can not only reduces the number of experiments but also helps in designing robust process and quality product [29]. The best approach to prepare your firm for this future is to spend time researching how you want AI to be used inside your corporation and learning about present AI technologies. AI/ML have the ability to revolutionize patient care by extracting new and crucial insights from the massive amounts of data created every day during the patient care. Companies of medical devices are incorporating these technologies into their products to help healthcare professionals and enhance patient care. For every biopharma business, reviewing marketing materials for regulatory reasons has been a required, but time-consuming, stage gate. The present medical, legal, and regulatory approval procedures for product promotional material are inefficient and unreliable, resulting in long cycle times. Despite the paucity of peer review of the literature at launch, promotional material is the single most essential source of information for newly authorized goods. This delays the delivery of authorized drugs to providers and patients. AI and machine learning have now been shown to drastically cut medical, legal, and regulatory review time while also enhancing content accuracy. This will increase the processes' speed and reliability, allowing medicines to reach the market faster.AI/ML based technologies are the future of the product lifecycle management in pharmaceutical industry.

References

1. McCarthy, J., What is artificial intelligence? Stanford University, Stanford, CA, pp. 64–70, 2007. Retrieved from http://jmc.stanford.edu/articles/whatisai/whatisai.pdf.
2. Tandel, H., Shah, D., Chavda, V., Nasal medication conveyance framework: An approach for brain delivery from essential to cutting edge. *Res. Rev. J. Med.*, 6, 14–27, 2016.
3. Chavda, V.P., Hossain, M.K., Beladiya, J., Apostolopoulos, V., Nucleic acid vaccines for COVID-19: A paradigm shift in the vaccine development arena. *Biologics*, 1, 337–356, 2021. https://doi.org/10.3390/biologics1030020.
4. Chavda, V.P., Kapadia, C., Soni, S., Prajapati, R., Chauhan, S.C., Yallapu, M.M., Apostolopoulos, V., A global picture: Therapeutic perspectives for COVID-19. *Immunotherapy*, 5, 351–371, 2022, doi: 10.2217/imt-2021–0168. https://doi.org/10.2217/imt-2021-0168.
5. Kolluri, S., Lin, J., Liu, R., Zhang, Y., Zhang, W., Machine learning and artificial intelligence in pharmaceutical research and development: A review. *AAPS J.*, 24, 19, 2022. https://doi.org/10.1208/s12248-021-00644-3.
6. Schuhmacher, A., Gatto, A., Kuss, M., Gassmann, O., Hinder, M., Big techs and startups in pharmaceutical R&D-a 2020 perspective on artificial intelligence. *Drug Discov. Today*, 26, 2226–2231, 2021. https://doi.org/10.1016/j.drudis.2021.04.028.
7. Schuhmacher, A., Brieke, C., Gassmann, O., Hinder, M., Hartl, D., Systematic risk identification and assessment using a new risk map in pharmaceutical R&D. *Drug Discov. Today*, 26, 2786–2793, 2021. https://doi.org/10.1016/j.drudis.2021.06.015.
8. Beran, D., Ewen, M., Chappuis, F., Reed, T., Hogerzeil, H., Pharmaceutical industry, non-communicable diseases and partnerships: More questions than answers. *J. Glob. Health*, 7, 2, 020301, 2017 Dec. doi: 10.7189/jogh.07.020301. PMID: 28959435; PMCID: PMC5804034.
9. Mikulic, M., Global pharmaceutical industry-statistics & facts, 2022. https://www.statista.com/topics/1764/global-pharmaceutical-industry/#topicHeader__wrapper (accessed May 25, 2022).
10. Chakraborty, P., Indian pharmaceuticals industry in global scenario: An appraisal. *J. Health Manag.*, 22, 424–429, 2020. https://doi.org/10.1177/0972063420937939.

11. Soni, G., Yadav, K.S., Gupta, M.K., QbD based approach for formulation development of spray dried microparticles of erlotinib hydrochloride for sustained release. *J. Drug Deliv. Sci. Technol.*, 57, 101684, 2020. https://doi.org/https://doi.org/10.1016/j.jddst.2020.101684.
12. Martin-Moe, S., Lim, F.J., Wong, R.L., Sreedhara, A., Sundaram, J., Sane, S.U., A new roadmap for biopharmaceutical drug product development: Integrating development, validation, and quality by design. *J. Pharm. Sci.*, 100, 3031–3043, 2011. https://doi.org/10.1002/jps.22545.
13. Yu, L.X., Pharmaceutical quality by design: product and process development, understanding, and control. *Pharm. Res.*, 25, 781–791, 2008. https://doi.org/10.1007/s11095-007-9511-1.
14. Garcia, F.A. and Vandiver, M.W., Throughput optimization of continuous biopharmaceutical manufacturing facilities. *PDA J. Pharm. Sci. Technol.*, 71, 189–205, 2017. https://doi.org/10.5731/pdajpst.2016.006882.
15. Yu, L.X., Amidon, G., Khan, M.A., Hoag, S.W., Polli, J., Raju, G.K., Woodcock, J., Understanding pharmaceutical quality by design. *AAPS J.*, 16, 771–783, 2014. https://doi.org/10.1208/s12248-014-9598-3.
16. Narayanan, H., Dingfelder, F., Condado Morales, I., Patel, B., Heding, K.E., Bjelke, J.R., Egebjerg, T., Butté, A., Sokolov, M., Lorenzen, N., Arosio, P., Design of biopharmaceutical formulations accelerated by machine learning. *Mol. Pharm.*, 18, 3843–3853, 2021. https://doi.org/10.1021/acs.molpharmaceut.1c00469.
17. Deokar, V., Sharma, A., Mody, R., Volety, S.M., Comparison of strategies in development and manufacturing of low viscosity, ultra-high concentration formulation for IgG1 antibody. *J. Pharm. Sci.*, 109, 3579–3589, 2020. https://doi.org/10.1016/j.xphs.2020.09.014.
18. Carracedo-Reboredo, P., Liñares-Blanco, J., Rodríguez-Fernández, N., Cedrón, F., Novoa, F.J., Carballal, A., Maojo, V., Pazos, A., Fernandez-Lozano, C., A review on machine learning approaches and trends in drug discovery. *Comput. Struct. Biotechnol. J.*, 19, 4538–4558, 2021. https://doi.org/https://doi.org/10.1016/j.csbj.2021.08.011.
19. Patel, L., Shukla, T., Huang, X., Ussery, D.W., Wang, S., Machine learning methods in drug discovery. *Molecules*, 25, 5277, 2020. https://doi.org/10.3390/molecules25225277.
20. Cloutier, T.K., Sudrik, C., Mody, N., Sathish, H.A., Trout, B.L., Machine learning models of antibody-excipient preferential interactions for use in computational formulation design. *Mol. Pharm.*, 17, 3589–3599, 2020. https://doi.org/10.1021/acs.molpharmaceut.0c00629.
21. Kruse, T., *Computational Design of Therapeutic Monoclonal Antibody Formulations*, pp. 155–170, Thesis Ph. D., Massachusetts Institute of Technology. Department of Chemical Engineering, Massachusetts Institute of Technology, USA, May 2019, https://dspace.mit.edu/handle/1721.1/127575 (accessed May 25, 2022).

22. Gentiluomo, L., Roessner, D., Frieß, W., Application of machine learning to predict monomer retention of therapeutic proteins after long term storage. *Int. J. Pharm.*, 577, 119039, 2020. https://doi.org/10.1016/j.ijpharm.2020.119039.
23. Bannigan, P., Aldeghi, M., Bao, Z., Häse, F., Aspuru-Guzik, A., Allen, C., Machine learning directed drug formulation development. *Adv. Drug Deliv. Rev.*, 175, 113806, 2021. https://doi.org/https://doi.org/10.1016/j.addr.2021.05.016.
24. Greenhill, S., Rana, S., Gupta, S., Vellanki, P., Venkatesh, S., Bayesian optimization for adaptive experimental design: A review. *IEEE Access*, 8, 13937–13948, 2020. https://doi.org/10.1109/ACCESS.2020.2966228.
25. Wilson, A., Fern, A., Tadepalli, P., J.L. Balcázar, F. Bonchi, A. Gionis, M. Sebag (Eds.), pp. 467–482 Springer Berlin Heidelberg, Berlin, Heidelberg, 2010.
26. Taticek, R. and Liu, J., F. Jameel, S. Hershenson, M.A. Khan, S. Martin-Moe (Eds.), pp. 31–46 Springer New York, New York, NY, 2015, https://doi.org/10.1007/978-1-4939-2316-8_3.
27. Zhong, R.Y., Xu, X., Klotz, E., Newman, S.T., Intelligent manufacturing in the context of industry 4.0: A review. *Engineering*, 3, 616–630, 2017. https://doi.org/https://doi.org/10.1016/J.ENG.2017.05.015.
28. Javaid, M., Haleem, A., Singh, R.P., Suman, R., Substantial capabilities of robotics in enhancing industry 4.0 implementation. *Cogn. Robot.*, 1, 58–75, 2021. https://doi.org/https://doi.org/10.1016/j.cogr.2021.06.001.
29. Arden, N.S., Fisher, A.C., Tyner, K., Yu, L.X., Lee, S.L., Kopcha, M., Industry 4.0 for pharmaceutical manufacturing: Preparing for the smart factories of the future. *Int. J. Pharm.*, 602, 120554, 2021. https://doi.org/10.1016/j.ijpharm.2021.120554.
30. FDA, Safeguarding pharmaceutical supply chains in a global economy, in: *House Committee on Energy and Commerce, Subcommittee on Health*, 2019b, https://www.fda.gov/news-events/congressional-testimony/safeguarding-pharmaceutical-supply-chains-global-economy.
31. Witkowski, K., Internet of things, big data, industry 4.0–innovative solutions in logistics and supply chains management. *Proc. Eng.*, 182, 763–769, 2017. https://doi.org/https://doi.org/10.1016/j.proeng.2017.03.197.
32. Jelsch, M., Roggo, Y., Kleinebudde, P., Krumme, M., Model predictive control in pharmaceutical continuous manufacturing: A review from a user's perspective. *Eur. J. Pharm. Biopharm.*, 159, 137–142, 2021. https://doi.org/https://doi.org/10.1016/j.ejpb.2021.01.003.

10

Artificial Intelligence and Machine Learning-Based Manufacturing and Drug Product Marketing

Kajal Baviskar[1], Anjali Bedse[2], Shilpa Raut[2] and Narayana Darapaneni[3]*

[1]Department of Pharmaceutical Chemistry, K. K. Wagh College of Pharmacy, Nashik, Maharashtra, India
[2]Department of Pharmaceutics, K. K. Wagh College of Pharmacy, Nashik, Maharashtra, India
[3]Data Science, Northwestern University School of Professional Studies, Chicago, IL, USA

Abstract
Artificial Intelligence (AI) and Machine Learning (ML) are the new drivers for the industry 4.0 revolution. Its use is becoming widespread across society. The dawn of AI and ML can also be witnessed in the pharmaceutical industry. The manufacturing sector has been significantly impacted by AI-ML. The ability of ML strategies to predict future events has allowed for the deciphering of complicated patterns in manufacturing patterns. This has opened the avenues for an intelligent decision support system in different manufacturing tasks like intuitive and continual inspection, fault detection, quality enhancement, process improvement, management of supply chain, and much more. ML approaches allow for the development of actionable intelligence to improve productivity without huge change in the required resources. AI and ML also have the potential to revolutionize marketing. It can assist in different aspects of marketing, like product cost, predictive analytics, market segmentation, etc. This chapter describes how AI and ML can be used in various aspects of pharmaceutical manufacturing and marketing. Different tools have been highlighted. Hurdles in the way of full-fledged applications of AI ML have also been mentioned.

**Corresponding author*: narayana.darapaneni@northwestern.edu

Vivek Chavda, Krishnan Anand and Vasso Apostolopoulos (eds.) Bioinformatics Tools for Pharmaceutical Drug Product Development, (197–232) © 2023 Scrivener Publishing LLC

Keywords: Artificial intelligence, machine learning, deep learning, neural networks, manufacturing, marketing, algorithms

Abbreviations

AI	Artificial Intelligence
ML	Machine Learning
DL	Deep Learning
ANN	Artificial neural network
PAT	Process Analytical Technology
QbD	Quality by Design
CNC	Computer Numerical Control
QSAR	Quantitative Structure-Activity Relationship
SVM	Support Vector Machines
RF	Random Forest
LDA	Linear Discriminant Analysis
QSPR	Quantitative Structure-Property Relationships
IoT	Internet of Things
NIRS	Near-Infrared Spectroscopy
CM	Continuous Manufacturing
CQA	Critical Quality Attributes
DNN	Deep Neural Network
PCA	Principal Component Analysis
ICA	Independent Component Analysis
PLS	Partial Least Squares
MKEICA	Multiway Kernel Entropy Independent Component Analysis
CIP	Cleaning In Place
IQAs	Intermediate Quality Attributes
DEM	Discrete Element Modelling
AHP	Analytic Hierarchy Process
VNS	Variable Neighborhood Search
CFD	Computational Fluid Dynamics

PSC	Pharmaceutical Supply Chain
RUL	Remaining Useful Life
PHM	Prognostics and Health Management
ELM	Extreme Learning Machines
CNN	Convolutional Neural Network
MSCNN	Multiscale Convolutional Neural Network
TFR	Time-Frequency Representation
DBN	Deep Belief Network
FNN	Fuzzy Neural Network
MES	Model Expert System
RWD	Real World Data
CRM	Customer Relationship Management

10.1 Introduction to Artificial Intelligence and Machine Learning

Over the years, industries have evolved rapidly with respect to technologies and automation. Industries have witnessed major progress in several areas. The advancement of electrical technology ushered in the second industrial revolution, enabling even greater output and more advanced machinery. The advancement and accessibility of computers as well as communication technologies, like computer networking, wireless communications and the internet, enabled the third industrial revolution [1]. The Fourth Industrial Revolution refers to the modern era of smart devices, storage technologies, and production facilities that can interface, trigger activities and monitor one another without the requirement for direct human intervention. This is generally referred to as "artificial intelligence."

The primary idea behind AI is to use learning to extend and complement systems' effectiveness and productivity for doing human jobs like problem-solving and decision-making. One of the important aspects of AI is machine learning [2]. ML is a subfield of AI that assists machines to train from data without being specifically programmed [3]. In order to provide accurate findings or make predictions based on that data, ML takes use of a significant quantity of structured as well as semi-structured data. Deep learning (DL) is a part of ML that can learn and model large amounts of informative data. The learning process can be supervised, semi-supervised,

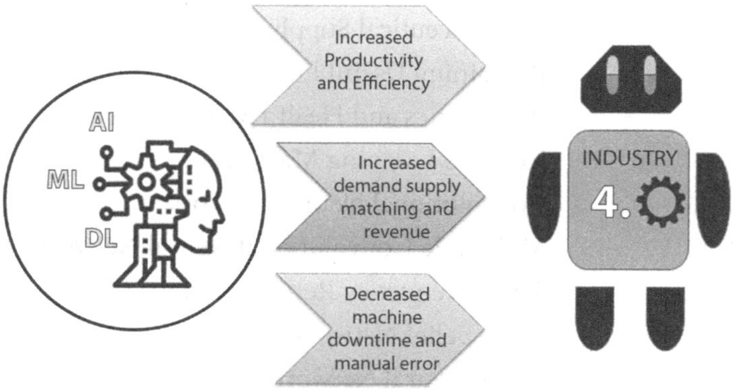

Figure 10.1 AI ML and Industry 4.0.

or unsupervised. Deep Learning's architecture is made up of numerous layers of hardware and GPU (Graphics processing units), which are referred to as artificial neural networks (ANNs). Industry integration of AI and ML promises benefits such as enhanced effectiveness and production, increased revenue, fewer machine downtimes, improved demand-supply matching, and reduced manual errors.

There have been tremendous advances in the pharmaceutical industry. The third industrial revolution was marked by enhanced Process Analytical Technology (PAT) and Quality by Design tools (QbD). Industry 3.0 is allowing for a better knowledge of how to acquire, analyze, and safeguard enormous amounts of data in the pharmaceutical production process. However, owing to AI and ML, revolution 4.0 can also be seen in pharmaceutical industries [1]. AI and ML are proliferating in the pharmaceutical industry. These have been contributing a lot in the pharmaceutical sector, since they enhance decision-making, maximize innovation, increase the efficiency of research and clinical trials, and develop valuable new tools for pharmaceutical industries. Figure 10.1 shows how AI-ML can boost Pharmaceutical Industries.

10.1.1 AI and ML in Pharmaceutical Manufacturing

Pharmaceutical manufacturing processes have seen dramatic changes. To improve the overall quality of the production process, Quality by Design (QbD) tools, and Process Analytical Technology (PAT) came into focus. Through process understanding, these tools offer a science-based approach to assure product quality. Quality errors in pharmaceutical manufacturing can have serious consequences, which is why they are closely monitored and regulated. When reviewing a product's acceptance, regulatory authorities are prone to checking the process's robustness and control. Failure to satisfy required quality standards could endanger years of effort and expenditure, especially since regulatory authorities may not accept process changes without persuasive documentation [4]. Hence, with manufacturing processes becoming more complex and an increased need for high quality and effective products, advanced manufacturing systems are trying to provide machines with human wisdom. Integration of AI and ML in manufacturing can be beneficial to the pharmaceutical industry. AI-assisted manufacturing processes not only provide economic advantages but can also offer advantages so as to design more rugged manufacturing processes.

AI may increase the efficiency of production, yielding more output and less waste. ML algorithms ensure that some activities are executed more precisely, as well as assist in the identification of areas where manufacturing processes can be further lowered, considerably improving production operations. Leading drug manufacturers have already integrated with or acquired AI technology. AI is useful for executing quality control, eliminating material waste, increasing manufacturing reuse, and forecasting maintenance. ML may assist in predicting and preventing over and undersupply, as well as addressing shortfalls and production line issues.

AI may provide opportunities to strengthen production efficiency and minimize waste. For example, a method that depends on human involvement to enter or manage data can be automated using CNC (computer numerical control). ML algorithms not only guarantee that activities are executed with high precision, but they also evaluate the process to see where it may be made simpler. This reduces material waste, accelerates manufacturing, and ensures that the product's critical quality attributes are constantly attained [5].

10.1.2 AI and ML in Drug Product Marketing

The marketing of pharmaceutical products has now shifted from traditional methods to digital marketing. Even customer's consumption of pharmaceuticals has shifted from traditional in-store to online shopping. AI can assist in a full examination of a product's core requirements from the customer's perspective, as well as analyze market needs, which aids in decision-making using prediction tools. AI does not only help to boost sales, but it can also forecast sales, which in turn avoids the expense of excess inventory or client loss due to shortages. AI can help to build innovative marketing techniques that will increase income and brand awareness. AI and advanced analytics applications are transforming businesses and marketplaces, allowing for greater performance and efficiency. The influence of AI on pharmaceutical sales and marketing, which rely heavily on human capabilities like knowledge and reasoning, can be profound. E-VAI is new revolutionary ML-based analytics to improve marketing results launched by Eularis for pharma companies. The platform demonstrates a significantly higher level of accuracy and comprehension of real-world driving impacts and synergistic effects as compared to traditional linear approaches [5–7].

10.2 Different Applications of AI and ML in the Pharma Field

As discussed in the introduction, AI and ML find various applications in the pharmacy field.

The section below highlights applications of AI and ML in different fields of pharmacy.

10.2.1 Drug Discovery

The process of drug discovery and development is complex, tedious, and financially exhausting. The usual research and development process takes place around 10–15 years. AI will be a promising tool that enables accurate and rapid recognition of leading compounds. Drugs that failed in clinical trials can be found for alternate therapeutic benefits using AI and ML. Quantitative Structure-Activity Relationship (QSAR) procedures such as decision trees, Support Vector Machines (SVMs), Random Forest (RF), and Linear Discriminant Analysis (LDA) have been applied to find new drug molecules and have developed into AI-based QSAR systems which may be leveraged for acceleration QSAR studies. Deep Chem, Deep Neural, Net QSAR, DeepTox, Neural Graph Fingerprints, ORGANIC and Potential Net are AI ML tools which have been utilized in drug discovery [8, 9].

10.2.2 Pharmaceutical Product Development

New chemical entity discovery is always followed by the inclusion of a new drug molecule into suitable pharmaceutical formulations with optimal delivery characteristics. In this circumstance, AI can be adopted rather than the traditional trial and error method. For example, a range of computational algorithms may resolve formulation design issues using Quantitative Structure-Property Relationships (QSPR), such as porosity, dissolution, stability problems, etc. Again, to choose the type, nature, as well as proportion of excipients depending on the physico-chemical properties of the drug, a decision-support program based on an AI algorithm can be used. This program utilizes a feedback process to check and change the overall process of product development [10].

10.2.3 Clinical Trial Design

Patients dropping out of clinical studies account for 30% of trial failures and require further recruitment to complete the experiment, wasting time and money. This may be prevented by keeping a tight eye on the participants and assisting them in sticking to the clinical trial protocol. AiCure created mobile technology to monitor regular medication consumption by schizophrenia patients in a Phase II trial, resulting in a 25% increase in patient adherence and the success of the clinical trial [11].

10.2.4 Manufacturing of Drugs

Looking at today's scenario of manufacturing, process controls and processes are usually separated. As a result, adjustments to control systems take longer to implement [1]. This problem could be solved by applying AI algorithms. The next section of this chapter elaborates on this application.

10.2.5 Quality Control and Quality Assurance

Product quality assurance may be achieved using a programmed platform for data entry, like an electronic lab notebook, and advanced, intelligent algorithms. Furthermore, Total Quality Management expert system's data mining and different knowledge innovation methods can be useful for making complex selections and developing technology for intelligent quality control [12].

10.2.6 Product Management

Product management involves market positioning, market prediction, and analysis, as well as for deciding product cost. With the use of e-commerce and the Internet of things (IoT), product management is becoming easier. The integration of AI promises many more advancements in this field. For example, AI techniques such as particle swarm optimization can be used to achieve a greater understanding of markets. It can assist in determining the product's marketing strategy based on reliable customer demand forecasting. AI tools involve customers and boost physician awareness. Furthermore, a customer entered keywords are examined by natural language processing technologies and correlated with the probability of purchasing the products [13, 14]. This application has been discussed in a further section of this chapter.

10.2.7 Drug Prescription

Errors in prescriptions are one of the most significant problems that customers and patients face. Because of various medication interactions, these mistakes might result in life-threatening occurrences. Patients or clients can use AI-powered knowledge bots as personalized self-service advisers. To avoid prescription errors, techniques like optical identification, graphic recognition, and picture classification using AI tools like CNN and YOLO are used [15].

10.2.8 Medical Diagnosis

AI has also made inroads into a medical diagnosis. DeepMind Health, a unit of Google, has invented ML algorithms that can detect distinctions among healthy and malignant cells in order to optimize radiation treatments [16].

10.2.9 Monitoring of Patients

For patient monitoring, physicians often have to evaluate vast amounts of complicated, diverse data in order to make life-critical choices. AI can be used to handle this data and analyze it effectively [17]. Remote patient monitoring is also possible by employing AI [18].

10.2.10 Drug Synergism and Antagonism Prediction

Prediction of drug synergism and antagonism are crucial for deciding on drug therapy. Instances can be cited in literature where AI has been applied to predict the same. For example, The Master Regulator Inference Algorithm successfully predicted 56% synergism utilizing 'Mater regulator genes'. Network-based Laplacian regularized least square synergistic medication combination as well as random forest may be utilized to determine synergism. Li *et al.* created a random forest-based synergistic medication combination model to predict synergistic anticancer drug combinations. Gene expression profiles were used to create this model [19].

10.2.11 Precision Medicine

There has been a change in recent years from a one-size-fits-all approach to therapeutic customization for individual patients. It relies on identifying a patient's health mechanisms, which is difficult. However, AI has emerged as a critical tool for deciphering patients' genetics and developing tailored medicines [20]. For instance, One Ring is a unique Parkinson's disease measuring system. ML system of which has been trained to simulate numerous Parkinson's movement symptoms, such as bradykinesia, dyskinesia, and tremor, in order to produce patient reports on a routine basis. This enables physicians to acquire information related to a patient's movement intensity with date and time, and it also assists in prescribing more effective treatments [21].

Applications discussed above have been briefed in Table 10.1.

10.3 AI and ML-Based Manufacturing

The manufacturing of pharmaceuticals involves many aspects which influence the product quality. There have been many advances in the field of pharmaceutical manufacturing. AI and ML can also be applied to pharmaceutical manufacturing. Figure 10.2 shows various aspects of Pharmaceutical Manufacturing in which AI-ML can be useful.

The use of AI-ML in various aspects of pharmaceutical manufacturing has been discussed below.

10.3.1 Continuous Manufacturing

In contrast to traditional batch production procedures, industries have begun to employ continuous manufacturing (CM). Production flexibility and efficiency may both be improved with continuous manufacturing. Here, units of the process are closely linked. At the start of the line, processing material is fed continually into the first unit of the process, whereas the finished product is released concurrently. The process control technique used on the CM lines includes relevant PAT tools which offer real-time information on the process level as well as product quality. Near-Infrared Spectroscopy (NIRS) is a common PAT tool because of its non-destructive, safe, and quick approach. Moreover, it does not require sample preparation. NIRS is now widely utilized for starting (raw) material identification, in-line process monitoring such as mixing, granule formulation, and drying, and process troubleshooting [4].

Table 10.1 Applications of AI–ML in pharma.

Sr. no.	Fields	Applications of AI and ML
1.	Drug discovery	• Molecular recognition with computers. • Search for hit and lead series patterns. • High-throughput checking. • Capacity to evaluate multiple candidates simultaneously. • Producing biopharmaceutical models. • Identification of promising molecules at later stages [8, 9].
2.	Pharmaceutical product development	• In R&D, boosting the value chain system. • Improving efficiency and production. • Lowering the cost [10].
3	Clinical trial design	• Clinical trial design using algorithms. • Proper monitoring of the patients [11].
4.	Drug manufacturing	• Substitute all manual tasks. • Continuous production. • BMR or real-time digital reporting tracking. • Simplified Pharmaceutical investigation records [1].
5.	Quality control and quality assurance	• Technology for intelligent quality control can be made. • Increasing quality standards with the smallest possible experiments [12].

(Continued)

Table 10.1 Applications of AI–ML in pharma. (*Continued*)

Sr. no.	Fields	Applications of AI and ML
6.	Product management	• Techniques like particle swarm optimization to achieve a greater understanding of markets. • Determining the product's marketing strategy. • Predicting consumer behavior [13, 14].
7.	Drug prescription	• AI-powered knowledge bots as a personalized self-service adviser. • Tools like CNN, YOLO used to avoid errors in prescription [15].
8.	Medical diagnosis	• Minimize the diagnosis errors. • Medical diagnosis for various clinical conditions [16].
9.	Patient monitoring	• Analyze large amounts of data related to patients. • Remote patient monitoring [17, 18].
10.	Drug synergism and antagonism prediction	• To predict potential synergistic and antagonistic activity. • Identification of the most efficient therapeutic combination [19].
11.	Precision medicine	• Analyze large and heterogeneous data sets. • Decision-making, classification, and pattern recognition [20, 21].

Advanced model-based control technologies are also seen as important for permitting continuous pharmaceutical manufacture since they promise to improve Critical Quality Attributes (CQA) control. Many robust physics-based models may be used to characterize various drug reactions [22, 23]. Through automated ML, AI combined with PAT may assist in the control of industrial processes as well as the overall development of the process [24]. Because they promise to improve CQA control, advanced model-based control technologies are seen as vital to permitting continuous pharmaceutical manufacture. However, these models have disadvantages such as complex architecture and hefty expenses. Data-driven

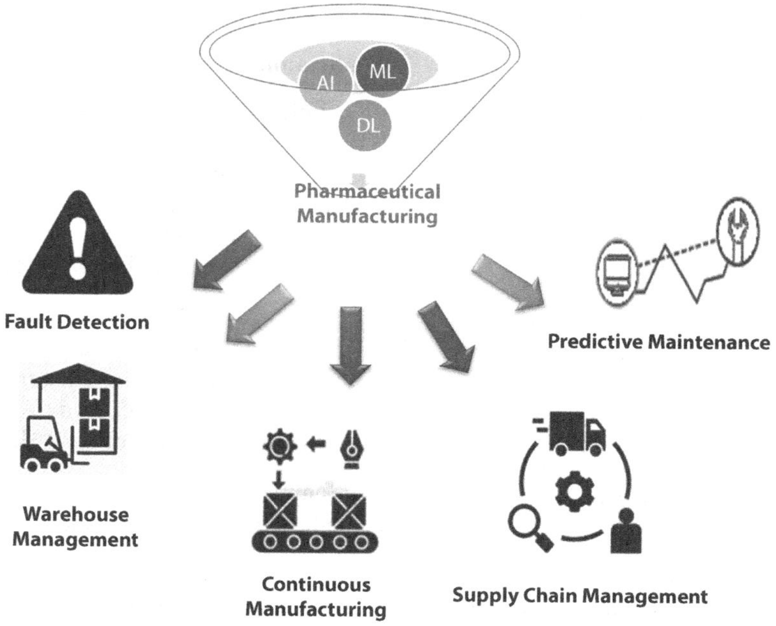

Figure 10.2 AI in pharmaceutical manufacturing.

models such as neural networks are frequently used in the chemical and biochemical processing sectors. RNNs (Recurrent Neural Networks) are a kind of ANN that uses hidden variables as a memory to record temporal relationships between control variables and system. RNNs serve as another source of control-oriented models by which dynamics of highly non-linear systems are captured adequately. It becomes comparatively simple to acquire and assess online because their creation is a data-driven process that yields increasingly efficient models with huge quantity of sensor and process information. This opens up new avenues for applying ML models or RNNs to allow continuous production of pharmaceuticals [25].

Rogge *et al.* used deep learning for continuous pharmaceutical solid dosage form production. Production process units included: feeding operations – wet-granulation – fluid-bed drying – screening and tableting. Researchers discovered that Deep Neural Networks (DNN) can learn from noisy PAT values and ANN predictions may be used to improve process knowledge and discriminate to identify critical process parameters. DNN may also be used as a backup source of information for internet monitoring. DNN offers process monitoring data even if one of the PAT sensors fails.

PAT, deep learning and process data science collaborate to create a proper monitoring framework for the continuous production line [4].

10.3.2 Process Improvement and Fault Detection

ML algorithms' predictive analytics capabilities can assist in the selection of the optimal set of parameters for a certain manufacturing process. This enables the manufacturing process to be improved and enhanced [26]. Fault detection is crucial in manufacturing, particularly when the operations are large-scale and intricate with a significant number of variables. During production, timely and precise identification of problems is critical since it lowers downtime and saves time. For flaw detection, ML methodologies such as artificial neural networks and fuzzy neural methods can be used [27]. There are several examples of AI-ML being used to detect faults during production.

Carter *et al.* utilized Passive Acoustic Emissions, and DL to find out a clogged fluidized bed distributor plate. Parts of a top-spray fluidized bed distributor plate, were actively covered to simulate blockages. Piezoelectric microphones were mounted on the vessel wall and positioned in the fluidized bed exhaust. Number of variables in time and frequency domain emerged from the monitoring data. These feature vectors were used by the ANN to train against each distributor plate obstruction circumstance. The deep learning model proved useful in a process control context during testing [28].

Colucci *et al.* used ML for online monitoring of quality of the product and failure in the process in pharmaceutical lyophilization process. ML algorithms were built using data from a non-invasive image sensor for real-time flaw identification and product quality monitoring. Principal Component Analysis (PCA) and Partial Least Square Regression were created and studied comparatively. 5 batches were collected under standard operational conditions for training of process reference model. Also, the classification capabilities of algorithms were evaluated by using five additional batches that simulated various forms of errors. The performance of the algorithms is greatly improved by combining data by using an infrared camera along with other varying parameters collected from the equipment's PLC and textural analysis performed on product images (RGB). The proposed algorithms are useful to handle batch heterogeneity while lowering off-spec products [29].

Batch operations are crucial in the pharmaceutical industry because they provide for greater production flexibility and the ability to react quickly to changing market conditions. When production circumstances in a batch process deviate from expectations, the quality of the product suffers, potentially leading to severe production failures. Non-Gaussian and nonlinear properties are seen in a large percentage of batch processes. A lot of studies on batch processes have been done. PCA, ICA (independent component analysis), and PLS (Partial Least Squares) are multivariate statistical (data-driven) tools to monitor the process that are becoming increasingly popular in this field. Peng and other researchers designed the Multiway Kernel Entropy Independent Component Analysis (MKEICA) algorithm for microbial fermentation process fault diagnosis with non-Gaussian and nonlinear coexistence [30]. The technique proposes the creation of a hybrid system that combines a ML-based fault detection method, a wireless communication model, and an ontology-based multi-agent system with cooperative control for monitoring of process [27, 28, 30].

10.3.3 Predictive Maintenance (PdM)

PdM assists maintenance personnel in anticipating problems and implementing corrective action on time. In PdM, ML flexibility can help with a variety of challenges, including unexpected failures. Data collection, data analysis, data modelling, and data prediction are the four processes in ML modelling. Smart sensors collect data from potentially malfunctioning components within an operational machine, revealing the machine's state and activity throughout its life cycle and detecting potential flaws. The data streaming approach is coupled with machine processing characteristics such as set points, configuration, and historical data to increase the accuracy and representation of data prediction. Data streaming is thoroughly investigated to uncover dependencies, as well as technological ideas connected to possible failure indications and the formulation of particular measures to address the projected failure. Data modelling is frequently used to identify flaws and to develop ML algorithms that serve as the foundation for predictive models. Before giving final clearance to the prediction models, the data prediction process goes through many steps to check failure detection accuracy [31]. Calzavara *et al.* used ML to forecast sprayer system failure in the Cleaning In Place (CIP) process for washing and cleaning the freeze-dryer [32]. To identify the manifold pump operating circumstances, the DBSCAN method (ML algorithm model) was used to create time-series data segmentation expedient. DBSCAN, which uses the process cycle number as a core characteristic, will prove to be the most successful time series clustering approach [30].

10.3.4 Quality Control and Yield

Manufacturing a pharmaceutical formulation in a timely manner while preserving quality is a demanding endeavor that requires a well-thought-out, scientific methodology. Pharmaceutical ingredients, excipients, associated interactions, unit activities, and equipment must all be detailed. Heuristics, decision trees, correlation, and first-principle models are all examples of how knowledge is used [24]. Data mining tools in the intelligent quality management system gives quality knowledge and the ability to find links between enterprise management processes. The proposed technique can help traditional quality systems to overcome the "knowledge bottleneck problem" and improve cooperative monitoring capabilities [33]. End-product testing may not provide as much assurance of product quality as process controls and preset material attributes do. For monitoring the relationship between process and quality, PAT was created to look at Intermediate Quality Attributes (IQAs) during the development of regulatory standards and to help with continual production improvement [34].

Goh *et al.* used Elman recurrent neural network to predict *in-vitro* dissolution release data of theophylline pellet formulations (matrix controlled-release). Applying this method, a tedious investigation to determine the appropriate pellet excipient ratio may be avoided [35].

Neuro-Fuzzy logic is a blended technique that integrates neural network learning using fuzzy logic's interpretive capabilities. In complex, multi-dimensional search spaces, Genetic Algorithms can be applied to find the best overall solution. For instance, throughout the manufacturing process, ramipril pills must be closely monitored, as the chemical product stability is influenced by mechanical stress, quantitative composition and compression specifications. Aksu *et al.* focused on the detailed examination of production data employing intelligent softwares and optimized the formulation [36]. Discrete Element Modelling (DEM) has been frequently used in the pharmaceutical sector to investigate powder segregation in binary mixtures, the impacts of modifying blade speed and shape, estimating the movement of tablets in the coating process, and assessment of residence time of the tablets beneath the spray zone [37].

10.3.5 Troubleshooting

The capacity assignment problem in the pharmaceutical industry is complicated by the fact that several factors must be considered at the same time, including machine throughput, process constraints, batch quantity, machine accessibility, machine effectiveness, workload balance, etc. As a result, this technique may be simplified and optimized using the heuristic strategy. The findings showed that the AHP (Analytic Hierarchy Process)-based technique proposed was both logical and practical. The usage of machines and the distribution of labor loads are far superior to the expert's results. For ease of usage, the method might be readily implemented as software. This will save time and make the completion of complicated tasks easier [38].

In the pharmaceutical industry, tablet film coating planning includes determining coating sequences on parallel machines for reducing both completion time and the number of jobs that are late. This difficulty is exacerbated by the fact that switching from one medicine to another necessitates a lengthy amount of cleaning and setup time, which varies depending on the previously coated drug. Chutamas *et al.* solved this issue using a variable arc exchange heuristic based on the Variable Neighborhood Search (VNS). The suggested heuristics were built from simple dispatching heuristics, such as the Earliest Due Date (EDD) and Longest Processing Time (LPT). A sequence of local-search operators, like 2OPT, RELOCATION, and SWAP, incrementally enhanced the initial solution. The outcomes of the predicted heuristic were comparable with the optimization model in terms of solution quality, with a difference of less than 5% for instances of 20 orders. In various respects, the proposed heuristic is advantageous to the production planner [39].

The CFD (Computational Fluid Dynamics) tool utilized Reynolds-Averaged Navier Stokes solver technology for the investigation impact of agitation and stress levels on equipment like stirred tanks enabling automation of pharmaceutical processes. Direct numerical simulations and large-eddy simulations, utilize sophisticated techniques to handle complex flow problems during manufacturing [37]. To minimize processing problem like capping of tablet in production process, ANNs and fuzzy models were used to investigate the relationship between equipment parameters and the capping problem [40].

10.3.6 Supply Chain Management

Pharmaceutical Supply Chain (PSC) management refers to the operations of monitoring, organizing, and executing the flow of a product from raw material sourcing to production and into the hands of the patient. It includes supply chain planning, risk management, quality management, and inventory management. Because of its complexity, the pharmaceutical business lags behind other industries in terms of operational performance. Effective pharmaceutical supply chain management serves to reduce potential risks to the pharmaceutical supply chain, such as drug counterfeiting and theft, and ensure that patients have timely access to pharmaceuticals. The PSC has lagged behind other industries in terms of operational effectiveness due to the complicated pharmaceutical processes. AI and analytics are expected to eliminate shortages, save costs, and improve transparency inside the PSC. PSC management can be improved significantly by using data analytics. Predictive solutions based on ML algorithms, in particular, have already shown a high degree of accuracy in getting precise estimates, assisting in the reduction of medicine shortages and excess inventory levels [41]. AI and ML may be used in a variety of supply chain management applications. The ML model may be used with the SVM to predict viable candidates for future customer-supplier collaborations. Product delivery in a short duration is a difficult endeavor. Planning ahead of time leads to higher storage costs and capital constraints. To address this problem, AI algorithms may be utilized to produce weekly demand estimates based on stock holding unit level over a six-month period. Past data from the last several years may be utilized to train the algorithm [42].

The period between placing a purchase order with a supplier and receiving it is known as "purchase lead time." Forecasting purchase lead time is an important function in the supply chain since it allows healthcare providers to avoid extended wait times. Estimating purchase lead time is a complex undertaking because of complicated manufacturing processes and the wide range of data. Nevertheless, AI has nevertheless helped to make great progress in this subject.

ML algorithms are being used to forecast future demand. With ML techniques, Oliveria *et al.* developed a system for lead time predicting in the PSC. Five algorithms were compared and contrasted. The findings of the experiment revealed that purchasing lead time may be predicted with great accuracy [43].

10.3.7 Warehouse Management

A lot of manual effort goes into the storage and delivery stage. Warehouse management is critical, especially for large pharmaceutical companies. There have been several advancements in warehouse management during the last two decades. Barcode technology is frequently used in inventory management to regulate stock levels. Integration of warehouse management systems with automatic identification technologies has been attempted [44]. Using genetic programming and unsupervised ML, Bandaru *et al.* built an intelligent framework for warehouse management. Pick-by-Light, Pick-by-Voice, and Pick-by-Vision techniques are used in modern AI warehouse management systems. The most common method is Pick-by-Voice, which makes use of voice messages instead of electronic or paper orders [45]. Each employee is provided with a microphone and headset as well as a wireless (belt-mounted) computer, in Pick-by-Voice technique, and is guided across the warehouse by the headset. The Eyes and hands of the worker are movable now that the clipboard is no longer required. The "pick by light" approach needs the installation of permanent shelf indicators. The indicator flashes to catch the attention and shows a number showing the number of items to be collected from that place. Each operator has its own work area, and all of the appropriate indicators glow up at the same time for each order. According to Lightning Pick Technologies this method produces quicker pick as compared to other operator-based method [46]. Classification of the inventory products is an important issue and a key operation in inventory management practices.

Dumitrescu *et al.* created AI-based models to maximize the utilization of wireless network sensors in pharmaceutical distribution centers. The approach combines a deep ANN -based learning model with the capacity to gather and centralize telemetry data from a sensor network in real-time. The prediction system, that depends on a rudimentary neural network and is used to improve warehouse processes, has demonstrated that it can decrease system as well as drug picking mistakes [47].

10.3.8 Predicting Remaining Useful Life

Predicting Remaining Useful life (RUL) is important for mechanical system Prognostics and Health Management (PHM). Maintenance programs may be established using an accurate RUL prediction to keep machines or components in proper working condition, avoiding unexpected system breakdowns. Data-driven and Model-based solutions have been obtained to attain this goal. Model-based solutions need precise modelling of the system's dynamics, which is difficult due to the rising complexity of mechanical systems as a result of fast industrial growth.

Understanding the detailed functioning mechanisms of mechanical systems is not needed for data-driven solutions. Instead, all that is necessary is the gathering of data from the systems, after which data-driven algorithms may be used to assess the condition of the systems. For RUL prediction, popular shallow ML and DL techniques can be utilized. In shallow-model-based RUL prediction, feature extraction and inference are commonly used. After extracting some significant data, ML methods such as ANNs, extreme learning machines (ELM), SVM, neural networks, and random forests can be used to predict the RUL. Without the need for manual feature extraction, DL can learn representative features from raw sensory input. Furthermore, it can integrate feature learning with RUL inference to improve RUL prediction generalization [48]. Using the LSTM technique, a very good result was obtained for RUL prediction [49, 50].

For RUL prediction of machine, Chen *et al.* suggested an attention-based DL architecture. A feature fusion framework was built to blend handmade and automatically learned features to improve RUL prediction performance [48]. A deep convolutional neural network (CNN) for the RUL prediction was proposed by Babu *et al.* [51].

To forecast the RUL, Zhu and researchers recommended using a multiscale convolutional neural network (MSCNN). To get Time-Frequency Representation (TFR), raw sensory data was first transformed using a wavelet transform. The TFR was then entered into MSCNN for the prediction of RUL. For the RUL prediction, Deutsch presented a deep belief network feed-forward neural network (DBN-FNN). The FNN was used to forecast RUL using the learnt features, while the DBN was utilized to learn representative features [51–53].

As discussed in above section, various AI-ML tools are now being used in Pharmaceutical Manufacturing. Tools have been summarized in Table 10.2.

10.3.9 Challenges

Without a doubt, AI-ML has the potential to transform pharmaceutical manufacturing, but doing so will require the adoption of modern manufacturing technologies as well as the resolution of legislative, technological, and logistical difficulties. While many pharmaceutical companies are familiar with the fundamental tools of PAT and QbD, fewer are prepared to take the next steps toward implementing advanced technology to enable smart manufacturing. One of the major reasons for the slow adoption of newer technology is the enormous institutional as well as regulatory expertise gained on old platform technologies.

(A) Regulatory Challenges

Current regulatory frameworks can be seen as a barrier to technological innovation. The sector may continue to adopt old practices due to a lack of regulatory precedent, even though new methods would minimize the regulatory burden and enhance quality in the long term. Another regulatory barrier is the time and effort necessary to file regulatory applications in many global jurisdictions with differing regulatory standards, especially for novel manufacturing technologies.

Table 10.2 AI ML tools for manufacturing.

Sr. no.	Tools	Details
1.	MKEICA	• Fault diagnosis of microbial pharmaceutical fermentation process [30].
2.	DEM	• Studies the effects of altering blade speed and shape on particle segregation in a binary mixture [37].
3.	CFD	• It Studies the • Agitation Impact • Levels of stress in equipment [37].
4.	ANNs along with fuzzy models	• Correlates between machine specifications and the capping issue for reducing capping of tablet in manufacturing process [34].
5.	Meta-classifier and tablet- classifier	• Forecast error in tablet production [54].
6.	Electronic Lab Notebook	• An automated data entry platform [55].
7.	Model Expert System (MES)	• A control system that receives minute-by-minute data using various sources and manages, monitors, and tracks diverse manufacturing information in real-time [7].
8.	Chemputer	• Synthesis and manufacturing of molecules [56].

(B) Technical Challenges

The existing manufacturing paradigm has technical limitations such as inflexible process settings, substantial offline testing (particularly for sterile products), and the necessity of regular human involvement in production operations.

(C) Logistical Challenges

Industry and regulators will have logistical hurdles in integrating AI-ML, and in certain cases, they may be fighting for the same limited resources.

To implement AI in pharmaceutical production, a variety of expertise beyond conventional biology, chemistry, and process engineering will be required [1].

10.4 AI and ML-Based Drug Product Marketing

Just like in other businesses, marketing is a crucial aspect of pharmaceuticals also. It involves tremendous analytics and statistics. AI ML can be viewed as a promising tool to assist in various aspects of marketing as shown in Figure 10.3. In marketing, AI and ML can be used right from product launch to market segmentation. Various tools as depicted in Table 10.2 can be used in pharmaceutical marketing field. The following section describes applications of AI ML in various aspects of marketing.

10.4.1 Product Launch

AI offers Real-World Data (RWD) to companies that may help them succeed in product launches and commercial success by managing targeted interactions with different stakeholders. Pharma industries are increasingly

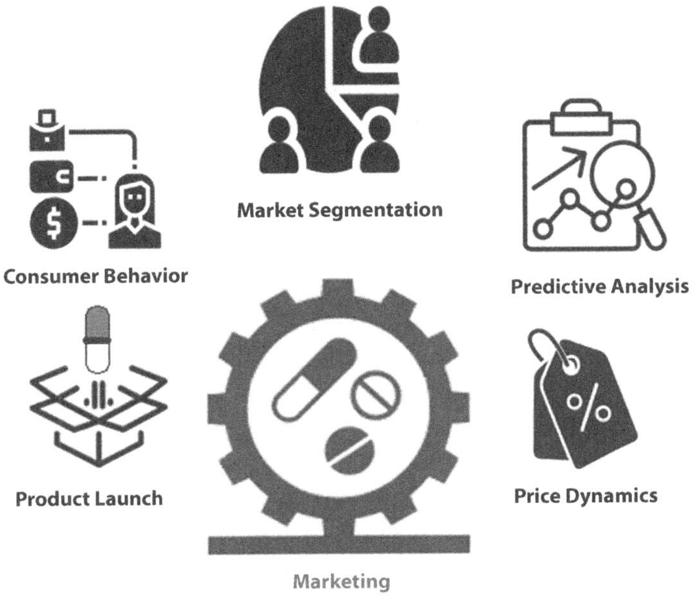

Figure 10.3 AI in drug product marketing.

using RWD to better recognize the value and effectiveness of products, as well as to rationalize the product's cost in a competitive market system. The AI-generated RWD gives a more accurate picture of the emerging standard of care as well as a more realistic assessment of the impact of a therapy on a larger patient group. Data-driven approaches are useful to plan for pricing and marketing strategies. Innovative optimization algorithms may strengthen confidence and help find more effective pricing opportunities, which could eventually translate into sales and profit. Incorporation of patient-centric approaches into sales and marketing strategies as well as AI-enabled effective e-commerce marketing solutions may help by anticipating behavior and advising on the best next steps to take, how to use channels, and how to maximize stakeholder involvement. ML and DL are consistently updated to identify changes and provide consistency to corporate strategy and sales techniques [57]. Lee *et al.* reported a Bass model and statistical and ML algorithms for the prelaunch prediction of new product demand. The diffusion process of products was explained by the Bass model, whereas two significant parameters of the Bass model were explained by statistical and ML algorithms before launch. A product attribute database was used an input and a product diffusion database was used as an output to develop prediction models. Statistical and ML-based regression algorithms are helpful to forecast the demand of the new product completely on the basis of product attributes and with no human intervention. This promotes successful pre-launch decision-making. The product database should be regularly updated and inclusive of highly homogeneous products for better predicting accuracy. Furthermore, the variables chosen as product attributes should not be exhaustive or constant [58, 59].

10.4.2 Real-Time Personalization and Consumer Behavior

A decision-making system based on data mining that employs a decision tree and an ANN is a hybrid approach to decide an organization's marketing strategies [60]. Innovative and effective use of search engines as a free advertising tool may assist industries in developing brands and achieving success in the e-commerce industry. Data insights provided by AI provide companies with additional real-time data to include marketing personalization on websites depending on-site visitor behavior. AI and ML can jointly collect personalized information about the purchasing preferences of patients. This enables users to choose personalized content in real-time. Personalized content can be prepared by immediately performing segmentation of the collected data. Age, gender, education, medication history, geolocation of patient and time of medication, behavior on websites, mobile devices, social media, email and others, and interests of the patient. Using statistical methods, previous sessions/medication data can be analyzed to forecast patient behavior [61].

Consumer behavior is the study of how people choose, utilize, and discard products and services. It gives useful data and insights on consumer emotions, perspectives, and preferences, all of which influence purchase decisions. This will allow marketers to better understand consumer needs, provide value products to customers, and generate income for the business. Data from social media and news, as well as previous sales and reviews, is analyzed by AI systems to determine what customers expect and on which things they are willing to spend more money. Customers' economic circumstances and spending capacity are also considered by these technologies. The nicest thing about these tools is that they are trustworthy and have estimate accurately future product demand and supply. This useful information may be used by enterprises to provide customized goods and services to the targeted locations. DL allows for the analysis of consumer behavior trends. Deep neural networks are used in DL to examine data and solve complicated problems faster than humans [62].

10.4.3 Better Customer Relationships

As the pharmaceutical industry become increasingly competitive, developing collaborative partnerships with stakeholders, physicians, patients, and is critical to the long-term demand for pharmaceutical services [63]. Customer relationship management (CRM) is a business approach for managing customers, clients, and sales that are being implemented by a variety of pharmaceutical industries.

This entails utilizing technology to streamline, automate and manage industry process. CRM aims to boost profits, revenue, and customer happiness [64]. CRM's main purpose is to collect enough information about a customer and then use it effectively enough to improve the customer's good experiences with the firm, resulting in more sales. The CRM system involves a number of procedures that continuously collect a big data. Using traditional systems, dealing of the massive data amounts is difficult. Incorrect data processing might potentially cause the automated process to stall. AI solutions help businesses better integrate and analyze client data, allowing them to predict, plan, and capitalize on new opportunities. AI techniques like data mining (subfield of data science) are suggested to overcome such problems. It is a mixture of AI, ML and DL.

The main roles of data mining are

1. Developing and predicting future models
2. Discovering new and hidden patterns
3. Extracting the useful information from the raw data from a database [65].

Various models of data mining, including association, classification, clustering, forecasting, regression, sequence finding, and visualization, can assist each of the CRM elements. For forecasting future client behaviors, the classification model is the most often used model in CRM [66]. The most commonly utilized data mining algorithms to address CRM difficulties and improve processes include SVM, Neural Network, Logistic Regression, and Decision Tree. Some examples of CRM tools developed by integrating AI-ML are enlisted below:

Marketo: It shortens the time for lead qualification.
SugarCRM: It can automatically search, optimize, and provide inputs to assist in collecting detailed business and personal profiles within seconds.
Salesforce: It is useful to provide predictions and recommendations based on customer data acquired [67].

10.4.4 Enhanced Marketing Measurement

Marketing measurement is important as it helps to know how marketing efforts are driving revenue and gives actionable insights to improve the results. The capacity to measure marketing has a favorable impact on the success of an organization. There are significant metrics for marketing measurement. Metrics refers to the ability to quantify economic performance using a large number of indicators. Metrics can be classified as financial or non-financial. As compared to traditional methods, ML inductive methods can be seen as a promising tool for enhancing marketing measurement [68].

10.4.5 Predictive Marketing Analytics

Predictive analytics is a method of data analysis concerned with gathering data and applying it to forecast trends and behavioral patterns. Predictive analytics is frequently used in marketing for reasons such as segmenting, targeting, getting hold of and keeping customers. It is also used in order to determine what types of ads to show and which would be the most effective.

The predictive analytics process involves data collection, data analysis, predictive modelling, deployment, model monitoring, etc. It is concerned with transforming massive amounts of data into knowledge that humans can comprehend and utilize. Predictive analytics has evolved from descriptive analytics, which seeks to forecast the future based on prior data. This approach employs advanced statistical techniques such as regression and decision trees [69].

However, besides statistical tools, ML methods can also be used in the predictive analysis [70]. In fact, ML is now an important part of predictive analytics. ML is viewed as a modernized version of predictive analytics. ML model's foundations are efficient pattern recognition and self-learning, which adapt spontaneously in response to varying patterns to allow necessary actions. Many businesses today rely on ML algorithms to gain a better understanding of their customers and possible revenue streams. Hundreds of current and newly created ML algorithms are used to generate high-end forecasts that guide real-time decisions while reducing the need for human participation [69].

Rebeiro *et al.* investigated the application of time series and data mining methods to predict sales of pharmaceutical distribution company products. Data mining techniques were used to evaluate past product sales data so as to find trends and do forecasting on the basis of the data's experience. The damped Pegels approach and the SMAPE precision measure were used to forecast sales for 357 medicines. The method was shown to be beneficial in the forecasting of product sales at the individual level, with results that were more accurate and reliable than the company's previous process. These prediction models created using neural network categorization can increase prediction model efficiency. They can be used to forecast drug demand and quantity. AI ML can be seen as a promising tool for predictive marketing analytics in the future [71, 72].

10.4.6 Price Dynamics

The ultimate price of the product is determined on the basis of market analysis and the costs incurred while developing the pharmaceutical formulation. AI can play an important role in product costing [73]. Improved data crunching, administration of the medicine access program, and identification of target patient populations in the country-specific drug access program can aid in the streamlining of brand marketing and advertising, as well as real-time cost analysis [24]. The software in ML examines large amounts of statistical data, such as product development expenses, market demand, inventory costs, production costs, and product prices of rivals. Based on this, algorithms can be developed to predict the product cost. Also, AI can assist in product cost reduction. AI lowers the overall clinical trials cost and contributes to better patient results by allowing for an earlier start with a proven medicine. It also lowers the cost of the production process and improves analytics through various computer software and algorithms. AI also reduces the R & D cost for large pharmaceutical corporations. Its competitor is an AI platform launched by Intelligence Node which is a retail competitive intelligence tool for analyzing rival pricing data and useful for retailers and brands to track the competition. Wise Athena and Navetti Price Point are two examples of software that allows users to determine their product's pricing. This type of software can also be adopted by pharma companies to aid in product costing [74].

10.4.7 Market Segmentation

Market segmentation involves splitting of the market into groups of customers with similar demands and purchasing behavior [75]. The primary goal of market segmentation in the marketing process is to allow a company to concentrate its marketing efforts on the most attractive opportunities. Organizations are vulnerable to losses without appropriate segmentation [76]. According to Charles W. Lamb and Carl McDaniel, choosing a market or product category to research is the first stage in segmenting markets, followed by selecting criteria for segmentation [77]. Substantiality, identifiability, accessibility, and responsiveness are four basic criteria to consider. Choosing segmentation descriptors is the next step. Descriptors specify which segmentation variables should be used. Profiling and analyzing the segment is the next step. Designing, implementing, and maintaining suitable marketing mixes is the final step (Table 10.3) [78].

However, traditional market segmentation approaches can be ineffective while analyzing big data. Big data clustering methods can be used to segment the market for massive data volumes. Different clustering algorithms, like centroid-based clustering, Distribution-based clustering, and density-based clustering can be used. Kamanthia *et al.* have proposed a business intelligence tool and a decision approach for market segmentation based on user behavioral science and geographic information. For segmentation, PCA was used, followed by the use of the k-mode clustering technique [79].

Table 10.3 AI ML tools for marketing.

Sr. no.	Tools	Applications
1.	Business intelligent Smart Sales Prediction Analysis	• Predict product sales in advance to avoid expenses associated with excess inventory or client loss due to shortages [80].
2.	In competitor	• Analyzes competitor pricing information. • Assists retailers and brands to observe the competition [74].
3.	Wise Athena and Navetti PricePoint	• Determination of the product cost [74].
4.	E-VAI	• AI platform for analysis and decision-making to improve marketing results [7].

10.4.8 Challenges

For marketing research, ML approaches hold a lot of potential, but still, there are many challenges which can come across for applying AI-ML in marketing. Though online survey platforms allow instant accession to responder's sample, but it raised issues regarding the integrity of the data collected [81]. Data quality issues like missing, incomplete, inconsistent, erroneous, duplicate, or obsolete data can be seen as the next hurdle [82]. When merging several dissimilar sources of data – which is typically a feature of digital data – that must be harmonized for a single study, it becomes more difficult to accurately monitor data quality. Again, data sparsity is a prevalent issue in ML applications which usually crops up as a part of the data-generating process [83]. Most of the information comes in form of unstructured data. These data have become a valuable asset as a result of the development of ML algorithms, resulting in new business models. However, so as to get its value, the unstructured data must first be turned into structured data through information extraction [82].

10.5 Future Prospects and Way Forward

Al, along with big data, is unquestionably the next big thing in pharma. For companies that are more adaptable and quicker to adopt, Al will almost certainly gain a strategic edge. Experts believe that integrating Al and ML will soon be required in order to compete in the industry. The transformation, on the other hand, will not occur overnight. Rather, it will happen gradually over the years. Al is likely to be integrated into most, if not all, pharmaceutical R & D operations by that time. As a result, the success rate of medication development should theoretically improve, and R & D efforts should be streamlined. Furthermore, Al might theoretically aid in properly identifying the subset of patients who will benefit from a specific medicine. This might significantly lower the failure rate and ensure a successful (and faster) launch. Pharma must become invested in the conversation by supporting the benefits of Al technology in order for Al to have a positive impact on patients and healthcare providers. Most of the top pharma companies are now adapting to AI and ML as these are promising tools to lower down overall product cost and to improve product yield and quality. Biotechnology based Pharma companies are especially investing in AI ML considering the complicated process in biotechnology research and manufacturing. AI ML assists in the analysis of consumer behavior and market need to forecast the products. AI and ML-based systems have been recently utilized in computer-assisted drug development attributed to superior data mining skills of these systems. This technique, however, has several downsides, such as the fact that a significant amount of data in data mining technology has a direct impact on the performance of both DL and ML methods. Also, the mechanism of DL models is still not clear, despite the fact that good DL approaches are capable of overcoming these obstacles. Furthermore, neural models of formation are used to alter various parameters, but only a few practical recommendations have been developed to improve these models [7, 37, 57, 58, 84].

10.6 Conclusion

The pharmaceutical industry has an emerging need for both novel technical strategies and fundamental scientific work, which enables the production of safe and effective pharmaceutical products. AI is increasingly being used in different sectors of society, including the pharmaceutical industry. It was discussed how AI and ML can be used in drug discovery, pharmaceutical product development, clinical trial design, drug manufacturing, quality control and quality assurance, product management, drug prescription, medical diagnosis, patient monitoring, drug synergism and antagonism prediction, and precision medicine.

Inventory management typically employs barcode technology to keep track of stock levels. Modern AI warehouse management systems utilize pick-by-light, pick-by-voice, and pick-by-vision approaches, Pick-by-Voice being the most frequent approach. In manufacturing, fault detection is critical, especially when operations are massive and complicated, with a big number of variables. ML approaches like ANNs and fuzzy neural methods can be used to detect flaws. ML inductive methodologies, when compared to traditional methods, might be considered a potential tool for improving marketing measurement. In PdM, ML flexibility can aid in the handling of a variety of issues, including unexpected failures. AI provides firms with real-world data (RWD) that may aid in product launches and commercial success by managing customized relationships with various stakeholders. Previous medication data can be analyzed using statistical approaches to predict patient behavior. The analysis of how consumers choose, acquire, and reject items and services is known as consumer behavior. The classification model is the most generally utilized model in CRM for projecting future customer behaviors. Data gathering, data analysis, predictive modelling, deployment, model monitoring, and so on are all part of the predictive analytics process. Hundreds of existing and newly developed ML algorithms are employed to provide high-end predictions that influence real-time choices while limiting the need for human involvement. The software in ML examines large amounts of statistical data, such as product development expenses, market demand, inventory costs, production costs, and competitors' product prices. The cost of a product may be predicted using algorithms. The market for massive data volumes may be segmented using big data clustering methodologies. Various clustering techniques can be utilized, including centroid-based clustering, distribution-based clustering, and density-based clustering. AI and ML have the potential to improve and manage all components of pharmaceutical manufacturing as well as marketing. However, there are numerous legal and technological barriers to fully adopting AI and ML in the pharmaceutical sector. Furthermore, because AI and ML rely on data, data quality and integrity can become a huge concern, particularly in the marketing sector, if data is not correctly handled.

References

1. Arden, N.S., Fisher, A.C., Tyner, K., Yu, L.X., Lee, S.L., Kopcha, M., Industry 4.0 for pharmaceutical manufacturing: Preparing for the smart factories of the future. *Int. J. Pharm.*, 602, 120554, 2021.
2. Rao, T.V.N., Gaddam, A., Kurni, M., Saritha, K., Reliance on artificial intelligence, machine learning and deep learning in the era of industry 4.0, in: *Smart Healthc. Syst. Des. Secur. Priv. Asp*, pp. 281–299, 2022.

3. Jarrahi, M.H., Artificial intelligence and the future of work: Human-AI symbiosis in organizational decision making. *Bus. Horiz.*, 61, 4, 577–586, 2018.
4. Rogers, A. and Ierapetritou, M., Challenges and opportunities in modeling pharmaceutical manufacturing processes. *Comput. Chem. Eng.*, 81, 32–39, 2015.
5. Damiati, S.A., Digital pharmaceutical sciences. *AAPS PharmSciTech.*, 21, 6, 1–2, 2020.
6. Ruan, Z. and Siau, K., Digital marketing in the artificial intelligence and machine learning age, 2019.
7. Paul, D., Sanap, G., Shenoy, S., Kalyane, D., Kalia, K., Tekade, R.K., Artificial intelligence in drug discovery and development. *Drug Discovery Today*, 26, 1, 80, 2021.
8. Mishra, V., Artificial intelligence: the beginning of a new era in pharmacy profession. *Asian J. Pharm. Free full text Artic. Asian J. Pharm.*, 12, 02, 72–76, 2018.
9. Mak, K.-K. and Pichika, M.R., Artificial intelligence in drug development: present status and future prospects. *Drug Discovery Today*, 24, 3, 773–780, 2019.
10. Mitchell, J.B., Artificial intelligence in pharmaceutical research and development. *Future Med. Chem.*, 10, 13, 1529–1531, 2018.
11. Krittanawong, C., Johnson, K.W., Tang, W.H.W., How artificial intelligence could redefine clinical trials in cardiovascular medicine: Lessons learned from oncology. *Per. Med.*, 16, 2, 87–92, 2019.
12. Zhao, C., Jain, A., Hailemariam, L. *et al.*, Toward intelligent decision support for pharmaceutical product development. *J. Pharm. Innov.*, 1, 1, 23–35, 2006.
13. Jalkala, A.M. and Keränen, J., Brand positioning strategies for industrial firms providing customer solutions. *J. Bus. Ind. Mark.*, 29, 3, 253–264, 2014.
14. Dou, W., Lim, K.H., Su, C., Zhou, N., Cui, N., Brand positioning strategy using search engine marketing. *MIS Q.*, 34, 2, 261–279, 2010.
15. De Carolis, B., de Rosis, F., Grasso, F., Rossiello, A., Berry, D.C., Gillie, T., Generating recipient-centered explanations about drug prescription. *Artif. Intell. Med.*, 8, 2, 123–145, 1996.
16. Amato, F., López, A., Peña-Méndez, E.M., Vaňhara, P., Hampl, A., Havel, J., Artificial neural networks in medical diagnosis. *J. Appl. Biomed.*, 11, 2, 47–58, 2013.
17. Davoudi, A., Malhotra, K.R., Shickel, B. *et al.*, Intelligent ICU for autonomous patient monitoring using pervasive sensing and deep learning. *Sci. Rep.*, 9, 1, 1–13, 2019.
18. Kantipudi, M.V.V., Moses, C.J., Aluvalu, R., Kumar, S., Remote patient monitoring using IoT, cloud computing and AI, in: *Hybrid Artificial Intelligence and IoT in Healthcare*, Intelligent Systems Reference Library, pp. 51–74, Springer, 2021.
19. Tsigelny, I.F., Artificial intelligence in drug combination therapy. *Brief. Bioinform.*, 20, 4, 1434–1448, 2019.

20. Álvarez-Machancoses, Ó, Galiana, E.J.D., Cernea, A., de la Viña, J.F., Fernández-Martínez, J.L., On the role of artificial intelligence in genomics to enhance precision medicine. *Pharmgenomics Pers. Med.*, 13, 105, 2020.
21. Meskó, B., The role of artificial intelligence in precision medicine. *Expert Rev. Precis. Med. Drug Dev.*, 2, 239–241, 2017.
22. Benyahia, B., Lakerveld, R., Barton, P.I., A plant-wide dynamic model of a continuous pharmaceutical process. *Ind. Eng. Chem. Res.*, 51, 47, 15393–15412, 2012.
23. Mesbah, A., Paulson, J.A., Lakerveld, R., Braatz, R.D., Model predictive control of an integrated continuous pharmaceutical manufacturing pilot plant. *Org. Process Res. Dev.*, 21, 6, 844–854, 2017.
24. Kalyane, D., Sanap, G., Paul, D. *et al.*, Artificial intelligence in the pharmaceutical sector: Current scene and future prospect, in: *The Future of Pharmaceutical Product Development and Research*, USA, pp. 73–107, Elsevier, 2020.
25. Wong, W.C., Chee, E., Li, J., Wang, X., Recurrent neural network-based model predictive control for continuous pharmaceutical manufacturing. *Mathematics*, 6, 11, 242, 2018.
26. Rai, R., Tiwari, M.K., Ivanov, D., Dolgui, A., Machine learning in manufacturing and industry 4.0 applications. *Int. J. Prod. Res.*, 59, 16, 4773–4778, 2021.
27. Nor, N.M., Hassan, C.R.C., Hussain, M.A., A review of data-driven fault detection and diagnosis methods: Applications in chemical process systems. *Rev. Chem. Eng.*, 36, 4, 513–553, 2020.
28. Carter, A. and Briens, L., An application of deep learning to detect process upset during pharmaceutical manufacturing using passive acoustic emissions. *Int. J. Pharm.*, 552, 1–2, 235–240, 2018.
29. Colucci, D., Prats-Montalbán, J.M., Ferrer, A., Fissore, D., On-line product quality and process failure monitoring in freeze-drying of pharmaceutical products. *Dry. Technol.*, 39, 2, 134–147, 2021.
30. Peng, C., Chunhao, D., Qiankun, Z., Fault diagnosis of microbial pharmaceutical fermentation process with non-Gaussian and nonlinear coexistence. *Chemom. Intell. Lab. Syst.*, 199, 103931, 2020.
31. Çınar, Z.M., Abdussalam Nuhu, A., Zeeshan, Q., Korhan, O., Asmael, M., Safaei, B., Machine learning in predictive maintenance towards sustainable smart manufacturing in industry 4.0. *Sustainability*, 12, 19, 8211, 2020.
32. Calzavara, G., Oliosi, E., Ferrari, G., A time-aware data clustering approach to predictive maintenance of a pharmaceutical industrial plant, in: *2021 International Conference on Artificial Intelligence in Information and Communication (ICAIIC)*, IEEE, pp. 454–458, 2021.
33. Wang, X., Intelligent quality management using knowledge discovery in databases. *2009 Int. Conf. Comput. Intell. Softw. Eng.*, pp. 1–4, 2009.

34. Gams, M., Horvat, M., Ožek, M., Luštrek, M., Gradišek, A., Integrating artificial and human intelligence into tablet production process. *AAPS PharmSciTech*, 15, 6, 1447–1453, 2014.
35. Goh, W.Y., Lim, C.P., Peh, K.K., Subari, K., Application of a recurrent neural network to prediction of drug dissolution profiles. *Neural Comput. Appl.*, 10, 4, 311–317, 2002.
36. Aksu, B., Paradkar, A., de Matas, M., Özer, Ö, Güneri, T., York, P., A quality by design approach using artificial intelligence techniques to control the critical quality attributes of ramipril tablets manufactured by wet granulation. *Pharm. Dev. Technol.*, 18, 1, 236–245, 2013.
37. Rantanen, J. and Khinast, J., The future of pharmaceutical manufacturing sciences. *J. Pharm. Sci.*, 104, 11, 3612–3638, 2015.
38. Engudomnukul, S., Prombanpong, S., Somboonwiwat, T., A heuristic approach to capacity assignment in pharmaceutical manufacturing production line, in: *Applied Mechanics and Materials*, Switzerland, pp. 1928–1933, Trans Tech Publ, 2014.
39. Pontrakul, C. and Jarumaneeroj, P., Heuristic based scheduling for tablets film coating process, in: *Proceedings of the 2018 2nd International Conference on Algorithms, Computing and Systems*, pp. 238–242, 2018.
40. Das, M.K. and Chakraborty, T., *ANN in Pharmaceutical Product and Process Development*, Academic Press, New York, 2016.
41. Nguyen, A., Lamouri, S., Pellerin, R., Tamayo, S., Lekens, B., Data analytics in pharmaceutical supply chains: state of the art, opportunities, and challenges. *Int. J. Prod. Res.*, 1–20, 2021.
42. Wenzel, H., Smit, D., Sardesai, S., A literature review on machine learning in supply chain management, in: *Artificial Intelligence and Digital Transformation in Supply Chain Management: Innovative Approaches for Supply Chains. Proceedings of the Hamburg International Conference of Logistics (HICL)*, vol. *27*, epubli GmbH, Berlin, pp. 413–441, 2019.
43. de Oliveira, M.B., Zucchi, G., Lippi, M., Cordeiro, D.F., da Silva, N.R., Iori, M., Lead time forecasting with machine learning techniques for a pharmaceutical supply chain, in: *Proceedings of the 23rd International Conference on Enterprise Information Systems (ICEIS), Online Streaming*, pp. 26–28, 2021.
44. Bandaru, S., Aslam, T., Ng, A.H.C., Deb, K., Generalized higher-level automated innovization with application to inventory management. *Eur. J. Oper. Res.*, 243, 2, 480–496, 2015.
45. Yang, J.X., Li, L.D., Rasul, M.G., Warehouse management models using artificial intelligence technology with application at receiving stage–A review. *Management*, 4, 6, 8, 2002.
46. Connolly, C., Warehouse management technologies. *Sens. Rev.*, 28, 2, 108–114, 2008.
47. Dumitrescu, B. and Gavrila, H., Models using artificial intelligence to optimize the use of wireless network sensors in pharmaceutical depots. I: Conception. *Tech. Sci.*, 3, 2, 189–200, 2018.

48. Chen, Z., Wu, M., Zhao, R., Guretno, F., Yan, R., Li, X., Machine remaining useful life prediction via an attention-based deep learning approach. *IEEE Trans. Ind. Electron.*, 68, 3, 2521–2531, 2020.
49. Zheng, S., Ristovski, K., Farahat, A., Gupta, C., Long short-term memory network for remaining useful life estimation, in: *2017 IEEE International Conference on Prognostics and Health Management (ICPHM)*, IEEE, pp. 88–95, 2017.
50. Zhang, J., Wang, P., Yan, R., Gao, R.X., Long short-term memory for machine remaining life prediction. *J. Manuf. Syst.*, 48, 78–86, 2018.
51. Sateesh Babu, G., Zhao, P., Li, X.-L., Deep convolutional neural network based regression approach for estimation of remaining useful life, in: *International Conference on Database Systems for Advanced Applications*, Springer, pp. 214–228, 2016.
52. Zhu, J., Chen, N., Peng, W., Estimation of bearing remaining useful life based on multiscale convolutional neural network. *IEEE Trans. Ind. Electron.*, 66, 4, 3208–3216, 2018.
53. Deutsch, J. and He, D., Using deep learning-based approach to predict remaining useful life of rotating components. *IEEE Trans. Syst. Man Cybern. Syst.*, 48, 1, 11–20, 2017.
54. Kraft, D.L., System and methods for the production of personalized drug products. U.S. Patent, 10, 189, 616, issued January 29, 2019.
55. Reklaitis, R., Towards intelligent decision support for pharmaceutical product development. *J. Pharma. Innov.*, 23–35, 2008.
56. Chan, H.C.S., Shan, H., Dahoun, T., Vogel, H., Yuan, S., Advancing drug discovery via artificial intelligence. *Trends Pharmacol. Sci.*, 40, 8, 592–604, 2019.
57. Naidoo, P., Bouharati, C., Rambiritch, V. *et al.*, Real-world evidence and product development: Opportunities, challenges and risk mitigation. *Wien. Klin. Wochenschr.*, 133, 15, 840–846, 2021.
58. Lee, H., Kim, S.G., Park, H., Kang, P., Pre-launch new product demand forecasting using the Bass model: A statistical and machine learning-based approach. *Technol. Forecast. Soc. Change*, 86, 49–64, 2014.
59. Sokele, M. and Moutinho, L., Bass model with explanatory parameters, in: *Innovative Research Methodologies in Management*, Switzerland, pp. 145–164, Springer, 2018.
60. Kumar, T.S., Data mining based marketing decision support system using hybrid machine learning algorithm. *J. Artif. Intell.*, 2, 03, 185–193, 2020.
61. Ma, L. and Sun, B., Machine learning and AI in marketing–Connecting computing power to human insights. *Int. J. Res. Mark.*, 37, 3, 481–504, 2020.
62. Davenport, T., Guha, A., Grewal, D., Bressgott, T., How artificial intelligence will change the future of marketing. *J. Acad. Mark. Sci.*, 48, 1, 24–42, 2020.
63. Kanyan, A., Andrew, J.V., Ali, J.K., Beti, M.M., Building customer relationship for gaining customer loyalty in the pharmaceutical industry. *J. Adv. Manage. Sci.*, 3, 4, 319–322, 2015.

64. John, W., Distribution structure in Indian Pharmaceutical Industry: Significance of Customer Relationship Management (CRM) and distributor relationships. *Pac. Bus. Rev. Int.*, 1, 3, 55–66, August 2016.
65. Mohana Krishna, I. and Fantin Irudaya Raj, E., *Artificial Intelligence in Business Management* [Internet], Archers & Elevators Publishing House, Banglore, 2021, Available from: https://books.google.co.in/books?id=5-1qEAAAQBAJ.
66. Ngai, E.W.T., Xiu, L., Chau, D.C.K., Application of data mining techniques in customer relationship management: A literature review and classification. *Expert Syst. Appl.*, 36, 2, 2592–2602, 2009.
67. Chatterjee, S., Ghosh, S.K., Chaudhuri, R., Nguyen, B., Are CRM systems ready for AI integration? A conceptual framework of organizational readiness for effective AI-CRM integration. *Bottom Line*, 32, 2, 144–157, 2019.
68. Solcansky, M. and Simberova, I., Measurement of marketing effectiveness. *Econ. Manage.*, 15, 755–759, 2010.
69. Ongsulee, P., Chotchaung, V., Bamrungsi, E., Rodcheewit, T., Big data, predictive analytics and machine learning, in: *2018 16th International Conference on ICT and Knowledge Engineering (ICT&KE)*, IEEE, pp. 1–6, 2018.
70. Surendro, K., Predictive analytics for predicting customer behavior, in: *2019 International Conference of Artificial Intelligence and Information Technology (ICAIIT)*, IEEE, pp. 230–233, 2019.
71. Ribeiro, A., Seruca, I., Durão, N., Sales prediction for a pharmaceutical distribution company: A data mining based approach, in: *2016 11th Iberian Conference on Information Systems and Technologies (CISTI)*, IEEE, pp. 1–7, 2016.
72. Senthilkumaran, U., Manikandan, N., Senthilkumar, M., Role of data mining on pharmaceutical industry-a survey. *Int. J. Pharm. Technol.*, 8, 3, 100–106, 2016.
73. Duran, O., Rodriguez, N., Consalter, L.A., Neural networks for cost estimation of shell and tube heat exchangers. *Expert Syst. Appl.*, 36, 4, 7435–7440, 2009.
74. De Jesus, A., AI for pricing–Comparing 5 current applications. *Emerj Artif. Intell. Res.*, 2, 2019.
75. Smith, B.D. and Awopetu, B., Mind-set and market segmentation in the pharmaceutical industry: An assessment of practice in the UK. *J. Pharm. Mark. Manage.*, 17, 3–4, 101–116, 2006.
76. McDonald, M., Christopher, M., Bass, M., Market segmentation, in: *Marketing*, pp. 41–65, Springer, London, 2003.
77. Lamb, C.W., Hair, J.F., McDaniel, C., *Marketing*, Cengage Learning, USA, 2012.
78. Sun, S., An analysis on the conditions and methods of market segmentation. *Int. J. Bus. Manage.*, 4, 2, 63–70, 2009.
79. Kamthania, D., Pawa, A., Madhavan, S.S., Market segmentation analysis and visualization using K-mode clustering algorithm for E-commerce business. *J. Comput. Inf. Technol.*, 26, 1, 57–68, 2018.

80. Mahajan, K.N. and Kumar, A., Business intelligent smart sales prediction analysis for pharmaceutical distribution and proposed generic model. *Int. J. Comput. Sci. Inform. Technol.*, 8, 407–412, 2017.
81. Goodman, J.K., Cryder, C.E., Cheema, A., Data collection in a flat world: The strengths and weaknesses of Mechanical Turk samples. *J. Behav. Decis. Mak.*, 26, 3, 213–224, 2013.
82. Gudivada, V., Apon, A., Ding, J., Data quality considerations for big data and machine learning: Going beyond data cleaning and transformations. *Int. J. Adv. Software*, 10, 1, 1–20, 2017.
83. Hair Jr., J.F. and Sarstedt, M., Data, measurement, and causal inferences in machine learning: Opportunities and challenges for marketing. *J. Mark. Theory Pract.*, 29, 1, 65–77, 2021.
84. Jämsä-Jounela, S.-L., Future trends in process automation. *Annu. Rev. Control*, 31, 2, 211–220, 2007.

11

Artificial Intelligence and Machine Learning Applications in Vaccine Development

Ali Sarmadi[1], **Majid Hassanzadeganroudsari**[2*] **and M. Soltani**[1,3†]

[1]*Centre for Biotechnology and Bioengineering (CBB), University of Waterloo, Waterloo, ON, Canada*
[2]*Institute for Health and Sport, Victoria University, Melbourne, VIC, Australia*
[3]*Department of Electrical and Computer Engineering, University of Waterloo, Waterloo, ON, Canada*

Abstract

Artificial Intelligence (AI) is a new branch of computer science that came in to field in the 1950s. Since then, much progress has been made where computers equipped with AI algorithms are capable of aiding humanity in a range of topics. One of the topics that humanity longs to receive help in is definitely medicine. In this chapter, the role of AI applications in monitoring large volumes of data (big data), identifying the patterns, and making predictions about the efficiency and performance of drugs and vaccines have been discussed. Moreover, the important findings and research are explained to reveal the interdisciplinary instinct of this field and draw an evolutionary storyline. This chapter discusses the ways that AI can help with vaccine development. Five major applications of AI in the field of vaccine development are addressed: (a) Prioritizing proteins as vaccine candidates; (b) Predicting binding scores of candidate proteins; (c) Predicting potential epitopes; (d) Design of multi-epitope vaccines; (e) Tracking RNA mutations of a virus. Finally, certain types of AI algorithms, machine learning, that are used to prioritize proteins and its applications are presented.

Keywords: Artificial intelligence, AI, vaccine development, machine learning, prioritizing proteins

**Corresponding author*: Majid.Hassanzadeganroudsari@vu.edu.au
†*Corresponding author*: msoltani@uwaterloo.ca

Vivek Chavda, Krishnan Anand and Vasso Apostolopoulos (eds.) Bioinformatics Tools for Pharmaceutical Drug Product Development, (233–254) © 2023 Scrivener Publishing LLC

11.1 Introduction

Artificial Intelligence (AI) is a new branch in computer science that aims to create intelligent machines. Because of the nascency of the AI, the definition and meaning of the word "intelligent" in the AI definition were considerable controversies. Even now, the importance of this word determines the approach of a scientist to this brand-new branch of technology. As of now, there are four different views about AI out there [1]. One can have a general overview of these definitions in Figure 11.1.

As it can be seen, depending on the application that one has in mind, four different approaches are available. The initiation of AI-called research and technologies are usually referred to as the works of Warren McCulloch and Walter Pitts in 1943 [2]. The basics of what was later called "Neural Network" was created this year in the concept of the perceptron. At that time, their work was based on three sources: elementary physiology and practice of the brain, an understanding of propositional logic, which was provided Russel and Whitehead works, and lastly, Turing's theory of computation. Their job was to propose a model of artificial neurons, where a neuron had on/off states: it was considered when it was "stimulated" by its nearby neurons [2]. McCulloch and Pitts claimed that any computable function could be calculated using a network of connected neurons and every logical connective (and, or, not, etc.). The idea of a network capable of learning to solve a problem also arises from their work. They suggested that, if we adequately define a network, it will be able to learn. In 1949, Donald Hebb proposed a simple of updating the connection strength between neurons, which is today known as "Hebbian Learning" and it is an influential model, even today [3]. A year later, two undergraduate Harvard students, named Marvin Minsky and Dean Edmonds, made the first

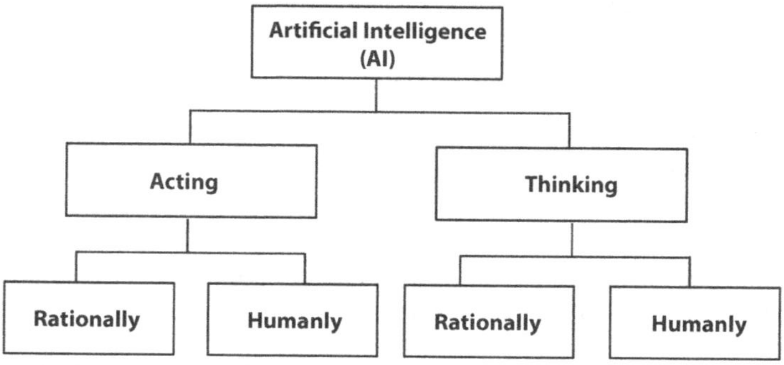

Figure 11.1 Different definitions of Artificial Intelligence.

neural network computers called Stochastic Neural Analog Reinforcement Calculator (SNARC) [4]. At the same time, one other important figure in the artificial intelligence field, Alan Turing was lecturing on this subject as early as 1947. His well-known agenda on this topic, which was written in 1950, is still a significant source that directs the research. The famous Turing's test, machine learning, genetic algorithms, and reinforcement learning were all introduced in that rich text, such as the child program idea. Turing's bright idea was why not to create a program that simulates a child's mind (and makes us learn what we desire) instead of trying to simulate an adult's mind.

1956 can be considered the official birth year of the field when John McCarthy [5], after receiving his Ph.D. in 1951 from Princeton, and working a few years there and Stanford, moved to Dartmouth College, the provenance of the discipline and started his carrier there. At this point, McCarthy, with the aid of some other prominent computer scientists, such as the Minsky as mentioned above, Claude Shannon, and Nathaniel Rochester, held a two-month workshop at Dartmouth and gathered those scientists interested in automata theory, neural nets, and the study of intelligence [6]. In the proposal of the workshop, these lines were noticeable:

"We propose that a 2-month, 10-man study of artificial intelligence be carried out during the summer of 1956 at Dartmouth College in Hanover, New Hampshire. The study is to proceed on the basis of the conjecture that every aspect of learning or any other feature of intelligence can in principle be so precisely described that a machine can be made to simulate it. An attempt will be made to find how to make machines use language, form abstractions and concepts, solve kinds of problems now reserved for humans, and improve themselves. We think that a significant advance can be made in one or more of these problems if a carefully selected group of scientists work on it together for a summer."

Major scientists attended the workshop, including Trenchard More from Princeton, Arthur Samuel from IBM, and Ray Solomonoff and Oliver Selfridge from MIT. But among them all, two of them achieved the most from the workshop: Allen Newell and Herbert Simon from Carnegie Tech (currently Carnegie Melon University). Before the workshop, they had already invented a program capable of solving logical problems, called Logical Theorist (LT). A short time after the workshop, Newell and Simon proposed another version of the program, which was able to solve most of the theorems in Chapter 2 of Russel and Whitehead's Principia Mathematica. Newell and Simon's work was so successful that the proof they provided for a theorem in the book with the aid of LT, was shorter than the one in the book, and Bertrand Russel himself admired the job that they had done.

However, besides this one, the Dartmouth workshop did not result in any other significant breakthrough in the field. But it had one effect for sure: It made the essential figures familiar with each other, and for the next 20 years, these people and their students were those who dominated this field [7]. To this point, we reviewed a very brief story of AI creation. Today, AI is much more than Newell and Simon's LT program or Minsky's neural network. It is now capable of many things that could not be even imagined in the 1940's and 50's. It can now get your description of an image, create that image for you, or segment an image into meaningful pieces, and categorize pictures that depict even fuzzy illustrations of diseases (say histopathology images of cancer-affected tissues). This last application of AI, meaning AI in medicine, is an auspicious one since, through that, humanity can be armed with the surgical precision of the computers against their oldest and fiercest enemies: diseases. Directing the research to this specific application, now that we have encountered a horrible global pandemic and suffered its consequences, seems to be more necessary and vital. Since the beginning of this disaster, the whole world has held its breath and waited for the vaccine's discovery. Moderna company, a company that made one of the first vaccines, soon after the release of its vaccine, revealed that AI was used in their research which resulted in the final product.

This chapter discusses the ways that AI can aid with vaccine development. Five major applications of AI in the field of vaccine development are addressed in this chapter:

1. Prioritizing Proteins as vaccine candidates
2. Predicting binding scores of candidate proteins
3. Predicting potential epitopes
4. Design of multi-epitope vaccines
5. Tracking the RNA mutations of a virus

In this chapter, AI and its application are mainly being utilized for the task "prediction". The role of AI applications in monitoring large volumes of data (big data), identifying the patterns, and making predictions in relation to the efficiency and performance of drugs and vaccines have been discussed in the following sections. Moreover, the important findings and research are explained to reveal the interdisciplinary instinct of this field and draw an evolutionary storyline.

11.2 Prioritizing Proteins as Vaccine Candidates

Developing safe and effective vaccines is still a challenge when encountering infectious diseases like HIV and malaria [8]. However, as it goes, new methods come into the field, and the technology of vaccine designation becomes more advanced. Reverse Vaccinology (RV) [9] is one of those methods mentioned above, which is a genome-based vaccine design approach. This method's task is essentially choosing vaccine candidates from the genome sequence [9]. This method showed considerable success in its first clinical trials [10], and in that regard, many research programs have been built upon it [11]. Various open-source versions of this method, in the form of a computer program, are out there and can be classified into two main categories: feature-input-based and algorithm-based.

The algorithmic type itself includes two main groups: rule-based filtering and Machine Learning (ML) based. In 2007, the first version ML-based version of RV program, named VaxiJen came into existence [12]. The next adaptation of the method was created by revising the ML method and editing the dataset [13, 14]. A crucial dissimilarity between VaxiJen and the method proposed by the two mentioned research teams, is that VaxiJen used physiochemical features, while the later method used biological characteristics. Another variation of RV programs was sprung from the development of the ANTIGENpro in 2010 [15]. Vaxign-ML program [16] is the latest version of RV ML-based programs. It is a sort of supervised ML classification exploited to predict bacterial protective antigens (BPAgs). In the research run by Ong *et al.*, several ML methods were examined to choose the best one among them. The best one (the one that utilizes XG-Boost) currently beats all of the aforementioned methods in terms of accuracy of the prediction.

After the spread of COVID-19, a scientific campaign began to produce high-quality vaccines to stop the outbreak of the disease. Using AI methods, particularly Deep Learning (DL) based approach, gradually entered the COVID related research. Yang, Bogdan, Nazarian [17] proposed a DL-based method for predicting potential vaccine subunits from the available SARS-Cov-2 spile protein sequence. The method is named deepVacPred. Moreover, the method was exercised to determine the linear Bcell epitopes, cytotoxic T lymphocytes (CTL) epitopes, and helper T lymphocytes (HTL) epitopes in the 26 subunit candidates and identified the top 11 of them to construct a multi-epitope vaccine for SARS-CoV-2 virus.

11.3 Predicting Binding Scores of Candidate Proteins

Molecular recognition plays a vital role in various biological functions and systems. Small-molecule ligands are crucial to key intracellular signaling pathways through inhibiting or triggering proteins. Ligand binding is an important topic in vaccine design, as the strength of a vaccine in inducing immunity heavily depends on it [18]. However, accurately calculating the protein-ligand interactions is a tough problem to solve. Some efficient computation methods already enable the researchers to search in the huge libraries of chemical compounds exploiting uncomplicated scoring functions and disregarding some partly essential matters such as protein flexibility, entropic and de-salvation effects. Achieving more accuracy needs using more complex theories like Molecular Dynamics (MD) which are extensively computationally expensive [19]. Therefore, if one can devise methods with high accuracy and low computational cost, it would be of much interest and that is exactly the field that ML methods are good at. ML in this discipline is mostly exploited to estimate the scoring functions and they do that task by learning the parameters and the structure of the model from data. Based on the duty that they fulfill, models in this subject can be categorized into three groups:

- Pose prediction models. These models are used to predict the correct binding structure of the protein ligands.
- Binding energy models. As the name suggests, these models are used to predict the binding energies of protein-ligand compounds.
- Virtual high-throughput screen. These models are used to differentiate binding ligands from non-binding ones.

These models usually accept three types of input features:

- 2D molecular structures
- 3D molecular structures
- Proteins

Both classical ML methods and more novel DL methods are exploited in the models. An illustration of this can be viewed in Table 11.1 [19].

Building these types of models, as much as any other data science investigation, relies on having access to an appropriate data source. Fortunately, many datasets on the internet are freely accessible to scholars. In that sense, three groups of datasets are recognizable:

Table 11.1 A summary of studies that have been done on protein—ligand scoring [19].

Study	Binary/ continuous	Protein	2D	3D	ML	DL	Data
Wallach, Dzamba, Heifets [20]	Binary	Yes	No	Yes	No	Yes	DUD-E, ChEMBL
Ramsundar, Kearnes, Riley, Webster, Konerding, Pande [21]	Binary	No	Yes	No	Yes	Yes	PCBA, MUV, DUD-E, TOX21
Gonczarek, Tomczak, Zaręba, Kaczmar, Dąbrowski, Walczak [22]	Binary	Yes	No	Yes	No	Yes	PDBBind, DUD-E, MUV
Wen, Zhang, Niu *et al.* [23]	Binary	Yes	Yes	No	No	Yes	DrugBank
Korotcov, Tkachenko, Russo, Ekins [24]	Binary	No	Yes	No	Yes	Yes	PubChem Bioassay
Gomes, Ramsundar, Feinberg, Pande [25]	Continuous	Yes	Yes	Yes	Yes	Yes	PDBBind
Ragoza, Hochuli, Idrobo, Sunseri, Koes [26]	Binary	Yes	No	Yes	No	Yes	DUD-E, ChEMBL
Stepniewska-Dziubinska, Zielenkiewicz, Siedlecki [27]	Continuous	Yes	No	Yes	No	Yes	PDBBind, Astek diverse set
Kundu, Paul, Banerjee [28]	Continuous	Yes	Yes	No	Yes	No	PDBBind, DUD-E
Mayr, Klambauer, Unterthiner *et al.* [29]	Binary	No	Yes	No	Yes	Yes	ChEMBL
Öztürk, Özgür, Ozkirimli [30]	Continuous	Yes	Yes	No	No	Yes	Kinase datasets [31, 32]

- Datasets including experimental structures
- Datasets containing data with known active compounds and binding energies
- Datasets covering various proteins and both active and inactive compounds

The first type of model that we mentioned before, meaning models intended for pose prediction, requires experimental complexes and hence, necessitates using the experimental structure datasets.

The Protein Data Bank database (PDB database) is a good exemplar of the first class of datasets. This database has been built in direct response to the need for experimental binding data. This database is usually updated annually and it includes systematically annotated protein-ligand complexes and relative experimental binding data. Since its creation, it has been used in many statistical and computational projects for developing scoring functions [33]. Mother Of All Databases (MOADB) is another project for gathering protein-ligand binding data, which is relatively huge in size. it includes about 23, 000 complexes and 8, 000 affinities [34].

While other datasets built for different purposes can be used for binding energy prediction, this task has its own instances of datasets. Binding DataBase (DB) is a freely accessible dataset containing experimental protein-small molecule interaction data. It is an anthology of over a million data records that are collected from scientific papers and US patents. Other than binding energies, the database collects features like temperature, pH, and buffer composition [35]. The Therapeutic Target Database (TTB) is another instance of a binding energy prediction dataset that encompasses protein-drug binding information and many expression profiles [36]. The same description is true about the DrugBank [37].

Datasets that can aid scholars in high-throughput must encompass a special property. To make a model that flawlessly purges the non-binding compounds, it is crucial to include inactive (or decoy) molecules in the dataset. Directory of Useful Decoy – Enhanced (DUD-E) consists of 102 unique proteins with an average of 124 active compounds and 50 decoy compounds for each target. The providers of the dataset used Bernis-Murcko frameworks to cluster the active sets to avoid chemotype basis [38]. DEKOIS 2 contains 81 benchmark datasets of 80 unique proteins and one that consists of separate datasets for two different known proteins binding pockets in a single protein. Four proteins are included in the datasets, which are the same as DUD-E and from BindingDB, the active sets are derived [39].

The Maximum Unbiased Validation (MUV) is generated by PubChem Bioassays [40], exploiting spatial statistics to ensure an unbiased dataset. MUV is a collection of 18 pairs of experiments. In order to be eligible for the dataset, the target must undergo a high-throughput screening (HTS) and a confirmatory screen (low-throughput dose-response experiment). A confirmatory bioassay was used to eliminate the possibility of experimental noise and artifacts that typically affect HTS screens [41]. A summary of the databases that we just discussed is observable in Table 11.2.

Table 11.2 A summary of databases available for binding scores.

Dataset name	Description	Link	Ref.
PDB	A database possessing experimentally acquired three-dimensional structures of proteins, nucleic acids and other biological macromolecules, with approximately 8000 records.	https://www.rcsb.org/	[33]
MOADB	Originally a smaller version PDB and it includes every high-quality example of ligand-protein binding	https://bindingmoad.org/	[42]
Community Structure-Activity Resource (CSAR)	Disseminated experimental datasets of crystal structures and binding affinities for diverse protein-ligand complexes	http://www.csardock.org/	[43]
BindingDB	A publicly online accessible database of measured binding affinities focusing on the interaction between proteins	https://www.bindingdb.org	[35]

(*Continued*)

Table 11.2 A summary of databases available for binding scores. (*Continued*)

Dataset name	Description	Link	Ref.
TTB	A pharmaceutical database providing information about known and explored therapeutic proteins and nucleic acid targets	http://db.idrblab.net/ttd/	[36]
DrugBank	A comprehensive database including information on drugs and drug targets	https://www.drugbank.com	[37]
Drug Target Commons (DTC)	A crowd-sourcing platform to improve the consensus and use of drug-target interactions	https://drugtargetcommons.fimm.fi/	[44]
DUD-E	A useful research tool encompassing 22, 886 active compounds and their affinities against 102 targets, an average of 224 ligands per target	http://dude.docking.org/	[38]
DEKOIS 2	A handy research tool for producing decoys based on a certain number of actives for any target.	Not an online tool	[39]
MUV	Includes several datasets and a software package for virtual screening	http://www.pharmchem.tu-bs.de/lehre/baumann/MUV.html	[41]

11.4 Predicting Potential Epitopes

Messenger RNA (mRNA) vaccines encipher the desired antigens from an mRNA string [45]. Explicitly, the mRNA's information is used in the cytoplasm to produce proteins responsible for triggering immune responses, including antigen-presenting cells (APCs) or antibodies and immunoglobulins [46]. Epitopes are an elementary but frequently looked-across facet for improving the effectuality of mRNA vaccines. This category can be split into B-cells and T-cells epitopes based on what part of the immune system is being actuated [47]. The mRNA vaccines, due to their effectiveness, are extensively used in the efforts of mankind the combat diseases since 1997 [48]. Epitopes appeared in the battle with COVID-19 and multiple peptide-based vaccines have been presented to prevent the spread of this disease, such as UB-612 [49] and NVX-CoV2373 [50].

Nevertheless, mRNA vaccines can also take advantage of the epitope-based designation attitude and both B-cell and T-cell can be exploited. The epitope features decide if the mRNA vaccine triggers an immune response and which kinds of responses will be activated. Epitope forecasting lets researchers find successful epitopes that simultaneously provide immunogenicity and cross-creativity for a targeted pathogen [51].

But how can AI and ML help in this process? From a bioinformatics point of view, epitope prediction methods can be categorized into sequence-based and structure-based [52]. An old-fashion but still a highly-used method for sequence-based methods is called motif search. This method consists of a neural network used to search for relationships and nonlinear data elucidation. One other widely used method in this sense is the Support Vector Machine (SVM) which is extensively used for epitope prediction and models like COBEpro, which forecasts linear B-cell epitope [53] and cleavage sites known as Pcleavage [54]. Hidden Markov models and quantitative similarity matrixes are other types of methods that are used in this sense. Also, some other less-known algorithms are exploited for epitope prediction. For example, Hu, He, Li [55] utilized NetMHCpan4.0 algorithm for predicting potential epitopes binding to HLA class I molecules in Causcasian and East Asian populations. ML methods in this field, have a long way to perfection point. Yet, binary classification is the prevalent approach and this issue, brings some difficulties to the action since there is a need for binarization of continuous biological quantities. Besides, we still cannot track the biological consequences of immunization using these techniques that are extremely effective on vaccine safety and success [56].

11.5 Design of Multi-Epitope Vaccine

It was after the spread of COVID-19 that the need for an accurate and at the same time, fast approach to developing vaccines was sensed since the virus was extending itself over the world with the basic reproduction number (R0) of 5.6. The classic method of vaccine design includes growing pathogens which itself contains multiple phases of isolating, inactivating, and injecting the virus that causes the disease it is known to be very time-consuming and it needs more than a year to be completed [17]. As such, researchers are currently working on alternative methods to skip the tedious process of pathogen growing and have created a design method without needing that part. Immunoinformatics and ML methods play a vital role in this new effort [57–59].

Generally speaking, the multi-epitope vaccines are built by various substantial protein fragments in overlaying epitopes. These parts are the vital parts of the virus that are responsible for inducing either cellular or humoral immune responses [60]. Now, a question that may arise is how can ML help design such vaccines?

The procedure of *in silico* vaccine design can be understood as opting for suitable parts of virus protein and then building them together as the final vaccine [61]. Each fragment is analyzed, and if it is recognized as having multiple eligibilities, it could be a subunit of the final vaccine. For example, a fine subunit should include various B-cell epitopes and T-cell epitopes and also, and it should possess antigenicity [62, 63]. This section is the very part that *in silico* methods, particularly ML methods can be taken advantage of. The procedures mentioned above are utilized to predict whether or not a particular subunit has particular merit. Traditional *in silico* methods can analyze a subunit for one merit at a time and this makes the whole process of multiepitope vaccine design tedious and time-consuming. DL-based methods make the task easier by making predicting the best subunit candidate, considering numerous merits at a time. DeepVacPred, as was mentioned earlier, is one of the DL-based solutions proposed to address this problem [17]. Various ML-based tools are available online and can be used for the mentioned purpose. BiPred-2.0 web server is an example of those online tools. BiPred-2.0[1] is a credible online tool that is trained by random forest algorithm and it enfolds a huge number of known linear B-cells.

[1]http://www.cbs.dtu.dk/services/BepiPred/

Table 11.3 Summary of online tools with application in multiepitope vaccine design.

Tool name	Method	Application
BiPred-2.0	Random forest	Recognizing various types of B-cells
ABCpred	RNN	Discriminating epitopes and nonepitopes
SVMtrip	SVM	Forecasting antigenic epitopes
BCPreds	SVM	Forecasting antigenic epitopes

ABCpred[2] is another online gadget that uses Recurrent Neural Networks (RNNs) to discriminate epitopes and nonepitopes and this would help a lot by improving the accuracy of the vaccine design process.

SVMtrip[3] and BCPreds[4] use SVM algorithm to forecast antigenic epitopes. The aforementioned tools details, in a nutshell, can be viewed in Table 11.3.

11.6 Tracking the RNA Mutations of a Virus

Structural investigations and biochemical experiments unfold many significant features of a virus. For example, surveying proteins in viruses can disclose many chief factors at disparate levels of a viral infectious circle, such as virus entry, replication, survival, and so on [64]. But viruses change over time due to their evolution. Forecasting evolution is a major target in virology, chiefly for pathogenic viruses [65]. Foretelling the evolution successfully and precisely will aid a lot in fields like vaccine design and maintenance, drug design, and surveillance of viral pathogens. The natural selection principle determines the evolutionary destiny of a viral population. Due to its essence, natural selection improves the adaptability of a population over time, performing some suitable mutations. It deletes lethal and disadvantageous mutations by purifying them from the population. Hence, as a virus continues its life trajectory, its fitness for living enhances [66].

---

[2]http://www.imtech.res.in/raghava/abcpred/

[3]http://sysbio.unl.edu/SVMTriP/

[4]http://ailab.ist.psu.edu/bcpred/

RNA viruses are those types of viruses that possess RNA in their genetic material. This RNA might be single or double-stranded. These kinds of viruses can use the presentment of RNA-dependent RNA polymerases for replication of their genomes or generate viral DNA that can be integrated into the host DNA [67]. RNA viruses' genetic capacity is very confined, so their repertoire of evolutionary paths in their life trajectory. But despite this limitation, RNA viruses display very serious challenges to evolutionary forecasting. Some of these challenges are genetic drift, mutation, and recombination. RNA viruses have high mutation rates (as huge as 1 mutation in 1000 bases) and many involvements in recombination and reassortment, enabling them to generate new genotypes from co-circulating RNAs [66]. The scenario that was just described is exactly the one currently on the scene about COVID-19, as it is evolving and has experienced several mutations so far [68]. As mentioned before, successful and non-lethal mutations improve the virus's fitness for living and, hence, make the combat with it, either through vaccines or drugs, harder. Therefore, the ability to forecast the mutations would be of great desire if it could be achieved.

Genome sequence analysis has been a field of interest exploiting ML and recently, DL, for a relatively long time (the whole process can be seen in Figure 11.2). So, much research has been done to predict the RNA viruses' future mutations. It is mentionable that either ML or DL analysis, like any other data science study, requires a relatively large amount of data on virus

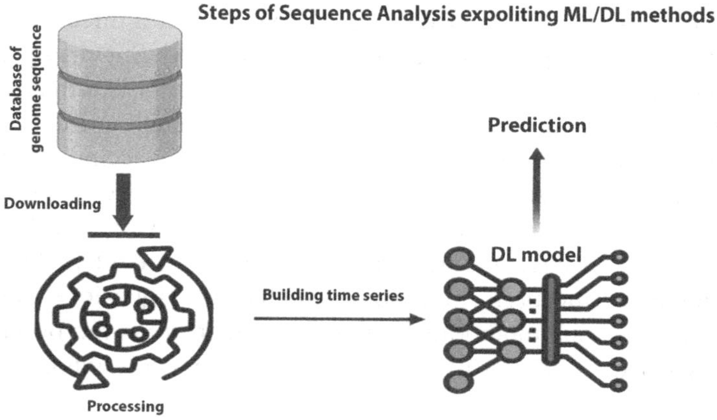

Figure 11.2 Total steps of sequence analysis using DL methods can be observed in the figure. First the complete genome sequence must be gathered from a reliable source. Then the data must be preprocessed. After that, the time series must be extracted from it and the input data is ready. At the next level, an appropriate DL method must be selected and it will do the forecasting work.

protein sequences. Thus, ML/DL methods are only applicable in the cases in that a sufficient amount of data is available. For example, Influenza is one of the cases in that its current existing data suffices. Its full genome data has been gathered and is accessible online[5] [69]. Possessing enough data, the prediction of mutations is executable but also challenging since the task is, in fact, predicting the future evolutionary path of a viral population. The study done by Yin, Luusua, Dabrowski, Zhang, Kwoh [70] is an illustrative example of mutation prediction. Their method was simply understanding the sequential mutations as time-series and hence, analyzing with an RNN. Since the protein sequence data of the virus is categorized by the year, researchers were able to construct a series, ordered by time and they have discriminated different variants of it using the k-means algorithm. Several experiments using a couple of classic ML methods (Logistic Regression (LR) and SVM) and DL RNN-based methods (LSTM, Gru, and the researchers' own custom method which is based on attention-mechanism named Tempel) and RNN-based methods outperformed the classic ML methods since they have a structural memory can memorize the information.

Sawmya, Saha *et al.* (2020) has applied the same approach on human coronavirus (hCov) genome sequence. Complete genome sequences of the hCov were gathered and accessible through GISAID initiative database (approximately 10, 000 high-quality genome sequence) [71]. The hCov genome sequence is available in the categorized form, both based on time and location (countries where the mutation took place). A time-series based on the date and location with the length of 300, 000 were made and used as the data. Then an RNN-based model, consisting of a 1-d convolutional layer and a RNN layer (the experiment was done using LSTM and bidirectional LSTM as RNN layer) was utilized to do the prediction. The result was significant and the accuracy of 94.98% and 95% were achieved using CNN-LSTM and CNN-bidirectional LSTM respectively. An interesting survey was carried out during the aforementioned investigation. The authors labeled the mutations that caused the number of death upper than the median of total COVID-19 death in different countries as severe mutations and those responsible for a number of death lower than the median as mild. Using this labeling, they performed a binary classification on different mutations exploiting both classic ML (lightGBM) and DL methods.

The same type of study, but into a broader domain, has been performed by Nguyen, Pathirana, Nguyen *et al.* [72]. The details of the deep learning method have not been mentioned in the paper but the results are

[5]http://www.ncbi.nlm.nih.gov/genomes/FLU/

considerable. The foretelling of the DL model in this study manifests that the mutation D614G in the virus spike protein, which was the subject of researchers' attention, won't probably make changes in protein secondary structure. The NCBI GenBank provided the data for this study[6].

Analyzing genome sequence, besides tracking mutations, can be suitable for applications like disease diagnosis too. Lopez-Rincon, Tonda, Mendoza-Maldonado *et al.* [73], utilizing Convolutional Neural Networks (CNNs), have devised an algorithm for recognizing COVID-19 from other virus strains with near-perfect accuracy.

Although AI provides an excellent opportunity for scientists, the human body is still so complex for AI models. And several critical issues must be considered regarding AI application in vaccine development. For instance, as the human body is so complex, the models cannot necessarily predict with reliability the impacts of the developed vaccine on the body. For example, the performance of ML algorithms depends on the training database. Moreover, ethics and AI ethics is a controversial topics to approach.

Conclusion

In this chapter, we discussed the application of AI, in the field of vaccine development. AI is a new branch of computer science that came in to field in the 1950s. Since then, lots of progress has been made in it and nowadays, computers, equipped with AI algorithms are capable of aiding humanity in lots of topics. One of the topics that humanity longs to receive help in is definitely medicine. Demonstrating the AI applications in vaccine development, we explained five certain applications: prioritizing proteins as vaccine candidates, predicting binding scores of candidate proteins, predicting potential epitopes, design of multi-epitope vaccines, and tracking the RNA mutations of a virus.

Regarding prioritizing proteins as vaccine candidates, certain types of AI algorithms, named machine learning algorithms, are used to prioritize proteins. These algorithms can learn the patterns in the data and use it to conclude things out of them, such as the eligibility of a protein for being used as a vaccine. Mentioning that, it is precisely the learning feature of the ML algorithms which becomes handy in predicting the binding scores of the proteins. Since the standard methods for this task, are either very simplified and miss many important details or very computationally expensive (like MD), a need for a method with reasonable computational

[6]https://www.ncbi.nlm.nih.gov/genbank/

cost and acceptable precision is embraced. ML methods by learning the feature of the proteins drawn from existing datasets of chemical compounds can approximate fairly accurate binding score functions. A table of accessible datasets in this field is presented in this chapter that summarizes each dataset's features and applications. A combination of classic methods like SVM with neural networks is used to predict potential epitopes to enhance the effectiveness of the mRNA vaccines. A certain type of neural network, Recurrent Neural Networks (RNNs), are also used in approximately the same manner to design multi-epitope vaccines. AI can also help the researchers to track and register the mutations that the RNA of a virus experience and check if the existing vaccines and drugs can affect the mutated version. This can be done by analyzing the genome sequence of the virus, finding viable and non-viable mutations, and analyzing the effectiveness of each new version with currently existing vaccines.

References

1. Müller, V.C. and Bostrom, N., Future progress in artificial intelligence: A survey of expert opinion, in: *Fundamental Issues of Artificial Intelligence*, pp. 555–572, Springer International Publishing, Switzerland, 2016.
2. McCulloch, W.S. and Pitts, W., A logical calculus of the ideas immanent in nervous activity. *Bull. Math. Biophys.*, 5, 4, 115–133, 1943.
3. Cooper, S.J. and Donald, O., Hebb's synapse and learning rule: A history and commentary. *Neurosci. Biobehav. Rev.*, 28, 8, 851–874, 2005.
4. Neocleous, C. and Schizas, C., Artificial neural network learning: A comparative review. *Methods and Application of Artificial Intelligence*, pp. 300–313, Springer, Berlin Heidelburg, 2022.
5. McCarthy, J., The inversion of functions defined by Turing machines. *Autom. Stud.*, 177, 181, 1956.
6. McCarthy, J., Minsky, M.L., Rochester, N., Shannon, C.E., A proposal for the dartmouth summer research project on artificial intelligence, August 31, 1955. *AI Mag.*, 27, 4, 12–12, 2006.
7. Russell, S. and Norvig, P., AI a modern approach. *Learning*, 2, 3, 4, 2005.
8. Organization WH, *MDG 6: Combat HIV/AIDS, malaria and other diseases*, World Health Organization, Geneva, 2014, http://www.who.int/topics/millennium_development_goals/diseases/en.
9. Rappuoli, R., Reverse vaccinology. *Curr. Opin. Microbial.*, 3, 5, 445–450, 2000.
10. Pizza, M., Scarlato, V., Masignani, V. *et al.*, Identification of vaccine candidates against serogroup B meningococcus by whole-genome sequencing. *Science*, 287, 5459, 1816–1820, 2000.

11. Dalsass, M., Brozzi, A., Medini, D., Rappuoli, R., Comparison of open-source reverse vaccinology programs for bacterial vaccine antigen discovery. *Front. Immunol.*, 10, 113, 2019.
12. Doytchinova, I.A. and Flower, D.R., VaxiJen: A server for prediction of protective antigens, tumour antigens and subunit vaccines. *BMC Bioinf.*, 8, 1, 1–7, 2007.
13. Bowman, B.N., McAdam, P.R., Vivona, S. *et al.*, Improving reverse vaccinology with a machine learning approach. *Vaccine*, 29, 45, 8156–8164, 2011.
14. Heinson, A.I., Gunawardana, Y., Moesker, B. *et al.*, Enhancing the biological relevance of machine learning classifiers for reverse vaccinology. *Int. J. Mol. Sci.*, 18, 2, 312, 2017.
15. Magnan, C.N., Zeller, M., Kayala, M.A. *et al.*, High-throughput prediction of protein antigenicity using protein microarray data. *Bioinformatics*, 26, 23, 2936–2943, 2010.
16. Ong, E., Wang, H., Wong, M.U., Seetharaman, M., Valdez, N., He, Y., Vaxign-ML: Supervised machine learning reverse vaccinology model for improved prediction of bacterial protective antigens. *Bioinformatics*, 36, 10, 3185–3191, 2020.
17. Yang, Z., Bogdan, P., Nazarian, S., An in silico deep learning approach to multi-epitope vaccine design: A SARS-CoV-2 case study. *Sci. Rep.*, 11, 1, 1–21, 2021.
18. Wang, D.D., Zhu, M., Yan, H., Computationally predicting binding affinity in protein–ligand complexes: Free energy-based simulations and machine learning-based scoring functions. *Briefings Bioinf.*, 22, 3, bbaa107, 2021.
19. Ellingson, S.R., Davis, B., Allen, J., Machine learning and ligand binding predictions: A review of data, methods, and obstacles. *Biochim. Biophys. Acta (BBA)-Gen. Subj.*, 1864, 6, 129545, 2020.
20. Wallach, I., Dzamba, M., Heifets, A., AtomNet: A deep convolutional neural network for bioactivity prediction in structure-based drug discovery. *arXiv preprint arXiv:1510.02855*, 2015, https://doi.org/10.48550/arXiv.1510.02855.
21. Ramsundar, B., Kearnes, S., Riley, P., Webster, D., Konerding, D., Pande, V., Massively multitask networks for drug discovery. *arXiv preprint arXiv:1502.02072*, 2015, https://doi.org/10.48550/arXiv.1502.02072.
22. Gonczarek, A., Tomczak, J.M., Zaręba, S., Kaczmar, J., Dąbrowski, P., Walczak, M.J., Interaction prediction in structure-based virtual screening using deep learning. *Comput. Boil. Med.*, 100, 253–258, 2018.
23. Wen, M., Zhang, Z., Niu, S. *et al.*, Deep-learning-based drug–target interaction prediction. *J. Proteome Res.*, 16, 4, 1401–1409, 2017.
24. Korotcov, A., Tkachenko, V., Russo, D.P., Ekins, S., Comparison of deep learning with multiple machine learning methods and metrics using diverse drug discovery data sets. *Mol. Pharmaceutics*, 14, 12, 4462–4475, 2017.
25. Gomes, J., Ramsundar, B., Feinberg, E.N., Pande, V.S., Atomic convolutional networks for predicting protein-ligand binding affinity. *arXiv preprint arXiv:1703.10603*, 2017, https://doi.org/10.48550/arXiv.1703.10603.

26. Ragoza, M., Hochuli, J., Idrobo, E., Sunseri, J., Koes, D.R., Protein–ligand scoring with convolutional neural networks. *J. Chem. Inf. Model.*, 57, 4, 942–957, 2017.
27. Stepniewska-Dziubinska, M.M., Zielenkiewicz, P., Siedlecki, P., Development and evaluation of a deep learning model for protein–ligand binding affinity prediction. *Bioinformatics*, 34, 21, 3666–3674, 2018.
28. Kundu, I., Paul, G., Banerjee, R., A machine learning approach towards the prediction of protein–ligand binding affinity based on fundamental molecular properties. *RSC Adv.*, 8, 22, 12127–12137, 2018.
29. Mayr, A., Klambauer, G., Unterthiner, T. *et al.*, Large-scale comparison of machine learning methods for drug target prediction on ChEMBL. *Chem. Sci.*, 9, 24, 5441–5451, 2018.
30. Öztürk, H., Özgür, A., Ozkirimli, E., DeepDTA: Deep drug–target binding affinity prediction. *Bioinformatics*, 34, 17, i821–i829, 2018.
31. Davis, M.I., Hunt, J.P., Herrgard, S. *et al.*, Comprehensive analysis of kinase inhibitor selectivity. *Nat. Biotechnol.*, 29, 11, 1046–1051, 2011.
32. Tang, J., Szwajda, A., Shakyawar, S. *et al.*, Making sense of large-scale kinase inhibitor bioactivity data sets: A comparative and integrative analysis. *J. Chem. Inf. Model.*, 54, 3, 735–743, 2014.
33. Liu, Z., Su, M., Han, L. *et al.*, Forging the basis for developing protein–ligand interaction scoring functions. *Acc. Chem. Res.*, 50, 2, 302–309, 2017.
34. Ahmed, A., Smith, R.D., Clark, J.J., Dunbar Jr., J.B., Carlson, H.A., Recent improvements to Binding MOAD: A resource for protein–ligand binding affinities and structures. *Nucleic Acids Res.*, 43, D1, D465–D469, 2015.
35. Gilson, M.K., Liu, T., Baitaluk, M., Nicola, G., Hwang, L., Chong, J., BindingDB in 2015: A public database for medicinal chemistry, computational chemistry and systems pharmacology. *Nucleic Acids Res.*, 44, D1, D1045–D1053, 2016.
36. Li, Y.H., Yu, C.Y., Li, X.X. *et al.*, Therapeutic target database update 2018: Enriched resource for facilitating bench-to-clinic research of targeted therapeutics. *Nucleic Acids Res.*, 46, D1, D1121–D1127, 2018.
37. Wishart, D.S., Feunang, Y.D., Guo, A.C. *et al.*, DrugBank 5.0: A major update to the DrugBank database for 2018. *Nucleic Acids Res.*, 46, D1, D1074–D1082, 2018.
38. Mysinger, M.M., Carchia, M., Irwin, J.J., Shoichet, B.K., Directory of useful decoys, enhanced (DUD-E): Better ligands and decoys for better benchmarking. *J. Med. Chem.*, 55, 14, 6582–6594, 2012.
39. Bauer, M.R., Ibrahim, T.M., Vogel, S.M., Boeckler, F.M., Evaluation and optimization of virtual screening workflows with DEKOIS 2.0–a public library of challenging docking benchmark sets. *J. Chem. Inf. Model.*, 53, 6, 1447–1462, 2013.
40. Wang, Y., Bryant, S.H., Cheng, T. *et al.*, Pubchem bioassay: 2017 update. *Nucleic Acids Res.*, 45, D1, D955–D963, 2017.
41. Rohrer, S.G. and Baumann, K., Maximum unbiased validation (MUV) data sets for virtual screening based on PubChem bioactivity data. *J. Chem. Inf. Model.*, 49, 2, 169–184, 2009.

42. Hu, L., Benson, M.L., Smith, R.D., Lerner, M.G., Carlson, H.A., Binding MOAD (mother of all databases). *Proteins: Struct. Funct. Bioinf.*, 60, 3, 333–340, 2005.
43. Dunbar Jr., J.B., Smith, R.D., Damm-Ganamet, K.L. *et al.*, CSAR data set release 2012: Ligands, affinities, complexes, and docking decoys. *J. Chem. Inf. Model.*, 53, 8, 1842–1852, 2013.
44. Tang, J., Ravikumar, B., Alam, Z. *et al.*, Drug target commons: A community effort to build a consensus knowledge base for drug-target interactions. *Cell Chem. Boil.*, 25, 2, 224–229. e222, 2018.
45. Verbeke, R., Lentacker, I., De Smedt, S.C., Dewitte, H., Three decades of messenger RNA vaccine development. *Nano Today*, 28, 100766, 2019.
46. Cai, X., Li, J.J., Liu, T., Brian, O., Li, J., Infectious disease mRNA vaccines and a review on epitope prediction for vaccine design. *Briefings Funct. Genomics*, 20, 5, 289–303, 2021.
47. Bosshard, H.R., Epitope mapping with peptides, in: *Peptides: Synthesis, Structures, and Applications*, B. Gutte (Ed.), p. 419, Springer, Switzerland, 1995.
48. Dolgin, E., The tangled history of mRNA vaccines. *Nature*, 597, 7876, 318–324, 2021.
49. Guirakhoo, F., Kuo, L., Peng, J. *et al.*, A novel sars-cov-2 multitope protein/peptide vaccine candidate is highly immunogenic and prevents lung infection in an adeno associated virus human angiotensin-converting enzyme 2 (AAV hACE2) mouse model. *BioRxiv*, 2020.
50. Tian, J.-H., Patel, N., Haupt, R. *et al.*, SARS-CoV-2 spike glycoprotein vaccine candidate NVX-CoV2373 elicits immunogenicity in baboons and protection in mice. *Nat. Commun.*, 12, 372, 2020.
51. Michel-Todó, L., Reche, P.A., Bigey, P., Pinazo, M.-J., Gascón, J., Alonso-Padilla, J., In silico design of an epitope-based vaccine ensemble for chagas disease. *Front. Immunol.*, 2698, 2019.
52. Patronov, A. and Doytchinova, I., T-cell epitope vaccine design by immunoinformatics. *Open Biol.*, 3, 1, 120139, 2013.
53. Sweredoski, M.J. and Baldi, P., COBEpro: A novel system for predicting continuous B-cell epitopes. *Protein Eng. Des. Sel.*, 22, 3, 113–120, 2009.
54. Bhasin, M. and Raghava, G., Pcleavage: An SVM based method for prediction of constitutive proteasome and immunoproteasome cleavage sites in antigenic sequences. *Nucleic Acids Res.*, 33, suppl_2, W202–W207, 2005.
55. Hu, W., He, M., Li, L., HLA class I restricted epitopes prediction of common tumor antigens in white and East Asian populations: Implication on antigen selection for cancer vaccine design. *PloS One*, 15, 2, e0229327, 2020.
56. Caoili, S.E.C., B-cell epitope prediction for peptide-based vaccine design: Towards a paradigm of biological outcomes for global health. *Immunome Res.*, 7, 2, 1, 2011.

57. Oany, A.R., Emran, A.-A., Jyoti, T.P., Design of an epitope-based peptide vaccine against spike protein of human coronavirus: An in silico approach. *Drug Des. Devel. Ther.*, 8, 1139, 2014.
58. Feng, Y., Qiu, M., Liu, L. *et al.*, Multi-epitope vaccine design using an immunoinformatics approach for 2019 novel coronavirus (SARS-CoV-2). *BioRxiv*, 2020.
59. Samad, A., Ahammad, F., Nain, Z. *et al.*, Designing a multi-epitope vaccine against SARS-CoV-2: An immunoinformatics approach. *J. Biomol. Struct. Dyn.*, 40, 1, 14–30, 2022.
60. Zhang, L., Multi-epitope vaccines: A promising strategy against tumors and viral infections. *Cell. Mol. Immunol.*, 15, 2, 182–184, 2018.
61. Mascola, J.R. and Fauci, A.S., Novel vaccine technologies for the 21st century. *Nat. Rev. Immunol.*, 20, 2, 87–88, 2020.
62. Purcell, A.W., McCluskey, J., Rossjohn, J., More than one reason to rethink the use of peptides in vaccine design. *Nat. Rev. Drug Discovery*, 6, 5, 404–414, 2007.
63. Callaway, E., Scores of coronavirus vaccines are in competition-how will scientists choose the best? *Nat. (Lond.)*, 2020.
64. Zeng, L., Li, D., Tong, W., Shi, T., Ning, B., Biochemical features and mutations of key proteins in SARS-CoV-2 and their impacts on RNA therapeutics. *Biochem. Pharmacol.*, 189, 114424, 2021.
65. Holmes, E.C., What can we predict about viral evolution and emergence? *Curr. Opin. Virol.*, 3, 2, 180–184, 2013.
66. Dolan, P.T., Whitfield, Z.J., Andino, R., Mapping the evolutionary potential of RNA viruses. *Cell Host Microbe*, 23, 4, 435–446, 2018.
67. Poltronieri, P., Sun, B., Mallardo, M., RNA viruses: RNA roles in pathogenesis, coreplication and viral load. *Curr. Genomics*, 16, 5, 327–335, 2015.
68. Wang, R., Hozumi, Y., Yin, C., Wei, G.-W., Mutations on COVID-19 diagnostic targets. *Genomics*, 112, 6, 5204–5213, 2020.
69. Bao, Y., Bolotov, P., Dernovoy, D. *et al.*, The influenza virus resource at the National Center for Biotechnology Information. *J. Virol.*, 82, 2, 596–601, 2008.
70. Yin, R., Luusua, E., Dabrowski, J., Zhang, Y., Kwoh, C.K., Tempel: Time-series mutation prediction of influenza A viruses via attention-based recurrent neural networks. *Bioinformatics*, 36, 9, 2697–2704, 2020.
71. Elbe, S. and Buckland-Merrett, G., Data, disease and diplomacy: GISAID's innovative contribution to global health. *Global Challenges*, 1, 1, 33–46, 2017.
72. Nguyen, T.T., Pathirana, P.N., Nguyen, T. *et al.*, Genomic mutations and changes in protein secondary structure and solvent accessibility of SARS-CoV-2 (COVID-19 virus). *Sci. Rep.*, 11, 1, 1–16, 2021.
73. Lopez-Rincon, A., Tonda, A., Mendoza-Maldonado, L. *et al.*, Classification and specific primer design for accurate detection of SARS-CoV-2 using deep learning. *Sci. Rep.*, 11, 1, 1–11, 2021.

12

AI, ML and Other Bioinformatics Tools for Preclinical and Clinical Development of Drug Products

Avinash Khadela[1], Sagar Popat[2], Jinal Ajabiya[3], Disha Valu[4], Shrinivas Savale[5] and Vivek P. Chavda[6]*

[1]Department of Pharmacology, L. M. College of Pharmacy, Ahmedabad, Gujarat, India
[2]Research and Development, Amneal Pharmaceutical Pvt. Ltd. Ahmedabad, Gujarat, India
[3]Department of Quality Assurance, L. M. College of Pharmacy, Ahmedabad, Gujarat, India
[4]Drug Product Development Lab, Intas Pharmaceutical Ltd. (Biopharma Division), Moraiya, Ahmedabad, Gujarat, India
[5]AIC-LMCP Foundation, L. M. College of Pharmacy, Ahmedabad, Gujarat, India
[6]Department of Pharmaceutics and Pharmaceutical Technology, L. M. College of Pharmacy, Ahmedabad, Gujarat, India

Abstract

In past few years, the pharma industry has seen a significant expansion in the digitalization of data. However, with digitalization comes the difficulty of acquiring, evaluating, and utilizing information to address complicated clinical situations. Traditional pharmaceutical research can be replaced by artificial intelligence (AI), which consists of a number of sophisticated tools and networks that can simulate the human mind and physiology. AI and machine learning (ML) play a significant role in medicinal development, including the prediction of pharmacological targets and the characteristics of small molecules. For the rapid creation of cellular and genetic therapeutics, AI- and ML-assisted dataset analysis presents a potent and promising route. This relatively young and fast developing discipline that is still in its infancy is evolving at an astounding pace. It is crucial, therefore, to

**Corresponding author*: Vivek7chavda@gmail.com; ORCID: https://orcid.org/0000-0002-7701-8597

Vivek Chavda, Krishnan Anand and Vasso Apostolopoulos (eds.) Bioinformatics Tools for Pharmaceutical Drug Product Development, (255–284) © 2023 Scrivener Publishing LLC

evaluate the creation of new algorithms, techniques, and tools, as well as the challenges, setbacks, and other obstacles emerging during their development, in order to support the growth of this very important sector. In this chapter, we present an overview of existing AI- and ML-based technologies and a peek of how AI and ML is reinventing preclinical and clinical drug research by showcasing real-world applications of AI and ML. In light of the hype and exaggeration surrounding AI and ML in drug development, we hope to give a realistic perspective by examining both the advantages and limitations of using AI and ML in drug research.

***Keywords*:** Deep learning, Bioinformatics tools, Preclinical and Clinical development, Artificial neural networks, Machine learning, Artificial intelligence

Abbreviations

AI	Artificial Intelligence
ML	Machine Learning
COVID-19	Coronavirus Disease 2019
SARS-CoV-2	Severe Acute Respiratory Syndrome Virus 2
ANN	Artificial Neural Networks
mRNA	Messenger Ribonucleic Acid
IR Spectroscopy	Infrared (IR) Spectroscopy
NIR	Near IR
MIR	Mid IR
FIR	Far IR
ATR-FTIR	Attenuated Total Reflectance Fourier Transform Infrared
MS	Mass Spectroscopy
PPI	Protein-Protein Interaction
NMR Spectroscopy	Nuclear Magnetic Resonance Spectroscopy
HPLC	High Performance Liquid Chromatography
GC	Gas Chromatography
DNA	Deoxyribonucleic Acid
RNA	Ribonucleic Acid
SDS-PAGE	Sodium Dodecyl Sulphate Polyacrylamide gel
QSAR	Quantitative Structure-Activity Relationship
SAR	Structure Activity Relationship
LD50	Lethal Dose (causing mortality on 50% of the population)
ED50	Effective Median Dose (producing desired efficacy in 50% population)

ADMET	Absorption, Distribution, Metabolism and Elimination
SVM	Support Vector Machine
RF	Random Forest Algorithm
MLR	Multiple Linear Regression
PCA	Principal Component Analysis
EMR	Electronic Medical Records
NLP	Natural Language Processing
EHR	Electronic Health Records
R&D	Research & Development
SERS	Surface Enhanced Raman Scattering
PDA	Photodiode array
DAD	Diode array detection
API	Atmospheric Pressure Ionization

12.1 Introduction

For the past three decades, clinical drug development process has not changed. This is mainly because of regulatory uncertainties, risk aversion, and skepticism toward technologies that are rapidly emerging but largely unproven namely artificial intelligence (AI), machine learning (ML) and wireless health monitoring devices and sensors. Moreover, a scarcity of meaningful biological data sources and advanced analytics to create hypothesis that could drive the development of novel medicines and diagnostic approaches. There is a need for novel strategies to test the new biomedical treatment approaches for evaluation of safety and efficacy. This is mainly because the conventional therapies/treatment approaches are only effective in limited population. The clinical trials, which are used for the development of new drug products and new therapeutic modalities, offer numerous opportunities for the applications of AI and ML techniques. Numerous elements of human sensory acuity have been improved by machine learning and artificial intelligence in order to identify clinically important correlations in imaging data [1]. The use of AI in clinical development of medicines amongst various drug development process of the pharmaceutical industry is highlighted in this chapter which reduced the human workload while also achieving the targets in a short period of time [2, 3].

To be successful in the pharmaceutical business, a greater degree of analytics is necessary. The objective is to increase our knowledge of human health by making more informed and prudent choices. Integrating human science with advances in data science and technology offers decision makers with more accuracy and relevance. It can alter how we accurately identify people and treat their health problems. How we might identify patients more quickly, may be even before they become patients. The demonstrated promise and enormous potential of employing AI and ML to expedite drug development while reducing costs and risks is a terrific innovation driver. We have the capacity to revolutionize the clinical development environment in ways that will benefit patients, sponsors, payers, and doctors by continuing to harness data, intelligence, analytics, and domain knowledge [4].

12.2 AI and ML for Pandemic

Recent outbreaks of "Coronavirus Disease 2019 (COVID-19)", caused by "severe acute respiratory syndrome virus 2 (SARS-CoV-2)", have impacted over two hundred nations and resulted in massive losses [5–7]. AI demonstrated superior performance in COVID-19 diagnosis, prognostic assessment, epidemic prediction, and medication development. During the COVID-19 pandemic, AI has the ability to greatly improve the efficacy of current medical and healthcare systems. The benefits of AI include high sensitivity and specificity in antigen/marker identification, rapid reporting, and consistent findings [8]. AI has made great strides in recent years, particularly in predictive machine learning models for medical treatment. Deep learning is a machine learning technique based on the intricate topologies of artificial neural networks (ANN). After giving adequate training data sets, deep learning demonstrates considerable discriminative performance and is necessary for generating predictions [9]. In medicine, technologies based on AI/ML attempt to enhance the quality of medical treatment, boost diagnostic accuracy, decrease possible mistakes or misses, and forecast outcomes by gleaning new insights from the massive quantity of patient-generated data [10]. Currently, several nations are still battling to limit the spread of COVID-19. Using AI techniques to assist with diagnosis, treatment, prognosis, prediction, evaluation of epidemic trends, surveillance, and public health decision-making may increase the efficacy and capacity of humans to combat the COVID-19 pandemic in the face of limited medical resources and rising healthcare demands [6, 11–14].

AI-generated predictions of viral structure have already saved scientists many months of testing. AI seems to have offered substantial assistance in this regard, despite the limitations imposed by so-called "continuous" rules and infinite combinatory predictions for the study of protein folding. The American new venture Moderna has distinguished itself by its expertise of messenger ribonucleic acid (mRNA)-based biotechnology, for which the study of protein folding is vital. With the assistance of bioinformatics, a key component of which is AI, it has substantially shortened the time necessary to build a prototype vaccination that can be tested on humans [15].

Using social media networks, AI systems that use natural language processing discover information regarding impending epidemics. In COVID-19 patients, machine learning (ML) algorithms are utilized to predict clinical outcomes such as death, risk for intubation, and risk for needing intensive care [16]. Artificial intelligence aids the creation and repurposing of medications and vaccines that may be useful in the fight against SARS-CoV-2 [17, 18].

The current advancements in AI and ML have considerably enhanced the therapy, medicine, testing, diagnosis, forecasting, contact tracing, and drug/vaccine development processes for the COVID-19 epidemic, and thus supporting the clinicians for decision making as well as reducing the need for human involvement in medical practice. However, the majority of models are not deployed sufficiently to demonstrate their real-world performance, yet they are enough to combat the SARS-CoV-2 pandemic [19].

12.3 Advanced Analytical Tools Used in Preclinical and Clinical Development

The need of discovering a new mode of therapy arises whenever any new disorder originates. Therapy may include the discovery of new chemical entities (or new biological entities) or modifying existing treatment which is present for a disorder nearly similar to the new one [20]. To discover a new chemical entity a process of drug development is to be followed which includes steps like: 1. Discovery of a lead molecule, 2. Pre-Clinical and Clinical Research, and 3. Review of Drug and Post-market safety monitoring.

To ensure that the molecule discovered is the one that is needed and it will provide desired therapeutic activity without causing any kind of side effects (or molecule with favorable risk/benefit potential), the molecule is subjected to different analytical techniques [21]. The chosen analytical technique should be accurate and precise in providing results and should also be able to detect the foreign molecule or impurities if generated along with the molecule [22]. The technique should be economical and easy to use in addition to being sensitive and selective. The method should be able to generate qualitative and quantitative results. The technique should also be helpful in structural analysis and purity analysis. Conventional analytical

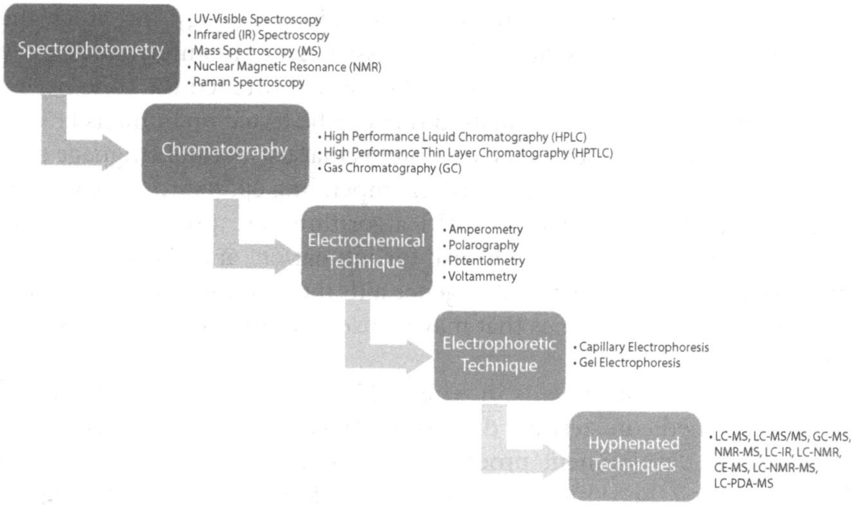

Figure 12.1 Successive use of conventional analytical tools in preclinical and clinical development of drug product (Adopted as per CC BY 4.0 License from [37]).

techniques for developing methods during preclinical and clinical drug development include various techniques (Figure 12.1) such as [23]:

1) Spectroscopic Techniques
2) Chromatographic Techniques
3) Electrochemical Techniques
4) Electrophoretic Techniques
5) Flow injection and Sequential Injection Analysis
6) Hyphenated techniques

12.3.1 Spectroscopic Techniques

These techniques mainly include the interaction of light or electromagnetic radiation with matter. There is a generation of spectra in the form of a result which gives information regarding the connection between the molecules within the matter. These technique can be majorly termed to be quantitative [24].

a. Ultraviolet (UV)-Visible Spectroscopy

Electrons within a molecule when subjected to UV (200-400 nm) or Visible radiation (400-800 nm), that some amount of radiation is transmitted while some radiation that is absorbed causes electrons to transform to an excited state. This is the basic principle of UV-Visible spectroscopy. It is an easy, cheap, simple, and rapid technique. The absorption of any molecule can be determined by this technique. Binary or Tertiary mixtures of different compounds can be analyzed using simultaneous estimation or derivatization where peaks that appear close to each other in the spectra can be resolved easily [25].

Recent advances in this technique include the characterization of metal nanoparticles and detecting the catalytic activity of polymeric microgels. The size and shape of metal nanoparticles can be easily determined and the kinetics of swelling and deswelling of microgels can also be monitored [26].

b. IR Spectroscopy

Infrared (IR) Spectroscopy is associated with the study of functional groups attached to the main structure of the molecule. It is also known as 'Fingerprinting' technique for a molecule as it serves as a unique identity for every different molecule due to its chemical bonding and atoms present within its structure. Vibrations and movements that occur between atoms within a molecule are detected by infrared radiation [27]. The frequency of radiation for the Near IR (NIR) region lies around 750 nm to 2500 nm, for Mid IR (MIR) region it is 2500 nm to 5000 nm while for Far IR (FIR) region it ranges from 50 μm to 1000 μm [28].

Current studies reveal that IR spectroscopy could be used as an important analytical tool to differentiate between viruses. Phosphate containing nucleic acid is detected around the region at 1240 cm^{-1} which increases within 1 or 2 days of infection and decreases after the 3rd day due to cell death. Attenuated Total Reflectance Fourier Transform Infrared (ATR-FTIR) is used for the diagnosis of Hepatitis B and Hepatitis C viruses. Differences in spectra of salivary samples infected with the virus are also useful to detect diseases like SARS-CoV-2 [29].

c. Mass Spectroscopy [MS]

This technique does not use any kind of radiation but the fragmentation of the parent molecule is the key working principle (Principle of ionization applying electrical charge (mass to charge ratio as unique attribute for a molecule)). Masses of generated daughter ions are helpful in the estimation of the molecular mass of the parent molecule. In modern-day, this technique is widely used in the discovery of clinical biomarkers. Clinical biomarkers are useful for lead molecule discovery for diseases like Diabetes and Cardiovascular disorders [30]. Accurate and precise structural analysis is one of the advantages of enhancing MS data resolution; as a consequence, we may acquire an improved biomolecular structure assessment in a consecutive and large-scale method. Furthermore, not only correct structural information but also the produced ion quantity is crucial factors in MS data. This advancement has made a significant contribution to a study field that studies biological processes as a scheme by monitoring the radical transformation in biological macromolecular dynamics. Consecutive variations in proteome activity in biochemical pathways are critical, and the magnitude of the changes is frequently used as a target for drug development or as a measure of therapeutic effectiveness [31]. To use this proteomic technique, the individual MS spectra obtained from each biomolecule in the complicated tissue specimens must be separated. MS is not limitless enough to accomplish all peak separations, thus we need to think about enhancing sample preparation and purification processes to make them appropriate for input into MS. The molecular information and spatial distribution of targeted molecules inside a tissue specimen are provided by imaging MS. MS-based clinical proteomics using clinical specimens and powerful bioinformatics can identify significant protein–protein interaction (PPI) networks and main protein players involved in disease subtype functioning processes. By combining these MS-based technologies, a seamless platform for drug discovery from compounds found in human clinical specimens can be created [32].

d. Nuclear Magnetic Resonance (NMR) Spectroscopy
With the application of magnetic field and radiofrequency, number of Hydrogen and Carbon can be estimated in a chemical moiety. The solid-state NMR can be useful in polymorphic studies, molecular structure, and prediction of packaging lattice in formulations like Hydrogel [33]. NMR provides a number of benefits and properties that are crucial in clinical metabolomics. Moreover, NMR spectroscopy is intrinsically extremely reliable, repeatable, unbiased, quantifiable, structurally, molecularly insightful, and needs minimal specimen processing and data interpretation. NMR may also be used to assess large cohorts, multi-site investigations, and longitudinal research [34].

e. Raman Spectroscopy
Scattered radiations detect the vibrational frequency of molecules and give information regarding crystal structure and polymorphism in this technique. Raman spectroscopy might offer a data-rich, non-invasive, non-destructive diagnostic tool to supplement the usage of traditional sample-based, rare, and destructive biochemical tests used to assess and confirm therapeutic cell quality [35]. Significantly, the accompanying are a few essential difficulties

that must be addressed. The identification of trustworthy biomarkers in biofluids is the first step that remains the "Gold standard" of diagnosis in oncology. The use of biomarkers in diagnosis necessitates collaboration between researchers in fundamental medicine, optical spectroscopy, and hospital doctors. Second, there are multicenter and large-scale clinical studies: large-scale trials should be undertaken according to established procedures to demonstrate the therapeutic benefits of SERS over alternative approaches. Third, SERS spectra feature artificial intelligence: despite the fact that SERS signals may have multiple strong peaks, analyzing the amplitude and wavelength changes directly is challenging [36]. Artificial intelligence-based illness diagnosis algorithms are required to quickly convert SERS spectra to a legible clinical standard. In 2021, three clinical studies using Raman spectroscopy and AI were filed. Overall, we expect SERS to make significant progress in the clinic during the next 5 years.

12.3.2 Chromatographic Techniques

These techniques are most widely used for the separation of a mixture of compounds and then individually determining them qualitatively or quantitatively. Screening of biological samples in therapeutic drug monitoring with the use of High-Performance Liquid Chromatography (HPLC) or identification of new drug molecule during the process of chemical synthesis using HPTLC, chromatographic techniques possess a wide range of applications in preclinical and clinical development. For detection of volatile gaseous samples, Gas chromatography (GC) technique can be employed [38].

Ion exchange chromatography, Affinity chromatography, and Size exclusion chromatographic techniques are widely used in industries for the purification of large volume biomaterials like monoclonal antibodies [39].

12.3.3 Electrochemical Techniques

These methods are employed for detecting drug molecules for therapeutic monitoring of drugs and clinical trials as they are easy to use and low on cost and less time consuming compared to spectroscopic or chromatographic methods. These techniques do not involve the use of large and complicated instrumentation and that is why are advantageous over other analytical methods. These include Voltametric Method, Polarographic method, Potentiometry, etc. [40]. Currently, these techniques are used for drug identification in molecular imprinted polymers that are used for the generation of artificial biomimetic receptors [41].

12.3.4 Electrophoretic Techniques

These techniques are majorly in use in the Biopharmaceutical industry as it involves the separation of cellular material like Deoxyribonucleic acid (DNA), Ribonucleic acid (RNA), or protein molecules, with the help of an electrical charge [42]. This separation occurs due to variation in molecular masses of these substances. It is also useful in detecting impurities present in monoclonal antibodies. Methods like Capillary Electrophoresis, Gel Electrophoresis, Sodium Dodecyl Sulphate Polyacrylamide Gel (SDS-PAGE) Electrophoresis, 2D Gel Electrophoresis, Western Blot, are widely employed in biopharmaceutical industries [43].

12.3.5 Hyphenated Techniques

These are the combination of spectroscopic, electrophoretic and chromatographic techniques that provide high throughput results. These techniques are interlinked by a bridge called 'Interface'. As the process remains fully automated it provides fast, accurate, and reproducible results. These techniques are of two types:

1. Double hyphenated
2. Triple hyphenated

Double hyphenated techniques include LC-MS, GC-MS, GC-IR, LC-IR, LC-NMR, etc. These are utilized for separation, identification, mass detection (LC-MS, LC-MS/MS) and quantitation. Biological screening of natural products can be achieved by these techniques. Triple hyphenated techniques include LC-PDA-MS, LC-NMR-MS, LC-DAD-API-MS, etc. For new molecule development, hyphenated techniques are preferred over conventional single techniques as separation and identification can be done together [44].

The software deployed with these advanced analytical technics for generation and recording of the results are getting smarter and utilize certain algorithms for data treatment, analysis and prediction. Various techniques come with the libraries of molecules, structures and properties that facilitate predictive analysis for identification and characterization (e.g. fingerprinting, fragmentation, etc.). The extensive data generated from the plethora of these advanced analytical techniques is analyzed by employing data science tools – AI and ML – to make 'go/no-go decisions' and critical decisions for the way forward in the preclinical and clinical development of the drug products.

12.4 AI, ML, and Other Bioinformatics Tools for Preclinical Development of Drug Products

Drug discovery can be described as planned and sequential process carried out to recognize a potential therapeutic drug molecule which can be used in medical emergencies (such as COVID-19) or in diseases lacking proper curative medical treatment (such as HIV) or to mitigate the adverse effects of currently available drug [45]. Drug discovery can be further divided into many steps starting from the identification of the targeted site or disease (target identification), confirmation of the molecular level target (target validation) based on which the type of drug molecule to be developed is justified i.e., small molecule or large biomolecule. Based on the target site and their properties, a molecule can be developed (lead identification) having proper efficacy and affinity for the target which can be carried out using various approaches such as serendipity, random approach, rationale approach or by drug metabolite study through tools like Quantitative structure-activity relationship (QSAR), molecular modelling, combinatorial chemistry and many more [46–51]. Last step of medicinal chemistry in drug discovery is lead optimization. Lead optimization is done by various *in-vitro* assay, pharmacophore and structure activity relation (SAR) studies. The main goal of lead optimization is to enhance the property or to identify the lead/molecule with maximum beneficiary properties. After proper optimization of lead, drug development process is initiated [45, 52].

Drug development process is further divided into two parts i.e., preclinical drug development stage and clinical development stage. Preclinical stage lays the foundation for the clinical studies of drug/drug product. During the preclinical studies various toxicity data with the therapeutic range, pharmacokinetic and pharmacodynamic studies, identification of lethal dose (LD50) and median effective dose (ED50) were carried out. To get the legal permission for clinical trials, investigational new drug application needs to be submitted to regulatory authority which needs adequate information on drug properties which can be known through pre-clinical studies. Pre-clinical studies play major role in finalization of drug for clinical trials [53].

Preclinical studies mainly emphasis on identifying pharmacodynamic and pharmacokinetic properties in the animals. To study the new drug molecules in animals is quite lengthy, tedious and sometimes causes unnecessary harm in the process. In few instances, it is also observed that the drug which proved safe in animals causes toxicity effects on human subjects [54]. So, to overcome the pain to animals and their shortcomings, to save the time and for faster and accurate results, various simulation softwares were developed. "*In-silico* Absorption, Distribution, Metabolism and Elimination (ADMET)" studies and physiological based pharmacokinetic studies form the basis of the data collection in pre-clinical trials. This section will touch upon the use of computational-based tools or software's which are used in pre-clinical drug development of pharmaceutical products.

12.4.1 Various Computational Tools Used in Pre-Clinical Drug Development

Successful discovery of single molecule as drug candidate needs billions of dollars and time of approximately one and half decades. On initial phase after lead optimization, activities and specificities of molecule are assessed, keeping pharmacokinetics and toxicities evaluation aside for later stage. However, it was highlighted that undesirable pharmacokinetic properties lead to unwanted efficacy and safety issue at later stage, which leads to failure of whole research [55]. Further, evaluation of ADMET properties in preclinical development phase is of utter importance in identifying the dose, to evaluate the toxicity, reducing the cost and increasing the success rate of clinical trials.

It is not possible to do *in-vitro* and *in-vivo* evaluation of every compound in animals in short time. Therefore, various *in-silico* models have come into existence which is replacing *in-vivo* methods to predict the various properties. *In-silico* model is based on molecular modelling (prediction based on 3D structure) which further works on structure or ligand-based methods [56, 57].

Many pharmaceutical giants have tied up with data science/AI based software-companies to brisk the drug development process (Table 12.1). Notable tie ups were of Pfizer and Novartis with IBM Watson, AstraZeneca and Johnson & Johnson with BenevoltenAI, Sanofi with Exscientia and many more [58]. All the *in-silico* models and QSAR based software work on the AI and stimulation. QSAR models are prominent mathematical models which are based on the molecular elucidation and identification of properties for the biological effect of the compound.

ML is generally based on the algorithms which are used for classification and regression-based modelling approaches (Table 12.2). Through algorithms, various tasks can be carried out which have useful finding in pre-clinical development.

Table 12.1 Bioinformatics tools used in pre-clinical drug development [59].

Sr. no.	Tools	Description
1.	QuantMap	Interrelationship between drugs, toxicity with other chemical entities to identify and mitigate the toxicity
2.	Connectivity mapping (Cmap)	Makes functional connection between drugs, genes, and disease to identify the role of drug
3.	SM2miR	It contains detailed information about miRNAs with its regulatory status which is helpful to interpret the functioning

Table 12.2 Use of ML algorithms in preclinical drug development [60].

Sr. no.	Category	Algorithms	Uses
1	Supervised	Support Vector Machine (SVM)	Binding affinity and position, physiochemical properties and ADMET properties prediction
		Random forest algorithm (Rf)	
		Multilayer perception	
		Multiple Linear Regression (MLR)	
2	Unsupervised	Principal Component Analysis (PCA)	Molecular pattern recognition
		Partial least square regression	
		Gaussian mixture models	

The future and the scope of the various modern computational techniques (AI/ML) depends on the database collection which can be used as training data, development of advanced model which can predict accurately and complete endpoint data collection. With the incomplete data, stimulation is hindered leading to less accurate outcome. With proper information and with the help of advanced logarithmic – mathematical tool the development of drug can be carried out in countable months saving time and resources.

AI/ML based algorithms are used for the drug toxicity prediction as well as prediction of its intrinsic pharmacodynamics activity [61]. Due to computer-predicted toxicity, many damaging and dangerous animal or clinical experiments may be avoided. *In silico* forecasting is low-cost, risk-free, and has a high throughput. Since human basic fundamental cellular data (mRNA) is often employed, the identification is mostly relied on system-level complexity; as a result, the technique is more universal than used by researchers doing test on single protein-related toxicity. In nutshell, as data size increases and accuracy improves, machine learning may become totally *In-silico* in pharmacological and computational biology findings, due to high efficient extraction and identification ability [62].

12.5 AI, ML, and Other Bioinformatics Tools for Clinical Development of Drug Products

For the past three decades, clinical drug development process has not changed. This is mainly because of regulatory uncertainties, risk aversion, and skepticism toward technologies that are rapidly emerging but largely unproven n1amely artificial intelligence (AI), machine learning (ML) and wireless health monitoring devices and sensors. Moreover, a scarcity of meaningful biological data sources and advanced analytics to create hypothesis that could drive the development of novel medicines and diagnostic approaches. The new strategies will be required to test the new biomedical treatment approaches for the evaluation of safety and efficacy of drugs and new modalities. This is mainly because conventional therapies are only effective in a limited population. However, the application of modern digital technologies, namely next-generation sequencing has increased our understanding of disease etiology in a large cohort of patients as well as the promise of generating personalized management therapies. For instance, the majority of new molecular entities approved by the United States Food and Drug Administration (USFDA) in recent years have been designed to target specific aberrations implicated in disease initiation and maintenance, which is a hallmark of precision medicine, that strives to personalized therapies based on the characteristics of an individual patients [63].

Table 12.3 Key terminologies and concepts related to machine learning in clinical drug development.

Terminologies	Definition/concept
Machine learning (ML)	A mathematical model that is able to improve its performance on a task by exposure to data.
Deep neural networks	ML models with one or more latent (hidden) layers allowing for the generation of non-linear output and complex interactions between layers. Deep neural networks power "deep learning," which enables tasks, such as image recognition, natural language processing (NLP), and complex predictions. Subtypes of deep neural networks are classified based on the relationship between hidden layers and include convolutional, recurrent, gated graph, and generative adversarial neural networks.
Training, test, and validation sets	Training set: Dataset from which the model learns the optimal parameters to accomplish the task. Test set: Dataset on which the performance of a trained, parameterized model is evaluated. Validation set: Dataset that is used to evaluate the model's performance during training. Differs from a test set in that it is used during training to establish hyperparameters of the model.
Supervised learning	A subset of ML in which the outcomes to be learned by the model ("labels") are provided in the training set. For example, teaching a model to identify breast cancer patients for study inclusion would require training the model on a training set containing labelled patients with and without breast cancer prior to validating that model on a new set of unlabeled patients with and without breast cancer.
Unsupervised learning	A subset of ML in which there are no pre-specified labels for the model to learn to predict; instead, models identify hidden patterns in the data.
Natural language processing (NLP)	A form of artificial intelligence that enables the understanding of language. Such modern NLP uses deep neural networks in which words and their relationships to each other are encoded in a set of highly dimensional vectors, enabling the model to parse the meaning of new pieces of text it is presented with.

Reprinted from "The role of machine learning in clinical research: transforming the future of evidence generation," by Weissler EH, 2021, Trials. 2021 22(1), 1-5. CC0 1.0.

It is imperative to get insights of the important concepts and principles of ML which are listed in Table 12.3.

Another pressing issue in drug research is the reporting of the outcomes of conventional clinical studies of average treatment effects, which may not easily translate into making tailored treatment decisions at the point of care [64]. On an average clinical trial take 6–7 years and a significant financial investment to establish the safety and efficacy of a drug molecule in human for a specific illness. However, just one out of every ten compounds that enter clinical trials is authorized, resulting in a considerable loss for the industry [65]. These failures might be attributed to inappropriate patient selection, a lack of technological needs, and bad infrastructure, and thus given the huge amount of digital medical data available, AI can be used to curb these failures [66]. Using new digital clinical endpoints and treatment response biomarkers amenable to close and efficient monitoring (e.g. circulating tumor DNA), improving safety and efficacy while reducing toxicity and adverse events, and greater insights into the patient journey using sensors, low-cost imaging are promising approaches to overcome these challenges [67–70].

ML and computer vision have improved numerous aspects of human visual perception to identify clinically meaningful patterns in, for instance, imaging data, and neural networks have been used for a variety of tasks ranging from medical image segmentation to clinical dataset generation, classification, and prediction [71]. Academic research laboratories, biotechnology-based organizations, and technology firms have been broadly investigating the use of AI and ML in three crucial areas. Firstly, machine-oriented learning to predict pharmacological characteristics of chemical molecules and identification of targets for drug discovery [72–74]. Secondly, using pattern recognition and segmentation techniques on medical images (for instance, retinal scans, pathology slides, and body surfaces, bones, and internal organs) to enable faster diagnosis and disease progression tracking along with computational augmentation of current clinical and imaging data sets using generative algorithms. Lastly, deep-learning techniques using multimodal data sources, namely genetic and clinical data, to find novel prediction models [75, 76].

12.5.1 Role of AI, ML, and Bioinformatics in Clinical Research

Preclinical research and observational studies lead to standard clinical studies and studies with pragmatic components that generate clinical registries and additional implementation work. While clinical research is crucial to improve healthcare and outcomes, it is difficult, labor-intensive, expensive, and it is prone to unforeseen errors and biases that might jeopardize its successful application, adoption, and acceptance [77]. AI and ML have the potential to improve clinical trial success, generalizability, patient-centricity, and efficiency. Numerous ML techniques for managing large and heterogeneous data sources, detecting complicated and occult patterns, and forecasting complex outcomes are available. As a result, ML can help with anything from preclinical drug development to pre-trial planning to

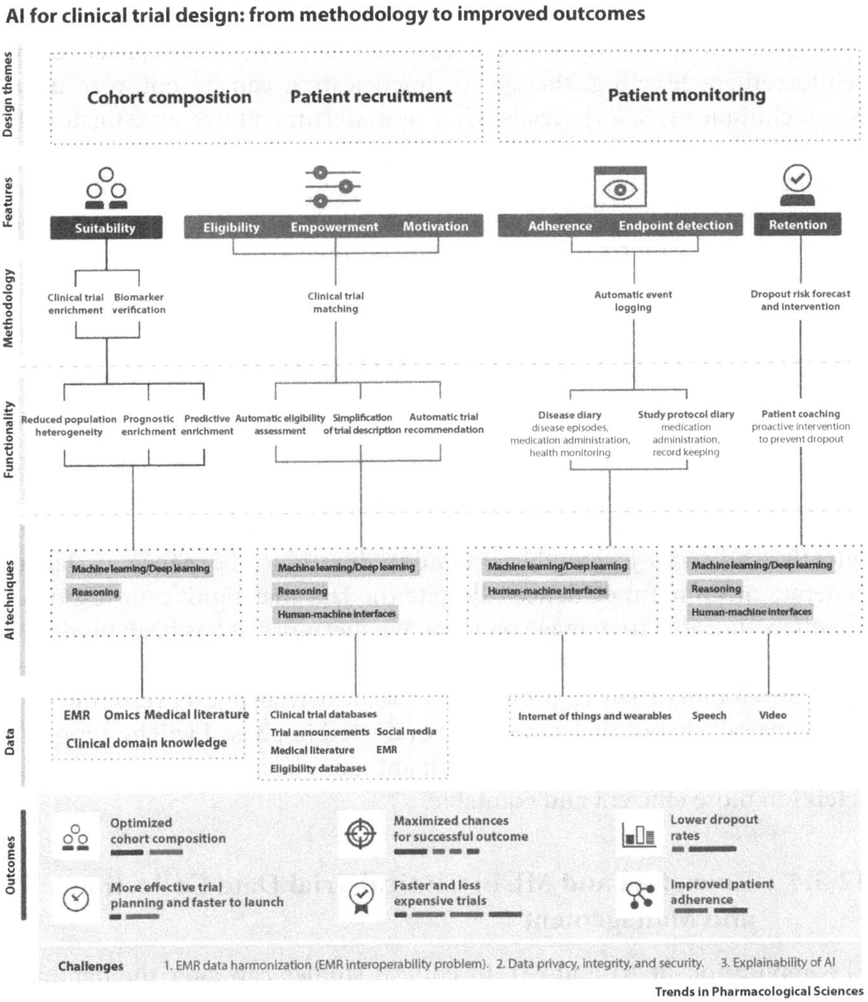

Figure 12.2 Implementation of AI in clinical trials (EMR: Electronic Medical Records) (Adopted under CC BY 4.0 License from [66]).

study execution to data management and analysis in clinical trials [57]. The implementation of AI in clinical trials has been illustrated in Figure 12.2.

12.5.2 Role of AI and ML in Clinical Study Protocol Optimization

When prospective medicinal substances reach the stage of human trials, ML can assist in increasing trial success from the beginning phase by applying simulation approaches to a large number of datasets from previous studies to optimize creation of a trial procedure. For example, as illustrated in approaches to "Alzheimer's illness" and "non-small cell lung cancer" using reinforcement learning, therapy regimen testing can be optimize using ML-techniques [78, 79]. Trials.AI, a new startup, allows investigators to submit protocols and uses NLP to highlight potential hazards and hurdles to effective study completion (namely as "inclusion/exclusion criteria" or "outcome measures"). This indicates clear opportunities to apply concepts of AI and ML to improve the efficacy and output of preclinical research and clinical study design.

12.5.3 Role of AI and ML in the Management of Clinical Trial Participants

Clinical trial participant management entails selecting target patient populations, recruiting patients, and retaining participants. Lack of patient pool because of higher drop-out rate and medication non-adherence frequently lead trials to lengthen intended duration or expense, or fail to generate meaningful evidences, despite the fact that significant resources are often allocated to manage patients. Furthermore, it has been predicted that between 33.6% and 52.4% of phase I–III clinical studies supporting drug development fail to progress to the next trial phase, resulting in a 13.8% overall chance that a medicine evaluated in phase I will be approved [80]. ML techniques can make participant identification, recruitment, and retention more efficient and equitable.

12.5.4 Role of AI and ML in Clinical Trial Data Collection and Management

The application of AI and ML in clinical studies can alter the data collecting, management, and analysis strategies as necessary (Figure 12.3).

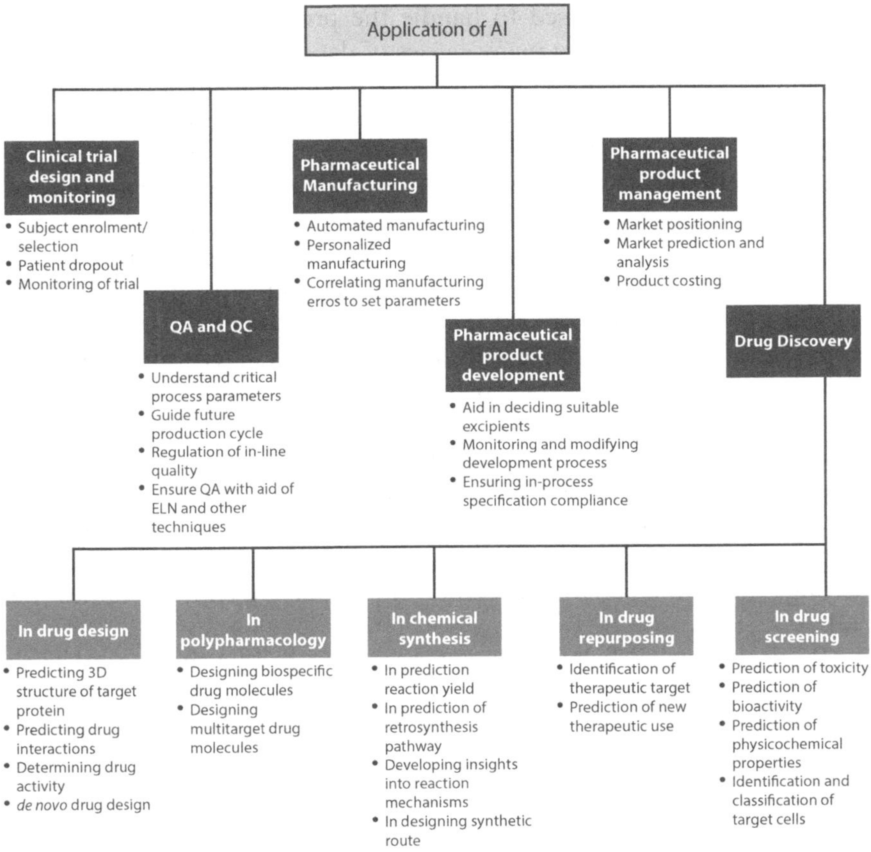

Figure 12.3 AI/ML application in product lifecycle management.

However, ML techniques can assist in addressing some of the pressing issues related to missing data and the collection of real-world data.

Automating data collection, whether in prospective trials or retrospective studies, is an appealing application of machine learning, specifically natural language processing (NLP), to study data management. This reduces the time, expense, and potential for error associated with human data extraction. Despite the fact that this application requires overcoming variable data formats and provenances, it has already demonstrated promising results in cancer, epilepsy, and depression [81–84]. ML can also be used to process these collected datasets. Identification of endpoints using ML-techniques compared to current manual approach is superior in terms of cost, complexity and time required as per the clinicians.

AI and ML can be used to handle the problem of missing data in numerous ways, including many causes of data missingness, data-related assumptions, goals, data collecting and intended analytic methodologies. Alternative objectives include directly imputing precise estimation of covariate values that are missing or averaging from possible multiple values to compute additional quantities of interest from a learning distribution. While the most recent methods are still evolving, and there is a need of precise systematic comparisons, baseline-raw data suggests that ML-techniques that are complex may not show superior outcomes compared to simple imputation methods, such as the population mean imputation [85]. Missing value algorithms are used to analyze sparse datasets namely registries, data extracted from electronic health records (EHR), ergonomic, and wearable devices [86–88].

Creation of hypothesis is completely based on dataset obtained from clinical trials and practices along with some registries and different ML-techniques are meant to perform such operations. Unsupervised learning, for example, can reveal phenotypic groupings in actual clinical settings that can be analyzed further in prospective clinical studies [89, 90].

There are several helpful ML-approaches to handle the clinical trials related datasets, but only limited techniques have been collected for improvisation of the quality of datasets. Since data acquisition and quality are considered the cornerstones of ML-techniques, conducting high-quality trials is crucial to enabling higher-level ML processing.

While traditional clinical studies and statistical approaches used in them are still widely used for generation of scientific data, enrichment with various AI approaches helps in improvisation of clinical research success. Since various ML techniques utilized in clinical research are improving quality of evidences generated, these techniques have the potential to save lives and alleviate suffering, generating an ethical imperative to look into this possibility. Application of ML in clinical studies now outnumber its actual use, owing to a lack of prospective studies on the relative effectiveness of ML versus traditional methodologies, as well as the time, energy, and cooperation required for change. Translucent discussion regarding the possible advantages and limitations of ML in clinical studies along with disseminating best practices must continue amongst academicians, government officials, and press in order to ensure the rational application of ML in the clinical trials.

12.6 Way Forward

Whenever human body encounters a new disease or disorder there arises a need to discover a therapy that can efficiently mitigate that particular disorder. Drug discovery is the first step in that direction which can associate the functioning of a synthetically or biotechnologically derived molecule to the disease by its therapeutic action to eradicate it from the human body [47, 49–51, 91, 92]. Further, the chemical moiety goes through pre-clinical and clinical trials and studies for safety and efficacy in target patients before getting approved for human use [93]. While going through all these processes a huge amount of data is generated which needs to be managed. Also there is a requirement for designing and integrating tools that can make the research work less challenging. Artificial Intelligence (AI) and machine learning (ML) are tools that can make research in preclinical and clinical development a smooth task.

AI is a mechanism that utilizes technology or computers to function as per the human brain and perform tedious tasks rapidly. AI instructs computers to master human behavior like judgment, calculation, reasoning, and problem-solving and also compile various subjects like logical thinking, technology, biology, psychology or philosophy, etc. [94]. It proves to help improvise the efficiency of research, reduce production costs and also meet human resource demand by reducing the time required for a particular process. AI uses a large amount of data, algorithms for pattern recognition, language processing, hardware platform, and computing vision to give precise results of the required analysis. ML comprises utilizing an algorithm that enhances its action by grasping existing information [95].

AI was coined by McCarthy in the 1950s and it gained popularity around the 1970s as it was used in MYCIN (AI program) to provide diagnostic decision support [96]. It is established that it takes 10 to 15 years in any kind of drug development and a majority of this time goes into clinical trials which also requires a huge amount of money. With the use of AI, the time to market and the cost of development can be significantly reduced [66].

AI and ML in preclinical and clinical development can be used to eliminate chemical/biological moieties which are less effective, right from the beginning and thus, ultimately saving high research costs and time. Chances to get desired results can be increased using targeted designing tools that accurately provide outcomes. AI can reduce the challenges and obstacles of conventional drug design methods and risk analysis. At the time when delivering therapeutic agents with desired activity and less safety concerns has become a challenge, AI comes into action to overcome this challenge. AI and ML algorithms can also help plan the research work. The tools that can aid in the synthesis of molecules, protein and peptide interactions, structure elucidation, prediction of toxicity, bioactivity prediction based on physicochemical properties, prognosis and diagnosis of a disease, monitoring release of drug from the formulation or device, QSAR, design of experiments, as well as data regulation and management are available. Applications of AI have tremendous potential to expand decision making, upgrade clinical processes, raise the patient outcome and lessen the cost of healthcare [97].

12.7 Conclusion

In the last decade, AI and ML have emerged as the disruptive technologies with the greatest potential to revolutionize R&D. This is due in part to breakthrough advancements in computer technology and the simultaneous elimination of earlier limits on the collection/processing of enormous amounts of data. In the meanwhile, the price of getting new treatments to market and to patients has grown exorbitant. It is obvious that AI and ML may enhance therapy, medicine, screening and prediction, forecasting, infection prevention and control, plus drug/vaccine research for the COVID-19 epidemic and minimize human involvement in medical practice. However, the majority of models are not deployed sufficiently to demonstrate their real-world performance, yet they are enough to combat the epidemic. ML has considerable potential for enhancing the efficacy and accuracy of clinical studies, but large limitations exist that must be overcome by addressing severe evidence gaps. The distinction between causality and correlation must be well understood, and it must be acknowledged that the growth of superior prediction skills does not make the scientific method obsolete. Credible inference still needs strong statistical judgement, which is especially important in drug development given the direct influence on patient's health and safety.

The adoption of AI technology offers significant potential for reducing the duration and expense of drug research. Although AI may not be a panacea for all drug development problems, it is undeniably a helpful tool when deployed in the appropriate context and with the appropriate data. The power of AI technologies will undoubtedly be utilized to complement human intellect and expand our capacities, perhaps altering the way we approach drug development, but they will not replace human intelligence.

References

1. Shah, P., Kendall, F., Khozin, S. *et al.*, Artificial intelligence and machine learning in clinical development: A translational perspective. *NPJ Digit. Med.* [Internet], 2, 1, 69, 2019, Available from: https://doi.org/10.1038/s41746-019-0148-3.
2. Weatherall, J., Khan, F.M., Patel, M. *et al.*, Chapter 10 - Clinical trials, real-world evidence, and digital medicine [Internet], in: *Ashenden Machine Learning, and Data Science in the Pharmaceutical Industry SKBT-TE of AI*, pp. 191–215, Academic Press, Elsevier, 2021, Available from: https://www.sciencedirect.com/science/article/pii/B9780128200452000118.
3. Bender, A. and Cortés-Ciriano, I., Artificial intelligence in drug discovery: What is realistic, what are illusions? Part 1: Ways to make an impact, and why we are not there yet. *Drug Discovery Today* [Internet], 26, 2, 511–524, 2021, Available from: https://www.sciencedirect.com/science/article/pii/S1359644620305274.
4. Weissler, E.H., Naumann, T., Andersson, T. *et al.*, The role of machine learning in clinical research: Transforming the future of evidence generation. *Trials* [Internet], 22, 1, 537, 2021, Available from: https://doi.org/10.1186/s13063-021-05489-x.
5. Chavda, V.P., Vora, L.K., Vihol, D.R., COVAX-19® Vaccine: Completely blocks virus transmission to non-immune individuals. *Clin. Complement. Med. Pharmacol.* [Internet], 1, 1, 100004, 2021, Available from: https://www.sciencedirect.com/science/article/pii/S2772371221000048.
6. Chavda, V.P., Vora, L.K., Pandya, A.K., Patravale, V.B., Intranasal vaccines for SARS-CoV-2: From challenges to potential in COVID-19 management. *Drug Discovery Today* [Internet], 26, 11, 2619–2636, 2021, Available from: https://www.sciencedirect.com/science/article/pii/S1359644621003317.
7. Chavda, V.P., Hossain, M.K., Beladiya, J., Apostolopoulos, V., Nucleic acid vaccines for COVID-19: A paradigm shift in the vaccine development arena. *Biologics*, 1, 3, 337–356, 2021.
8. Wang, L., Zhang, Y., Wang, D., Tong, X., Liu, T., Zhang, S., Huang, J., Zhang, L., Chen, L., Fan, H., Clarke, M., Artificial intelligence for COVID-19: A systematic review. *Front Med. (Lausanne)*, 8, 704256, 2021.
9. Abdulaal, A., Patel, A., Charani, E., Denny, S., Mughal, N., Moore, L., Prognostic modeling of COVID-19 using artificial intelligence in the United Kingdom: Model development and validation. *J. Med. Internet Res.*, 22, 8, e20259, 2020.
10. Hwang, T.J., Kesselheim, A.S., Vokinger, K.N., Lifecycle regulation of artificial intelligence- and machine learning-based software devices in medicine. *JAMA*, 322, 23, 2285–2286, 2019.
11. Dogan, O., Tiwari, S., Jabbar, M.A., Guggari, S., A systematic review on AI/ML approaches against COVID-19 outbreak. *Complex Intell. Syst.*

[Internet], 7, 5, 2655–2678, 2021, Available from: https://doi.org/10.1007/s40747-021-00424-8.
12. Chavda, V.P. and Apostolopoulos, V., Mucormycosis – An opportunistic infection in the aged immunocompromised individual: A reason for concern in COVID-19. *Maturitas* [Internet], 58, 58–61, 2021, Available from: https://www.sciencedirect.com/science/article/pii/S0378512221001365.
13. Chavda, V.P., Feehan, J., Apostolopoulos, V., A veterinary vaccine for SARS-CoV-2: The first COVID-19 vaccine for animals. *Vaccines (Basel)*, 9, 6, 631, 2021 Jun 10.
14. Chavda, V.P., Patel, A.B., Vihol, D. *et al.*, Herbal remedies, nutraceuticals, and dietary supplements for COVID-19 management: An update. *Clin. Complement. Med. Pharmacol.* [Internet], 2, 1, 100021, 2022.
15. Chauhan, G., Madou, M.J., Kalra, S., Chopra, V., Ghosh, D., Martinez-Chapa, S.O., Nanotechnology for COVID-19: Therapeutics and vaccine research. *ACS Nano* [Internet], 14, 7, 7760–7782, 2020, Available from: https://doi.org/10.1021/acsnano.0c04006.
16. Khemasuwan, D. and Colt, H.G., Applications and challenges of AI-based algorithms in the COVID-19 pandemic. *BMJ Innov.* [Internet], 7, 2, 387 LP – 398, 2021, Available from: http://innovations.bmj.com/content/7/2/387.abstract.
17. Chavda, V.P., Gajjar, N., Shah, N., Dave, D.J., Darunavir ethanolate: Repurposing an anti-HIV drug in COVID-19 treatment. *Eur. J. Med. Chem. Rep.* [Internet], 3, 100013, 2021, Available from: https://www.sciencedirect.com/science/article/pii/S2772417421000133.
18. Chavda, V.P., Kapadia, C., Soni, S. *et al.*, A global picture: Therapeutic perspectives for COVID-19. *Immunotherapy* [Internet], pp. 351–371, 2022, 10.2217/imt-2021-0168. Available from: https://doi.org/10.2217/imt-2021-0168.
19. Lalmuanawma, S., Hussain, J., Chhakchhuak, L., Applications of machine learning and artificial intelligence for Covid-19 (SARS-CoV-2) pandemic: A review. *Chaos Solitons Fractals* [Internet], 139, 110059, 2020, Available from: https://www.sciencedirect.com/science/article/pii/S0960077920304562.
20. Newman, D.J. and Cragg, G.M., Natural products as sources of new drugs over the nearly four decades from 01/1981 to 09/2019. *J. Nat. Prod.* [Internet], 83, 3, 770–803, 2020, Available from: https://doi.org/10.1021/acs.jnatprod.9b01285.
21. Hughes, J.P., Rees, S., Kalindjian, S.B., Philpott, K.L., Principles of early drug discovery. *Br. J. Pharmacol.* [Internet], 162, 6, 1239–1249, 2011, Available from: https://pubmed.ncbi.nlm.nih.gov/21091654.
22. Betz, J.M., Brown, P.N., Roman, M.C., Accuracy, precision, and reliability of chemical measurements in natural products research. *Fitoterapia* [Internet], 82, 1, 44–52, 2011, Available from: https://pubmed.ncbi.nlm.nih.gov/20884340.
23. Siddiqui, M.R., AlOthman, Z.A., Rahman, N., Analytical techniques in pharmaceutical analysis: A review. *Arab. J. Chem.* [Internet], 10, S1409–S1421,

2017, Available from: https://www.sciencedirect.com/science/article/pii/S1878535213001056.

24. Schermann, J.-P., *2 - Spectroscopy* [Internet], J-PBT-S Schermann and M of BBB (Eds.), pp. 59–128, Elsevier, Amsterdam, 2008, Available from: https://www.sciencedirect.com/science/article/pii/B9780444527080500034.
25. Görög, S. and Szántay, C., *Spectroscopic methods in drug quality control and development* [Internet], Second E, JCBT-E Lindon of S and S (Eds.), pp. 2640–2650, Academic Press, Oxford, 2010, Available from: https://www.sciencedirect.com/science/article/pii/B978012374413500066X.
26. Begum, R., Farooqi, Z.H., Naseem, K. *et al.*, Applications of UV/Vis spectroscopy in characterization and catalytic activity of noble metal nanoparticles fabricated in responsive polymer microgels: A review. *Crit. Rev. Anal. Chem.*, 48, 6, 503–516, 2018.
27. Colthup, N.B., *Infrared spectroscopy* [Internet], Third E, RABT-E Meyers of PS and T (Eds.), pp. 793–816, Academic Press, New York, 2003, Available from: https://www.sciencedirect.com/science/article/pii/B0122274105003409.
28. Scotter, C.N.G., *Infrared spectroscopy | Near-infrared* [Internet], Second E, P. Worsfold, A. Townshend, Poole CBT-E of AS (Eds.), pp. 415–426, Elsevier, Oxford, 2005, Available from: https://www.sciencedirect.com/science/article/pii/B0123693977002776.
29. Kitane, D.L., Loukman, S., Marchoudi, N. *et al.*, A simple and fast spectroscopy-based technique for COVID-19 diagnosis. *Sci. Rep.* [Internet], 11, 1, 16740, 2021, Available from: https://doi.org/10.1038/s41598-021-95568-5.
30. Crutchfield, C.A., Thomas, S.N., Sokoll, L.J., Chan, D.W., Advances in mass spectrometry-based clinical biomarker discovery. *Clin. Proteomics.*, 13, 1, 2016.
31. Iwamoto, N. and Shimada, T., Recent advances in mass spectrometry-based approaches for proteomics and biologics: Great contribution for developing therapeutic antibodies. *Pharmacol. Ther.* [Internet], 185, 147–154, 2018, Available from: https://www.sciencedirect.com/science/article/pii/S0163725817303042.
32. Nakayama, N., Bando, Y., Fukuda, T. *et al.*, Developments of mass spectrometry-based technologies for effective drug development linked with clinical proteomes. *Drug Metab. Pharmacokinet.* [Internet], 31, 1, 3–11, 2016, Available from: https://www.sciencedirect.com/science/article/pii/S1347436715000774.
33. El Hariri El Nokab, M. and van der Wel, P.C.A., Use of solid-state NMR spectroscopy for investigating polysaccharide-based hydrogels: A review. *Carbohydr. Polym.* [Internet], 240, 116276, 2020, Available from: https://www.sciencedirect.com/science/article/pii/S0144861720304501.
34. Letertre, M.P.M., Giraudeau, P., de Tullio, P., Nuclear magnetic resonance spectroscopy in clinical metabolomics and personalized medicine: Current challenges and perspectives. *Front. Mol. Biosci.* [Internet], 8, 698337, 2021, Available from: https://pubmed.ncbi.nlm.nih.gov/34616770.

35. Rangan, S., Schulze, H.G., Vardaki, M.Z., Blades, M.W., Piret, J.M., Turner, R.F.B., Applications of raman spectroscopy in the development of cell therapies: State of the art and future perspectives. *Analyst* [Internet], 145, 6, 2070–2105, 2020, Available from: http://dx.doi.org/10.1039/C9AN01811E.
36. Xi, X. and Liang C., Perspective of future SERS clinical application based on current status of raman spectroscopy clinical trials. *Front Chem.*, 9, 665841, 2021 Jul 20.
37. Sharma, S., Singh, N., Ankalgi, A.D., Rana, A., Ashawat, M.S., Modern trends in analytical techniques for method development and validation of pharmaceuticals: A review. *J. Drug Deliv. Ther.* [Internet], 11, 1-s SE-Review, 2021, Available from: http://jddtonline.info/index.php/jddt/article/view/4515.
38. Loos, G., Van Schepdael, A., Cabooter, D., Quantitative mass spectrometry methods for pharmaceutical analysis. *Philos. Trans. A. Math. Phys. Eng. Sci.* [Internet], 374, 2079, 20150366, 2016, Available from: https://pubmed.ncbi.nlm.nih.gov/27644982.
39. Tuzimski, T. and Petruczynik, A., Review of chromatographic methods coupled with modern detection techniques applied in the therapeutic drugs monitoring (TDM). *Molecules*, 25, 17, 4026, 2020 Sep 3.
40. Aboul-Enein, H.Y., Sibel A. Ozkan: Electroanalytical methods in pharmaceutical analysis and their validation. *Chromatographia* [Internet], 75, 13, 811, 2012, Available from: https://doi.org/10.1007/s10337-012-2268-7.
41. Cui, B., Liu, P., Liu, X., Liu, S., Zhang, Z., Molecularly imprinted polymers for electrochemical detection and analysis: Progress and perspectives. *J. Mater. Res. Technol.* [Internet], 9, 6, 12568–12584, 2020, Available from: https://www.sciencedirect.com/science/article/pii/S2238785420316574.
42. Lino, C.A., Harper, J.C., Carney, J.P., Timlin, J.A., Delivering CRISPR: A review of the challenges and approaches. *Drug Delivery* [Internet], 25, 1, 1234–1257, 2018, Available from: https://pubmed.ncbi.nlm.nih.gov/29801422.
43. Řemínek, R. and Foret, F., Capillary electrophoretic methods for quality control analyses of pharmaceuticals: A review. *Electrophoresis* [Internet], 42, 1–2, 19–37, 2021, Available from: https://doi.org/10.1002/elps.202000185.
44. Patel, K.N., Patel, J.K., Patel, M.P., Rajput, G.C., Patel, H.A., Introduction to hyphenated techniques and their applications in pharmacy. *Pharm. Methods* [Internet], 1, 1, 2–13, 2010, Available from: https://pubmed.ncbi.nlm.nih.gov/23781411.
45. Sinha, S. and Vohora, D., *Drug Discovery and Development: An Overview*, Elsevier Inc., Amsterdam, 2018.
46. Vivek, C., Patel, C., Bhadani, J., Metabolomics: At a glance. *Res. Rev. A J. Drug Formul. Dev. Prod.*, 4, 1, 23–30, 2017.
47. Chavda, V., Thalkari, Y., Marwadi, S., New strategies in drug discovery [Internet]. *Comput. Bioinform.*, 25–48, 2021, Available from: https://doi.org/10.1002/9781119654803.ch2.

48. Chavda, V., Sheta, S., Changani, D., Chavda, D., New bioinformatics platform-based approach for drug design [Internet]. *Comput. Bioinform.*, 101–120, 2021, Available from: https://doi.org/10.1002/9781119654803.ch6.
49. Anand, K., Ramesh, M., Singh, T. *et al.*, One-step synthesis of picolinohydrazides from fusaric acid: DFT, structural characterization and molecular inhibitory studies on metastatic tumor-derived exosomal and non-exosomal proteins. *J. Mol. Struct.* [Internet], 1255, 132442, 2022, Available from: https://www.sciencedirect.com/science/article/pii/S0022286022001156.
50. Chavda, V.P., Ertas, Y.N., Walhekar, V. *et al.*, Advanced computational methodologies used in the discovery of new natural anticancer compounds. *Front. Pharmacol.*, 12, 702611, 2021.
51. Chavda, V.P., Patel, A.B., Mistry, K.J., Suthar, S.F., Wu, Z.X., Chen, Z.S., Hou, K., Nano-drug delivery systems entrapping natural bioactive compounds for cancer: Recent progress and future challenges. *Front Oncol.*, 12, 867655, 2022 Mar 29.
52. Deore, A.B., Dhumane, J.R., Wagh, H.V., RBS. The stages of drug discovery and development process. *Asian J. Pharm. Res. Dev.*, 7, 6, 62–67, 2019.
53. Chi, L.H., Burrows, A.D., Anderson, R.L., Can preclinical drug development help to predict adverse events in clinical trials? *Drug Discovery Today*, 27, 1, 257–268, 2022.
54. Van Norman, G.A., Limitations of animal studies for predicting toxicity in clinical trials. *JACC Basic Transl. Sci.*, 4, 7, 845–854, 2019.
55. Caldwell, G.W., Yan, Z., Tang, W., Dasgupta, M., Hasting, B., ADME optimization and toxicity assessment in early- and late-phase drug discovery. *Curr. Top. Med. Chem.*, 9, 965–980, 2009.
56. Wu, F., Zhou, Y., Li, L., Shen, X., Chen, G., Computational approaches in preclinical studies on drug discovery and development. *Front. Chem.*, 8, 1–32, 2020.
57. Réda, C., Kaufmann, E., Delahaye-Duriez, A., Machine learning applications in drug development. *Comput. Struct. Biotechnol. J.* [Internet], 18, 241–252, 2019, Available from: https://pubmed.ncbi.nlm.nih.gov/33489002.
58. Paul, D., Sanap, G., Shenoy, S., Artificial intelligence in drug discovery and development. *Drug Discovery Today*, 26, 80–93, 2021.
59. Gill, S.K. and Christopher, A.F., Emerging role of bioinformatics tools and software in evolution of clinical research. *Perspect. Clin. Res.*, 7, 3, 115–122, 2016.
60. Vijayan, R.S.K., Kihlberg, J., Cross, J.B., Poongavanam, V., Enhancing preclinical drug discovery with artificial intelligence. *Drug Discovery Today*, 27, 4, 967–984, 2022.
61. Wu, Y. and Wang, G., Machine learning based toxicity prediction: From chemical structural description to transcriptome analysis. *Int. J. Mol. Sci.* [Internet], 19, 8, 2358, 2018, Available from: https://pubmed.ncbi.nlm.nih.gov/30103448.

62. Pastur-Romay, L.A., Cedrón, F., Pazos, A., Porto-Pazos, A.B., Deep artificial neural networks and neuromorphic chips for big data analysis: Pharmaceutical and bioinformatics applications. *Int. J. Mol. Sci.*, 17, 8, 1313, 2016 Aug 11.
63. Jørgensen, J.T. and Hersom, M., Companion diagnostics-a tool to improve pharmacotherapy. *Ann. Transl. Med.*, 4, 24, 482, 2016.
64. Rothwell, P.M., Factors that can affect the external validity of randomised controlled trials. *PLoS Clin. Trials* [Internet], 1, 1, e9–e9, 2006, Available from: https://pubmed.ncbi.nlm.nih.gov/16871331.
65. Hay, M., Thomas, D.W., Craighead, J.L., Economides, C., Rosenthal, J., Clinical development success rates for investigational drugs. *Nat. Biotechnol.* [Internet], 32, 1, 40–51, 2014, Available from: https://doi.org/10.1038/nbt.2786.
66. Harrer, S., Shah, P., Antony, B., Hu, J., Artificial intelligence for clinical trial design. *Trends Pharmacol. Sci.* [Internet], 40, 8, 577–591, 2019, Available from: https://www.sciencedirect.com/science/article/pii/S0165614719301300.
67. Bettegowda, C., Sausen, M., Leary, R.J. *et al.*, Detection of circulating tumor DNA in early- and late-stage human malignancies. *Sci. Transl. Med.*, 6, 224, 224ra24, 2014.
68. Patel, S., Park, H., Bonato, P., Chan, L., Rodgers, M., A review of wearable sensors and systems with application in rehabilitation. *J. Neuroeng. Rehabil.* [Internet], 9, 1, 21, 2012, Available from: https://doi.org/10.1186/1743-0003-9-21.
69. Shah, P., Yauney, G., Gupta, O. *et al.*, Technology-enabled examinations of cardiac rhythm, optic nerve, oral health, tympanic membrane, gait and coordination evaluated jointly with routine health screenings: An observational study at the 2015 Kumbh Mela in India. *BMJ Open*, 8, 4, e018774, 2018.
70. Eckardt, J.-N., Wendt, K., Bornhäuser, M., Middeke, J.M., Reinforcement learning for precision oncology. *Cancers (Basel).* [Internet], 13, 18, 4624, 2021, Available from: https://pubmed.ncbi.nlm.nih.gov/34572853.
71. Krizhevsky, A., Sutskever, I., Hinton, G.E., ImageNet classification with deep convolutional neural networks [Internet], in: *Advances in Neural Information Processing Systems*, Conference proceedings and it is a Part of Advances in Neural Information Processing Systems 25 (NIPS 2012), F. Pereira, C.J. Burges, L. Bottou, K.Q. Weinberger (Eds.), Curran Associates, Inc., 2012, Available from: https://proceedings.neurips.cc/paper/2012/file/c399862d3b9d6b76c8436e924a68c45b-Paper.pdf.
72. Zhang, Y., Ye, T., Xi, H., Juhas, M., Li, J., Deep learning driven drug discovery: Tackling severe acute respiratory syndrome coronavirus 2. *Front. Microbiol.*, 12, 739684, 2021 Oct 28.
73. Chen, H., Engkvist, O., Wang, Y., Olivecrona, M., Blaschke, T., The rise of deep learning in drug discovery. *Drug Discovery Today* [Internet], 23, 6, 1241–1250, 2018, Available from: https://www.sciencedirect.com/science/article/pii/S1359644617303598.

74. Dara, S., Dhamercherla, S., Jadav, S.S., Babu, C.H.M., Ahsan, M.J., Machine learning in drug discovery: A review. *Artif. Intell. Rev.* [Internet], 55, 3, 1947–1999, 2022, Available from: https://doi.org/10.1007/s10462-021-10058-4.
75. Alipanahi, B., Delong, A., Weirauch, M.T., Frey, B.J., Predicting the sequence specificities of DNA- and RNA-binding proteins by deep learning. *Nat. Biotechnol.* [Internet], 33, 8, 831–838, 2015, Available from: https://doi.org/10.1038/nbt.3300.
76. Rajkomar, A., Oren, E., Chen, K. *et al.*, Scalable and accurate deep learning with electronic health records. *NPJ Digit. Med.* [Internet], 1, 1, 18, 2018, Available from: https://doi.org/10.1038/s41746-018-0029-1.
77. Fogel, D.B., Factors associated with clinical trials that fail and opportunities for improving the likelihood of success: A review. *Contemp. Clin. Trials Commun.* [Internet], 11, 156–164, 2018, Available from: https://pubmed.ncbi.nlm.nih.gov/30112460.
78. Romero, K., Ito, K., Rogers, J.A. *et al.*, The future is now: Model-based clinical trial design for Alzheimer's disease. *Clin. Pharmacol. Ther.*, 97, 3, 210–214, 2015.
79. Zhao, Y., Zeng, D., Socinski, M.A., Kosorok, M.R., Reinforcement learning strategies for clinical trials in nonsmall cell lung cancer. *Biometrics* [Internet], 67, 4, 1422–1433, 2011, Available from: https://pubmed.ncbi.nlm.nih.gov/21385164.
80. Wong, C.H., Siah, K.W., Lo, A.W., Estimation of clinical trial success rates and related parameters. *Biostatistics* [Internet], 20, 2, 273–286, 2019, Available from: https://doi.org/10.1093/biostatistics/kxx069.
81. Han, J., Chen, K., Fang, L. *et al.*, Improving the efficacy of the data entry process for clinical research with a natural language processing-driven medical information extraction system: Quantitative field research. *JMIR Med. Inform.*, 7, 3, e13331, 2019.
82. Fonferko-Shadrach, B., Lacey, A.S., Roberts, A. *et al.*, Using natural language processing to extract structured epilepsy data from unstructured clinic letters: Development and validation of the ExECT (extraction of epilepsy clinical text) system. *BMJ Open*, 9, 4, e023232, 2019.
83. Savova, G.K., Danciu, I., Alamudun, F. *et al.*, Use of natural language processing to extract clinical cancer phenotypes from electronic medical records. *Cancer Res.*, 79, 21, 5463–5470, 2019.
84. Malke, J.C., Jin, S., Camp, S.P. *et al.*, Enhancing case capture, quality, and completeness of primary melanoma pathology records via natural language processing. *JCO Clin. Cancer Inform.*, 3, 1–11, 2019.
85. Liu, Y. and Gopalakrishnan, V., An overview and evaluation of recent machine learning imputation methods using cardiac imaging data. *Data*, 2, 1, 8, 2017.
86. Phung, S., Kumar, A., Kim, J., A deep learning technique for imputing missing healthcare data. *Annu. Int. Conf. IEEE Eng. Med. Biol. Soc. IEEE Eng. Med. Biol. Soc. Annu. Int. Conf.*, vol. 2019, pp. 6513–6516, 2019.

87. Qiu, Y.L., Zheng, H., Gevaert, O., A deep learning framework for imputing missing values in genomic data. *bioRxiv* [Internet], 406066, 2018, Available from: http://biorxiv.org/content/early/2018/09/03/406066.abstract.
88. Luo, Y., Szolovits, P., Dighe, A.S., Baron, J.M., 3D-MICE: Integration of cross-sectional and longitudinal imputation for multi-analyte longitudinal clinical data. *J. Am. Med. Inform. Assoc.*, 25, 6, 645–653, 2018.
89. Ngufor, C., Warner, M.A., Murphree, D.H. *et al.*, Identification of clinically meaningful plasma transfusion subgroups using unsupervised random forest clustering. *AMIA ... Annu. Symp. Proceedings. AMIA Symp.*, vol. 2017, pp. 1332–1341, 2017.
90. Tomic, A., Tomic, I., Rosenberg-Hasson, Y., Dekker, C.L., Maecker, H.T., Davis, M.M., SIMON, an automated machine learning system, reveals immune signatures of influenza vaccine responses. *J. Immunol.*, 203, 3, 749–759, 2019.
91. Chavda, V.P., Chapter 4 - Nanobased nano drug delivery: A comprehensive review, in: *Micro and Nano Technologies*, S.S. Mohapatra, S. Ranjan, N. Dasgupta, R.K. Mishra, SBT-A Thomas of T.N.D., D.S. (Eds.), pp. 69–92, Elsevier, Amsterdam, 2019.
92. Chavda, V.P., Nanotherapeutics and nanobiotechnology, in: *Applications of Targeted Nano Drugs and Delivery Systems*, pp. 1–13, Elsevier, Amsterdam, 2019.
93. Javaid, M., Haleem, A., Singh, R.P., Suman, R., Artificial intelligence applications for industry 4.0: A literature-based study. *J. Ind. Integr. Manage.* [Internet], 07, 01, 83–111, 2021, Available from: https://doi.org/10.1142/S2424862221300040.
94. Hong, N., Liu, C., Gao, J. *et al.*, State of the art of machine learning-enabled clinical decision support in intensive care units: Literature review. *JMIR Med. Inform.*, 10, 3, e28781, 2022.
95. Zhang, C. and Lu, Y., Study on artificial intelligence: The state of the art and future prospects. *J. Ind. Inf. Integr.* [Internet], 23, 100224, 2021, Available from: https://www.sciencedirect.com/science/article/pii/S2452414X21000248.
96. Yin, J., Ngiam, K.Y., Teo, H.H., Role of artificial intelligence applications in real-life clinical practice: Systematic review. *J. Med. Internet Res.*, 23, 4, e25759, 2021.
97. Gupta, R., Srivastava, D., Sahu, M., Tiwari, S., Ambasta, R.K., Kumar, P., Artificial intelligence to deep learning: Machine intelligence approach for drug discovery. *Mol. Divers.* [Internet], 25, 3, 1315–1360, 2021, Available from: https://pubmed.ncbi.nlm.nih.gov/33844136.

Part III

BIOINFORMATICS TOOLS FOR HEALTHCARE SECTOR

13

Artificial Intelligence and Machine Learning in Healthcare Sector

Vivek P. Chavda[1], Kaushika Patel[2], Sachin Patel[3] and Vasso Apostolopoulos[4*]

[1]Department of Pharmaceutics and Pharmaceutical Technology, L M College of Pharmacy, Ahmedabad, Gujarat, India
[2]Department of Pharmaceutical Technology, L.J. Institute of Pharmacy, L J University, Ahmedabad, Gujarat, India
[3]Formulation & Development–OSD, Amneal Pharmaceuticals Pvt. Ltd, Ahmedabad, Gujarat, India
[4]Institute for Health and Sport, Victoria University, Melbourne, VIC, Australia

Abstract
Artificial Intelligence (AI) and Machine learning (ML) are the emerging areas that have a major potential to boost the healthcare services. AI/ML modalities have been integrated into multiple domains of clinical practice, biomedical research, and healthcare administration. The key categories involved are screening and daily fitness monitoring, diagnostic services in radiology, pathology, and gastroenterology, and assistance in clinical decision-making and palliative care. Nevertheless, the large-scale integration of AI/ML in healthcare faces formidable challenges such as increased installation and maintenance costs, medical errors with a potential to harm patients, gaps in AI-related ethical frameworks, unemployment and decreased capacity building among the human workforce. Currently, numerous entrepreneurial ventures have been developed in the context of innovation in healthcare AI/ML. Their products and services range from vitals' monitoring to advanced diagnostics. In a nutshell, AI/ML may play a crucial role in resolving the issues pertaining to complexity and up surging data in healthcare system. Altogether, AI/ML is a part of modern healthcare, whose further implementation is subject to comprehensively addressing relevant challenges.

Keywords: Artificial intelligence, machine leaning, AI/ML, healthcare, healthcare services, digital health, diagnosis, machine learning

**Corresponding author*: Vasso.Apostolopoulos@vu.edu.au

Vivek Chavda, Krishnan Anand and Vasso Apostolopoulos (eds.) Bioinformatics Tools for Pharmaceutical Drug Product Development, (287–314) © 2023 Scrivener Publishing LLC

Abbreviations

AI	Artificial Intelligence
ML	Machine Learning
IT	Information Technology
COVID19	Corona Virus Disease 2019
DNNs	Deep Neural Networks
CT	Computed Tomography
CXR	Chest x-ray
WSI	Whole-slide imaging
OCT	Optical coherence tomography
AMD	Age-related macular degeneration
ANN	Artificial neural networks
ECG	Electrocardiograms
EMR	Electronic medical records
FDA	Food drug administration
NLP	Natural language processing
RPA	Robotic process automation
TB	Tuberculosis
ICU	Intensive care unit
R&D	Research and development
HER	Electronic health record

13.1 Introduction

Artificial intelligence (AI) pertains by definition to a construct mimicking human intelligence intending to reduce human workload. AI has major potential to positively affect healthcare services. To date, diverse AI tools have been integrated into research and/or clinical practice related to both non-communicable (cancer, cardiovascular and neurological diseases) and communicable diseases [1].

AI is based on programming language enabling compatibility of its applications with the existing computational systems. Hence, these programs can be integrated into the information technology (IT) infrastructure of healthcare services and in devices used by patients, physicians, and researchers [2].

AI helps in prior detection and prognosis, treatment as well as the consequences with evaluation and clinical decision making. AI is raised in assisting the use of high-risk medications, such as vancomycin (antibiotic) which has a narrow therapeutic index, and requires close monitoring and records whilst patient administration [3].

Data provided by AI aids doctors and medical supervisors to provide accurate diagnoses and treatment plans. Tracking the spread of infectious diseases can be predicted by AI [4]. AI has played a crucial role in managing epidemics and pandemics including COVID-19. During COVID outbreak, 63 million deaths were reported worldwide but due to scientific consciousness and the use of AI tools, the COVID-19 pandemic was easy to deal with. Through this, and the impact AI has had in the healthcare sector, questions are raised and there are concerns that AI doctors one day will replace human doctors. AI sometimes removes the need for human decisions and hence proved that AI has become successful and grown in mimicking human intelligence [5].

The inclusion of machine learning into clinical healthcare promises the application of tools based on algorithms functioning independent of physicians and are ultimately of crucial help to healthcare workers. Commercial companies are emphasizing the use of ML in medical decision making in terms of the timely and analysis of data in the absence of physicians which is one of the major next generation requirements in the healthcare field. The algorithms used in ML might be a suitable substitution for physicians in the interpretation of images, especially in radiology and anatomy [6].

13.2 The Exponential Rise of AI/ML Solutions in Healthcare

There is an immense rise in the use of AI and related tools in healthcare systems. AI is bringing a standard shift in healthcare as it mimics human intelligence. AI is carrying ease of work towards humans and shares a major part in doing some major work which is time-consuming if human efforts are intended [7].

The transformation can be shown in eight ways:

1) **Keeping well**

   AI in healthcare reduces time and also reduces human efforts, works more efficiently and at a lower cost. We have achieved the threshold in the healthcare sector on the basis of the potential of AI.

2) **Early detection**
The failure of early diagnosis of disease by humans is rare. In addition, according to the American cancer society, mammograms of the cancer may depict false positive results predicting 1 to 2 healthy women in world with cancer [8]. AI however, enables 30 times faster detection with 99% accuracy.
3) **Diagnosis**
AI technology in combination with machine learning and system neuroscience builds powerful algorithms that mimic the human brain and is successful in the diagnosis of the disease that is comparable to the human diagnosticians [7].
4) **Decision making**
With the use of AI, appropriate and timely decisions may be taken, followed by, precise actions that enables identification of the risk to patients and accurate decisions can be made which can save patients' life with deadly diseases [9].
5) **Treatment**
AI provides great disease management for chronically ill patients who are at risk of adverse episodes. With better coordinated plans, AI improves patient compliance for the management of long-term treatment plans. Robots have also been used in executing certain operations in addition to their use in legs and rehabilitation [10].
6) **End of Life care**
Due to the lack of conversation, conditions like dementia or cardiovascular disorders, lead to premature death. As such, robots are used to remove the loneliness and coordinate with the patient [10].
7) **Research**
AI has also been implicated in the discovery and development of new drug molecule. AI may also be utilized to potentially curb the tenure and investment cost for the marketing of drugs [11].
8) **Training**
The training related to AI can be executed anywhere with the help of smart phones. Incorporating AI in difficult situations can help to resolve it, even during travelling. In recent years there is an immense growth in AI and we are developing knowledge of AI due to the COVID-19 pandemic [12].

Researchers have spent many hours to build improved technologies to alleviate the COVID-19 pandemic. Prominently AI/ML was used in the interpretation of COVID-19. AI was able to screen, predict the result in a better way giving timely responses and achieving the milestone in the establishment of AI in the healthcare field [5].

With the involvement of AI technology, drug candidates can be designed using computational chemistry techniques with the help of different software programs, enabling millions of drug compounds to be screened in a matter of days. As such, the time for the discovery of new drugs is drastically reduced. In the drug discovery process, the primary goal is to identify a specific medicine that treats required diseases by binding with a specific target molecule prevalent in that disease. Computational techniques and machine languages, have transformed research and development in Rapid drug Discoveries [13].

AI has overcome the obstacles by detecting novel interactions with small proteins. In fact, different digital tools are now available that continuously monitor the heartbeat, blood pressure and other vitals. In this modern era, we the humans are incomplete without a system that mimics the Human Intelligence which is known as Artificial intelligence [14].

ML as a subset of AI focuses on three important domains of healthcare namely medical imaging, natural language processing of medical documents and genetic information. These areas furthermore assist in the diagnosis, detection and prediction of diseases. Advancement in the digital technology may serve as a vital tool for the healthcare professionals in improving patient compliance towards treatment [15].

13.3 AI/ML Healthcare Solutions for Doctors

A three-tiered influence of AI is witnessed in medicine. Firstly, it influences clinicians, primarily through an accelerated and accurate interpretation of the image. Secondly, it influences health systems through improved workflow and reduced medical errors. Thirdly, it affects patients, as it allows them to handle their data for health promotion [16]. In the future, almost every sort of healthcare specialist will prefer AI technology, particularly ML [16]. Deep neural networks (DNNs) are primarily used to recognize patterns in pathology slides, medical scans, retinal pictures, skin lesions, endoscopy, electrocardiograms, vital signs, and faces [16]. Radiology is one field that has received much attention for AI/ML applications [17]. Several studies have compared the AI algorithms with doctors, for example, the CT (computed tomography) scans for the head (in case of brain hemorrhage, trauma, and acute neurological events) [18–20], CXR (Chest X-ray) scans (in case of metastatic nodules in lungs and multiple events) [21], breast cancer density diagnosis by mammography [22], and wrist X-rays (prospective study) [23]. According to a few retrospective studies, the Deep Learning of digitized pathology slides has the potential to increase interpretation accuracy and speed [16]. For example, AI has shown promising results in the pathological examination of breast cancer and its metastasis [24–26], brain tumors [27], and lung carcinoma [28]. Unfortunately, pathologists have been more skeptical than radiologists in embracing scan digitization [29]. The use of glass slides instead of digital images remains common in the field together with whole-slide imaging (WSI) to examine a whole sample of the tissue on a slide [29]. Gastroenterologists often face challenges in detecting small adenomatous or sessile polyps during colonoscopy. There have been reports on the clinical validation of AI in gastroenterology that have shown improved speed and accuracy during a real-time colonoscopy [30, 31].

DNNs' diagnostic accuracy is compared to dermatologists' for algorithms that classify skin cancer (skin cancers, melanoma, and skin lesions) using image analysis [32–34]. Quite dismally, these studies were not performed in a clinical context, where a clinician would conduct a physical examination and be responsible for providing an accurate diagnosis. Despite these issues, primary care clinicians identify the majority of skin lesions, and issues with inaccuracy have been emphasized. It would be a big breakthrough if AI can successfully encourage competent dermatologists. Several studies have compared the performance of algorithms and ophthalmologists in diagnosing various eye disorders. These include diabetic retinopathy [35–37], cataracts (congenital) [38], retinal diseases (OCT, optical coherence tomography) [39], macular degeneration [40], retinopathy of prematurity [41], and diabetic retinopathy and age-related macular degeneration (AMD) [42]. The accuracy of interpretation based on ANN was comparable with that of ophthalmologists in rare eye conditions, such as congenital cataracts and retinopathy of prematurity [41]. Electrocardiograms (ECG) and echocardiograms are the two most common images used by cardiologists in practice. DNNs have been used to assess these [43, 44]. The machine-read ECGs that relies on the rules-based algorithms mostly render inaccurate interpretations [45]. On the contrary, high sensitivity (93%) and specificity (90%) have been achieved using the deep learning-based diagnosis of heart attacks [46]. A DNN and six cardiologists assessed more than sixty-four thousand one-lead ECGs (>29,000 patients) for arrhythmia. The accuracy was comparable across fourteen electrical conduction disturbances [47]. A DNN and cardiologists categorized a limited group of 267 patient studies into 15 conventional views for echocardiography. The algorithm's overall accuracy for single still images was 92 percent, whereas for certified echocardiographers' accuracy was 79 percent. This, however, does not represent the actual reading of studies, which are video loops in motion [43]. The classification of pulmonary artery hypertension, cardiac amyloid, and hypertrophic cardiomyopathy is highly accurate for more than eight thousand echocardiograms included in a retrospective study [44]. In the field of mental health, digital tracking of mood and depression through interactive chatbots, sensors, facial recognition, voice, speech, and keyboard interaction, are among the techniques in development [48–52]. Prediction of depression diagnosis for electronic medical records documentation has been reported through social media, such as Facebook posts [53]. ML has been used to characterize depression [54–56], predict suicide [54, 57–59], antidepressant medication [60], and psychosis bouts in patients suffering from schizophrenia [61]. AI has its utility in various clinical settings and clinicians. These include neurologists (stroke facilitation, diagnosis of electroencephalograms) [62], anesthesiologists (helps them monitor oxygen levels while performing the surgery) [63], oncologists (in searching appropriate clinical trials) [64], breast cancer patients (pre-empting surgery) [65], and congenital disease diagnosis through facial recognition [66].

13.4 AI/ML Solution for Patients

AI has the potential to affect millions of patients and is now being employed in medicine to improve healthcare by ramping up processes and improving their accuracy. This has paved the way for improved healthcare in general [67]. ML evaluates patients' electronic medical records (EMR) and pathology slides, assisting in the patient diagnosis and treatment options [68]. Early accomplishments including radiological image processing, ChatBots, smartwatches, smartphones, and diagnostic tools have fueled interest in AI applications in healthcare [16, 69–77]. For example, AI has been used to aid in the diagnosis and evaluation of dementia patients and their families [78]. Further, AI is looked upon as the future of diabetes care in patients as it will enable a fundamental change in diabetes care, different from prevalent management strategies and more towards data-driven precision care [79]. Further, the FDA has approved smartwatch algorithms for detecting atrial fibrillation, and recording ECG and its interpretation (based on the heart rate of the user at rest and while performing physical activity [69–71]. There are speculations that the widespread use of such algorithms, particularly among low-risk, young people who wear smartwatches, which may result in a large number of false-positive atrial fibrillation diagnoses and unnecessary medical investigations. However, these smartwatches have an in-built DL algorithm that is capable of reading the ECG and accurately detecting fluctuations in the blood-potassium levels. This information is critical in patients diagnosed with renal diseases. Furthermore, ear infections, skin lesions and rashes, retinal illnesses (age-related macular degeneration and diabetic retinopathy), and migraine headaches are among the conditions for which AI-based smartphone tests are being developed. AiCure, for example, is a smartphone app that uses AI to track medicinal adherence (NCT02243670). Here, patients record their videos while consuming the prescribed medicine. Some other apps calculate calorie content in a food item using image recognition. To increase trust levels, efforts are directed to employ AI nearest-neighbor analysis for finding matches for connecting patients with desired doctors [72, 73]. Thus, AI-based technological intervention aids in disseminating critical information on patient health credit to its user-friendly approach.

While there is a hype regarding these new technologies, not much research has been done on "how AI could be used safely in clinical practice?" Notably, there has been a negligible involvement with patients, who would be affected by AI in healthcare applications. This is worrisome as patient anxieties regarding AI could be a major impediment to the widespread adoption and usage of these tools. Reportedly, public perception of non-medical AI varies, with elements including media coverage and prior experiences. These cumulatively affect public opinion on non-medical AI [80]. These factors emphasize the significance of patient engagement in ensuring that these technologies are incorporated into healthcare in a way that builds public trust and alleviate common patient concerns, which could lead to "AI Winter" [81–83].

Furthermore, because patients are the main beneficiaries of most of these AI innovations, it is critical to understand their priorities, values, and needs. It is important to ensure that these advancements are well-received, developed, and implemented in an ethical manner that aids in improved patient outcomes. Even though patients do not engage with AI technologies directly, they are the ones who are most at risk posed by the unethical implementation of technology [84]. There is an ethical need to guarantee that patient needs and values are included in the implementation plans to the extent that they are willing to accept the AI application-associated risks in healthcare. Proactive patient participation, as in other fields of medical research, is a critical element of the ethical implementation of AI healthcare [85].

In medicine, AI/ML applications make use of massive amounts of clinical data and computing power to aid evidence-based decision-making [16]. This introduces additional ethical concerns about data use transparency, data stewardship accountability, and potential disparities in AI implementation [86]. Presently, relatively insufficient research has been conducted to characterize the perspectives of patients and other stakeholders on AI applications in healthcare. Furthermore, the few studies that have looked at patient perspectives have only included a limited set of AI tools. This limits their usefulness as a predictor of patient participation with additional AI applications in healthcare [10, 87]. Patient participation in particular AI applications is a significant aspect of the process of research and development. However, the analysis of wider public opinions on AI-assisted healthcare is not facilitated by such engagement. This is critical for implementation design, health policy development, and innovation priority setting.

Several patient concerns could dampen interest in AI/ML uses in healthcare. For example, patients are concerned about AI's safety, dangers to patient choice, possible hikes in healthcare expenses, bias in the source of data, and data security, among other things. Therefore, acceptance of AI by patients is predicated on reducing these potential risks, and addressing these challenges proactively is crucial for the growth of ethical innovation and the long-term viability of AI applications in healthcare [75].

Recently there is an increasing insistence on applying ML to procure refined interferences along the care continuum. ML implements SMS alerts and relevant, subtle content that promises timely actions and hence is essential in the field of research [7].

13.5 AI Solutions for Administrators

AI has numerous administrative applications in the healthcare sector. In comparison to patient care, the use of AI in medical settings is less revolutionary. However, AI in hospital administration can be substantially efficient. Clinical documentation, processing claims, management of medical records and revenue cycle are some of the preferred uses for AI/ML in patient care. ML application of AI is used for payment and claims administration in healthcare, wherein it pairs data from distinct databases. The providers and insurers must verify the submitted claims for their accuracy. To ascertain and sort out the errors in codes eliminate inaccurate claims saving money, time and resources for all the parties concerned [88].

It is no wonder that the diagnostic implications of AI in healthcare using the concept of ML has received the most attention as it has the potential to bring many significant improvements to the healthcare administration in the future. AI-enabled technologies have the potential to reduce administrative and clinical burnout whilst also enhancing overall employee satisfaction. Intelligent data capture software can now automatically learn identification, classification, and extraction of information related to patients from the documentation. Further, these documents are indexed for incorporation into the records of the patients. All this is possible due to the progress in natural language processing (NLP) and unsupervised machine learning. Consequently, there will be a decline in the requirement for administrators for direct handling of data, which in turn, will minimize the risks concerning errors or omissions for data entry. The issue of cybersecurity can be addressed by organizations will simplifying and strengthening their cybersecurity operations using advanced security technologies. This will enable them to focus on updating internal security rules and processes. Further, AI may be able to assist in resolving the persistent issue of data interoperability [89].

RPA (robotic process automation) refers to software robots with ML capabilities that enable automation of everything from patient admissions to billing. Human language can be comprehended and processed using NLP. The administrative documentation operations, such as transcript and patient-case summary preparation can be automated using NLP. Prior authorization, processing of bills and claims, and provider productivity are the key areas where AI might improve administrative procedures. Prior authorization deals with the identification of the medical and pharmacological benefits of the patients as well as their health plan. Here, it becomes crucial to determine which medications or health services need prior authorization for extracting benefits for each patient's particular health plan. Finally, it includes seeking approval for patient documentation collection and provision. As several hospitals and providers handle a huge number of prior authorizations on daily basis, AI-powered NLP and RPA may enable automation of these. Claims processing and billing are cost- and time-extensive. RPA can be employed for entering, processing, and adjusting the claims, which makes them reliable and simpler. Further, clinical notes can be converted into standardized codes using NLP. AI can be a promising approach in eliminating manual tasks, such as documentation of patients' summaries and chart notes, noting prescriptions and testing orders, etc., which divert the providers from the direct care of the patients. AI-based automation is expected to improve provider productivity rendering improved patient care. Therefore, AI improves productivity, patient care, and provider efficiency while lowering administrative costs [90].

ML serves to resolve the issues pertaining to claims and payment administration by feasibly matching data across the different databases. It helps the Insurers in the verification of the authenticity of the claims. Reliable identification, accurate analysis, correct codes and incorrect claims saves all parties involved i.e. health insurers, governments and providers alike , a great deal of time, money and effort [7].

For example, the AI platform from Olive (https://oliveai.com/) enables the automation of the most time-consuming processes in the healthcare industry. Anything from checking eligibility to claims (unadjudicated) and migration of data is automated. This allows the administrators to focus on higher-level responsibilities providing an improved patient experience. Further, to improve the patient experience, the Cleveland

Clinic (http://my.clevelandclinic.org/) is employing AI to collect data from abundant administrative and health-record data points. This, in turn, helps individuals customize their healthcare regimens.

13.6 Factors Affecting the AI/ML Implementation in the Healthcare Sector

AI is highly capable in healthcare sector in scientific work, but there are only a few, mostly minor, authentic AI applications in the preventative, diagnostic and treatment domains [91]. Our selection and study of success criteria for AI adoption attempt to bridge the gap between considerable academic AI developments in recent years and the comparatively low practical use in healthcare. Today, private and governmental entities may already exploit AI implementation based on recognized results, driving the applicability from scientific development to real-world. Additional success criteria might include trustworthy methods, data management rules and risk level evaluations. Because the success elements are interconnected, future research should focus on their optimal interaction to fully use the potential of AI in real-world applications.

13.6.1 High Cost

Plenty of time and resources are required to create a machine that can work like humans or in a better way and can cost a huge amount of money. Artificial intelligence needs to operate on the latest software and hardware, and requirements, thus making it costlier. Even its repair and maintenance have large expenses [92]. AI-based software programs need regular up-gradation to cope with changing environment. It needs to become smarter day by day. In case of a severe breakdown of the system, the process of recovering the lost codes and reinstalling the system requires a huge amount [93].

Company	Cost required	To set up
Apple	$200 million	SIRI
Amazon	$26 million	Alexa

Similarly, AI methods are also used in clinical practice and even in the self-management of diabetes. AI is used to design patterns for either high or low blood sugar levels in diabetes patients. The devices which have such kind of system in it are also costlier to purchase. One of these is Glucometer a small portable machine used to measure glucose in the blood [94]. The price of it is Rs. 500 which is quite not affordable for every person. Recently, a device called Pulse Oximetry was used extensively during the COVID-19 pandemic. It was used to measure the oxygen level of the blood. It was sold at a much higher rate during that pandemic [5].

13.6.2 Lack of Creativity

AI can learn over time from its experiences however, AI cannot be creative in its approach. It cannot create its own algorithms or codes. Errors in the machine cannot be solved by themselves. AI requires human input. AI is not capable to learn to think out of the box [95]. It works effectively and efficiently even better than human beings but one cannot build human intelligence in a machine [96]. Humans can use data around them and can use their minds to make decisions. Whereas, AI needs a huge amount of data for processing something as simple as editing a text. AI can help in designing or creating but cannot compete with the human brain. Their ability is just limited to the person who programs and commands them. Therefore, creativity and imagination are not the forte of AI [97].

13.6.3 Errors Potentially Harming Patients

Any error in the ML/AI system can cause a threat to a patient's life. Self-destruction of machines may happen if the input of data is in the wrong hands and the results might be hazardous for humans. Say, for example, the patient may take a wrongly recommended drug or a tumor can be missed by a radiological scan or it might allocate a hospital bed wrongly which is already occupied by one of the patients which lead to discomfort for that patient, this all occurs due to error in AI's system [98]. Patients react differently when an error occurs either due to software or provider. A single AI system's error can take thousands of patient's life, instead, there might be a limited number of patients who may get injured by a single doctor's mistake [7].

13.6.4 Privacy Issues

It is a serious problem related to patient data. On one side, researchers are attempting to protect the data of the patient but on the other side, hackers find ways to get access [99]. Even giant companies like Google have privacy data issues. AI can predict information about a patient using past details. AI also has a function called "Clearview face recognition", through which it captures the user's photo so that whenever next time the patient visit and if he/she may not have come up with their details, that function can be useful just by recognizing the user by taking his/her photo and thus can retrieve all the information belonging to them [100]. But hackers exploit the photo of the user in multiple apps. One such app is DeepFake in which anyone can put the face of the person on the body of the other. This is then prone to various malpractices [101].

13.6.5 Increase in Unemployment

AI seems to have an impact on the unemployment rate. AI displace the work of doctors from the tasks which they were performing previously [102]. A lot of money has been already spent on developing AI system so why would someone appoint laborers for a particular job as they are getting their work done within less time and even more efficiently than a person (labor) do. McKinsey predicted that AI will replace at least 30% of human labor by 2030. Human interference has decreased as AI is replacing the majority of repetitive tasks with robots. Also, we know machines are much better at working than humans [103].

13.6.6 Lack of Ethics

Machines like humans can never make a bond with other people. Machines do not have any emotions or moral values [104]. They can't even understand how the patients feel when ill. Humans have effective communication skills. Humans can transfer knowledge, understand the data, and can judge the quality of any given data [105].

13.6.7 Promotes a Less-Effort Culture Among Human Workers

AI is automating the majority of its work. Humans are getting addicted to these inventions which can cause problems for future generations. To make our work easier and faster, we thereby get dependent on such systems and have become lazier [106]. Physical activity gets reduced; eyesight problems, weight gain, and mental stress are different perspectives of getting dependent on machines.

13.7 AI/ML Based Healthcare Start-Ups

From the available domains for AI/ML applications, one with tremendous significance is the healthcare sector. AI is associated with many of current most significant healthcare innovations. For example, AI assisted in the recovery from the global impact of the COVID-19 pandemic through early detection of COVID-19 for patient assistance and repurposing of the drug. The need for Healthtech start-ups is increasing rapidly. With greater access to technology, increasing digital health and wellness awareness amongst

Table 13.1 AI/ML based healthcare start-ups in India.

Start-ups	**Website**	**Product developed**	**Application in healthcare**
NIRAMAI Health Analytix (health tech startup)	https://www.niramai.com/	Thermalytix: AI-based high-resolution thermal sensor	Early detection of breast cancer in clinical settings
qure.ai	https://www.qure.ai/	-	Interpretation of radiology images and scans using deep learning algorithms, provide community solutions for tuberculosis (TB), public health, and COVID-19
HealthifyMe (Platform for digital health and wellness)	https://www.healthifyme.com/	Ria: AI-based virtual assistant	Provides fitness, health and nutrition solutions, and recommends diet to its users, tracks their calorie intake and furnish health guidance
PharmEasy (Smartphone-based application)	https://pharmeasy.in/	-	Uses ML and big data tools to connect users with pharmacies for quick and easy medical delivery

(Continued)

Table 13.1 AI/ML based healthcare start-ups in India. (*Continued*)

Start-ups	**Website**	**Product developed**	**Application in healthcare**
SigTuple Technologies	https://sigtuple.com/	AI platform and Automated digital microscope	Ophthalmology and pathology: AI-based automation of medical data
OncoStem Diagnostics	https://www.oncostem.com/	CanAssist: Statistical models based on data support vector machines are used for assigning risk scores for tumor patients. Five cancer biomarkers, and patients' clinical and pathological data are used for risk score assignment.	Assessment of tumor aggressiveness and identification of recurrence risk characteristics
Artelus	https://artelus.com/	AI-based (deep learning) contactless diabetic retinopathy screening system	Performs an eye examination in < 3 minutes

(*Continued*)

Table 13.1 AI/ML based healthcare start-ups in India. (*Continued*)

Start-ups	**Website**	**Product developed**	**Application in healthcare**
Tricog	https://www.tricog.com/	InstaECG: cloud-connected cardiac device	Quick (within 10 minutes) interpretation and analysis of ECG reports
		InstaEcho: cloud-connected cardiac device	Quick and accurate diagnosis of echocardiogram
Quotient Health	https://www.quotientbd.com/	-	Use ML to reduce the cost of supporting EMR [electronic medical records] systems to obtain improved care at a lower cost.
KenSci	https://www.kensci.com/	-	Use ML to predict illness and treatment to help physicians and payers intervene earlier, predict population health risk by identifying patterns and surfacing high risk markers and model disease progression and more.

(*Continued*)

Table 13.1 AI/ML based healthcare start-ups in India. (*Continued*)

Start-ups	**Website**	**Product developed**	**Application in healthcare**
Quantitative Insights	https://www.quantinsights.com/	-	Use ML to improve the speed and accuracy of breast cancer diagnosis with its computer assisted breast MRI workstation Quantx.
Orderly Health	https://orderlyhealth.com/	-	Use ML to develop as "an automated, 24/7 concierge for healthcare" via text, email, Slack, video-conferencing
MD Insider	https://mdinsider.com/		Use ML to better match patients with doctors.
Beta Bionics	https://www.betabionics.com/	-	With the help of ML develops a wearable "bionic" pancreas it calls the iLet, which manages blood sugar levels around the clock in those with Type 1 diabetes."

(*Continued*)

Table 13.1 AI/ML based healthcare start-ups in India. (*Continued*)

Start-ups	Website	Product developed	Application in healthcare
BERG	https://www.berghealth.com/	-	Interrogative Biology platform employs ML for disease mapping and treatments in oncology, neurology and other rare conditions

the consumers, and investors pouring in, the ground for modern healthcare is under creation. As demand for remote healthcare rises, the industry's playing field is unlocked for upheaval. The desire for a positive change with high financial returns has found takers between both the founders of medical start-ups and investors and the industry's future seems bright.

Many major tech businesses and start-ups are working hard to improve natural language processing to eliminate the requirement for keyboards and human scribes during clinic visits [107]. Augmedix, Google, Microsoft, Suki, DeepScribe, Robin Healthcare, Saykara, Sopris Health, Tenor.ai, Carevoice, Notable, Orbita, and Sensely are among the firms operating in this field. Some of the companies that have introduced AI-based healthcare in India include NIRAMAI Health Analytix, qure.ai, HealthifyMe, PharmEasy, SigTuple Technologies, and OncoStem Diagnostics, Artelus, and Tricog. Many start ups have also been invented based on ML concept like Quotient Health, KenSci, Quantitative Insights, Orderly health and many others. Few of the start-ups are described below in Table 13.1.

13.8 Opportunities and Risks for Future

AI/ML offers several opportunities for the future growth in the healthcare sector. For example, PathAI (https://www.pathai.com/) has developed machine and deep learning algorithms, which help pathologists to diagnose cancer more precisely. PathAI aims to provide patients with error-free diagnoses and effective treatments. Various AI interventions in healthcare are as follows:

13.8.1 Patient Mobility Monitoring

In a hospital, multiple patients may have been admitted to an intensive care unit (ICU) and are under the watch of limited nursing staff. So, it will be difficult for nurses to take care of multiple patients hence, this factor will affect the treatment of patients. Monitoring their activities is important. So, researchers installed sensors equipped with Machine learning algorithms in ICU to track patient mobility and give notifications to the staff when patients are in trouble [108].

13.8.2 Clinical Trials for Drug Development

Drug development and its trial incur huge costs and time with significantly lower success rates [109]. The success rates for the clinical trials of the developed drugs are soaring due to poor selection of the patient cohort and criteria for their recruitment together with ineffective patient monitoring [110]. AI techniques have matured to t1 the point that they can be used in real-world situations to help human decision-makers. AI can upgrade clinical trial success rates by transforming critical aspects of study design from planning to execution, therefore reducing pharma Research and Development (R&D) costs. AI developments can be utilized to revamp crucial steps and in clinical trial design for improving trial success rates [110].

13.8.3 Quality of Electronic Health Records (EHR)

Traditionally, clinicians either prefer to note down or would type patient-related information, inviting human error. With the use of AI and speech recognition technology, however, interaction with the patient can be documented more precisely in near-real-time [111].

13.8.4 Robot-Assisted Surgery

Al-supported robots assist surgeons to make more accurate movements. Many hospitals use AI to conduct abdominal surgeries and also have developed robotic technology to perform surgery on the brain and to suture blood vessels [112].

As every coin has two sides, there are associated risks due to AI in the healthcare sector also along with the benefits. As summarized in above sections the risk components involved are privacy issues, unemployment due to lack of job, ethical implications, safety concern due to involvement of machines, algorithmic bias predicting greater likelihood of disease on the basis of gender or race despite of being not the causal factor and lack of transparency as deep learning algorithms used for image analysis are virtually impossible to interpret or explain [7].

13.9 Conclusion and Perspectives

Digital technologies like AI and ML are the future within the healthcare sector due to the exciting and progressive opportunities they have to offer in the area. The simultaneous understanding of various disciplines like informatics, biology, chemistry and computer science enable the profound understanding of genetic and environmental factors contributing to the emergence of complex diseases. AI/ML has potential to play pivotal roles in the evolution of precision medicine, which is recognized worldwide as a need of advancement in healthcare. Even though prior endeavors for diagnosis and therapeutic proposals have been arduous, it is believed that AI will eventually surmount that domain as well. AI in collaboration with ML has made significant breakthroughs in imaging processing due to the fact that scan analysis is often done using machines. Incorporating ML to develop a reliable method of understanding the genomic landscape interlinks across genes to bestow to inherent cancer risk could contribute immensely in the improvement of patient healthcare on an individual level. AI-based applications, such as speech and text recognition find their way into recording clinical notes and communicating with patients. The most difficult hurdle for AI in the majority of healthcare set-ups is assuring their acceptance in everyday clinical practice. Regulatory approval, EHR integration, standardization and consistency of products introduced, clinician-friendly, regular up-gradation, and purchase by public or private domains, are important considerations for the clinical success and acceptance of AI-based applications. Given the fact that AI-based technologies are still in their infancy with limited applications, they need to make a yet longer journey to realize the above-mentioned goals. Further, AI technologies will boost clinical efforts for patient care rather than substitute clinicians. Human healthcare professionals may gradually involve in the procedures and job designs that count on inherent human skills, such as persuasion, compassion and broad view integration. Conclusively, AI and ML will become an integral component of the healthcare system at all levels.

The exhaustive data collection possible with AI will benefit the healthcare professionals in the accurate diagnosis and the treatment of complex diseases in the future. The in-depth knowledge of genetic variation contributing to individual susceptibility enables both the patients and doctors to make early lifestyle changes for the preventive measures. Additionally it will allow the physicians to predict most suitable prognostics and diagnostics relevant for a particular patient, making the treatment time and cost effective, while improving patient output and compliance in the long run. Just as AI started Turing decoding the riddle machine, it would become possible to decrypt the secrets of the human body and genomics with the assistance of AI and machine learning. Being one of the most promising and consequential technologies to impact human societies, it will require continuous watch and implementation of thoughtful policy in the upcoming years.

References

1. Miller, D.D. and Brown, E.W., Artificial intelligence in medical practice: The question to the answer? *Am. J. Med.*, 131, 2, 129–133, 2018.
2. Tahri Sqalli, M. and Al-Thani, D., On how chronic conditions affect the patient-AI interaction: A literature review. *Healthcare*, 8, 3, 313, 2020.
3. Wang, Z., Ong, C.L.J., Fu, Z., AI models to assist vancomycin dosage titration. *Front. Pharmacol.*, 13, 801928, 2022.
4. Agrebi, S. and Larbi, A., Use of artificial intelligence in infectious diseases, in: *Artificial Intelligence in Precision Health*, pp. 415–438, 2020.
5. Islam, M.N., Inan, T.T., Rafi, S., Akter, S.S., Sarker, I.H., Islam, A.K.M.N., A systematic review on the use of AI and ML for fighting the COVID-19 pandemic. *IEEE Trans. Artif. Intell.*, 1, 3, 258–270, 2020.
6. Char, D.S., Shah, N.H., Magnus, D., Implementing machine learning in healthcare — Addressing ethical challenges. *N. Engl. J. Med.*, 378, 11, 981–983, 2018.
7. Davenport, T. and Kalakota, R., The potential for artificial intelligence in healthcare. *Future Healthc. J.*, 6, 2, 94–98, 2019.
8. Kenner, B.J., Abrams, N.D., Chari, S.T. *et al.*, Early detection of pancreatic cancer. *Pancreas*, 50, 7, 916–922, 2021.
9. Lu, K. and Liao, H., A survey of group decision making methods in healthcare Industry 4.0: Bibliometrics, applications, and directions. *Appl. Intell.*, 1–25, 2022.
10. Stai, B., Heller, N., McSweeney, S. *et al.*, Public perceptions of artificial intelligence and robotics in medicine. *J. Endourol.*, 34, 10, 1041–1048, 2020.
11. Gupta, R., Srivastava, D., Sahu, M., Tiwari, S., Ambasta, R.K., Kumar, P., Artificial intelligence to deep learning: Machine intelligence approach for drug discovery. *Mol. Diversity*, 25, 3, 1315–1360, 2021.

12. Zhang, K., Liu, X., Shen, J. *et al.*, Clinically applicable AI system for accurate diagnosis, quantitative measurements, and prognosis of COVID-19 pneumonia using computed tomography. *Cell*, 181, 6, 1423–1433, e1411, 2020.
13. Erickson, B.J., Korfiatis, P., Akkus, Z., Kline, T.L., Machine learning for medical imaging. *RadioGraphics*, 37, 2, 505–515, 2017.
14. Esmaeilzadeh, P., Use of AI-based tools for healthcare purposes: A survey study from consumers' perspectives. *BMC Med. Inf. Decis. Making*, 20, 1, 170, 2020.
15. Toh, C.P. and Brody, J., Applications of machine learning in healthcare, in: *Smart Manufacturing - When Artificial Intelligence Meets the Internet of Things*, 2021.
16. Topol, E.J., High-performance medicine: The convergence of human and artificial intelligence. *Nat. Med.*, 25, 1, 44–56, 2019.
17. Wang, X., Peng, Y., Lu, L., Lu, Z., Bagheri, M., Summers, R.M., ChestX-Ray8: Hospital-scale chest x-ray database and benchmarks on weakly-supervised classification and localization of common thorax diseases, in: *2017 IEEE Conference on Computer Vision and Pattern Recognition (CVPR)*, pp. 3462–3471, 2017.
18. Arbabshirani, M.R., Fornwalt, B.K., Mongelluzzo, G.J. *et al.*, Advanced machine learning in action: Identification of intracranial hemorrhage on computed tomography scans of the head with clinical workflow integration. *NPJ Digital Med.*, 1, 1, 9, 2018.
19. Chilamkurthy, S., Ghosh, R., Tanamala, S. *et al.*, Deep learning algorithms for detection of critical findings in head CT scans: A retrospective study. *Lancet*, 392, 10162, 2388–2396, 2018.
20. Titano, J.J., Badgeley, M., Schefflein, J. *et al.*, Automated deep-neural-network surveillance of cranial images for acute neurologic events. *Nat. Med.*, 24, 9, 1337–1341, 2018.
21. Eapen, G.A., Singh, R., Kalra, M.K. *et al.*, Deep learning in chest radiography: Detection of findings and presence of change. *PLoS One*, 13, 10, e0204155, 2018.
22. Lehman, C.D., Yala, A., Schuster, T. *et al.*, Mammographic breast density assessment using deep learning: Clinical implementation. *Radiology*, 290, 1, 52–58, 2019.
23. Nam, J.G., Park, S., Hwang, E.J. *et al.*, Development and validation of deep learning–based automatic detection algorithm for malignant pulmonary nodules on chest radiographs. *Radiology*, 290, 1, 218–228, 2019.
24. Liu, Y., Kohlberger, T., Norouzi, M. *et al.*, Artificial intelligence–based breast cancer nodal metastasis detection: Insights into the black box for pathologists. *Arch. Pathol. Lab. Med.*, 143, 7, 859–868, 2018.
25. Steiner, D.F., MacDonald, R., Liu, Y. *et al.*, Impact of deep learning assistance on the histopathologic review of lymph nodes for metastatic breast cancer. *Am. J. Surg. Pathol.*, 42, 12, 1636–1646, 2018.

26. Ehteshami Bejnordi, B., Veta, M., Johannes van Diest, P. *et al.*, Diagnostic assessment of deep learning algorithms for detection of lymph node metastases in women with breast cancer. *JAMA*, 318, 22, 2199–2210, 2017.
27. Capper, D., Jones, D.T.W., Sill, M. *et al.*, DNA methylation-based classification of central nervous system tumours. *Nature*, 555, 7697, 469–474, 2018.
28. Coudray, N., Ocampo, P.S., Sakellaropoulos, T. *et al.*, Classification and mutation prediction from non–small cell lung cancer histopathology images using deep learning. *Nat. Med.*, 24, 10, 1559–1567, 2018.
29. Acs, B. and Rimm, D.L., Not just digital pathology, intelligent digital pathology. *JAMA Oncol.*, 4, 3, e253–e261, 2018.
30. Mori, Y., Kudo, S-e, Misawa, M. *et al.*, Real-time use of artificial intelligence in identification of diminutive polyps during colonoscopy. *Ann. Intern. Med.*, 169, 6, 357–366, 2018.
31. Wang, P., Xiao, X., Glissen Brown, J.R. *et al.*, Development and validation of a deep-learning algorithm for the detection of polyps during colonoscopy. *Nat. Biomed. Eng.*, 2, 10, 741–748, 2018.
32. Yang, S.J., Berndl, M., Michael Ando, D. *et al.*, Assessing microscope image focus quality with deep learning. *BMC Bioinform.*, 19, 1, 77, 2018.
33. Esteva, A., Kuprel, B., Novoa, R.A. *et al.*, Dermatologist-level classification of skin cancer with deep neural networks. *Nature*, 542, 7639, 115–118, 2017.
34. Haenssle, H.A., Fink, C., Schneiderbauer, R. *et al.*, Man against machine: Diagnostic performance of a deep learning convolutional neural network for dermoscopic melanoma recognition in comparison to 58 dermatologists. *Ann. Oncol.*, 29, 8, 1836–1842, 2018.
35. Abràmoff, M.D., Lavin, P.T., Birch, M., Shah, N., Folk, J.C., Pivotal trial of an autonomous AI-based diagnostic system for detection of diabetic retinopathy in primary care offices. *NPJ Digital Med.*, 1, 1, 695–698, 2018.
36. Kanagasingam, Y., Xiao, D., Vignarajan, J., Preetham, A., Tay-Kearney, M.-L., Mehrotra, A., Evaluation of artificial intelligence–based grading of diabetic retinopathy in primary care. *JAMA Netw. Open*, 1, 5, e182665, 2018.
37. Gulshan, V., Peng, L., Coram, M. *et al.*, Development and validation of a deep learning algorithm for detection of diabetic retinopathy in retinal fundus photographs. *JAMA*, 316, 22, 2402–2410, 2016.
38. Long, E., Lin, H., Liu, Z. *et al.*, An artificial intelligence platform for the multihospital collaborative management of congenital cataracts. *Nat. Biomed. Eng.*, 1, 2, 1553–1560, 2017.
39. De Fauw, J., Ledsam, J.R., Romera-Paredes, B. *et al.*, Clinically applicable deep learning for diagnosis and referral in retinal disease. *Nat. Med.*, 24, 9, 1342–1350, 2018.
40. Burlina, P.M., Joshi, N., Pekala, M., Pacheco, K.D., Freund, D.E., Bressler, N.M., Automated grading of age-related macular degeneration from color fundus images using deep convolutional neural networks. *JAMA Ophthalmol.*, 135, 11, 1170–1176, 2017.

41. Brown, J.M., Campbell, J.P., Beers, A. *et al.*, Automated diagnosis of plus disease in retinopathy of prematurity using deep convolutional neural networks. *JAMA Ophthalmol.*, 136, 7, 803–810, 2018.
42. Kermany, D.S., Goldbaum, M., Cai, W. *et al.*, Identifying medical diagnoses and treatable diseases by image-based deep learning. *Cell*, 172, 5, 1122–1131. e1129, 2018.
43. Madani, A., Arnaout, R., Mofrad, M., Arnaout, R., Fast and accurate view classification of echocardiograms using deep learning. *NPJ Digital Med.*, 1, 1, 6, 2018.
44. Zhang, J., Gajjala, S., Agrawal, P. *et al.*, Fully automated echocardiogram interpretation in clinical practice. *Circulation*, 138, 16, 1623–1635, 2018.
45. Willems, J.L., Abreu-Lima, C., Arnaud, P. *et al.*, The diagnostic performance of computer programs for the interpretation of electrocardiograms. *N. Engl. J. Med.*, 325, 25, 1767–1773, 1991.
46. Strodthoff, N. and Strodthoff, C., Detecting and interpreting myocardial infarction using fully convolutional neural networks. *Physiol. Meas.*, 40, 1, 015001, 2019.
47. Hannun, A.Y., Rajpurkar, P., Haghpanahi, M. *et al.*, Cardiologist-level arrhythmia detection and classification in ambulatory electrocardiograms using a deep neural network. *Nat. Med.*, 25, 1, 65–69, 2019.
48. Cao, B., Zheng, L., Zhang, C. *et al.*, DeepMood: Modeling mobile phone typing dynamics for mood detection, in: *Proceedings of the 23rd ACM SIGKDD International Conference on Knowledge Discovery and Data Mining*, pp. 747–755, 2017.
49. Mohr, D.C., Riper, H., Schueller, S.M., A solution-focused research approach to achieve an implementable revolution in digital mental health. *JAMA Psychiatry*, 75, 2, 113–114, 2018.
50. Barrett, P.M., Steinhubl, S.R., Muse, E.D., Topol, E.J., Digitising the mind. *Lancet*, 389, 10082, 1877, 2017.
51. Firth, J., Torous, J., Nicholas, J. *et al.*, The efficacy of smartphone-based mental health interventions for depressive symptoms: A meta-analysis of randomized controlled trials. *World Psychiatry*, 16, 3, 287–298, 2017.
52. Fitzpatrick, K.K., Darcy, A., Vierhile, M., Delivering cognitive behavior therapy to young adults with symptoms of depression and anxiety using a fully automated conversational agent (Woebot): A randomized controlled trial. *JMIR Ment. Health*, 4, 2, e19, 2017.
53. Eichstaedt, J.C., Smith, R.J., Merchant, R.M. *et al.*, Facebook language predicts depression in medical records. *Proc. Natl. Acad. Sci.*, 115, 44, 11203–11208, 2018.
54. Schnyer, D.M., Clasen, P.C., Gonzalez, C., Beevers, C.G., Evaluating the diagnostic utility of applying a machine learning algorithm to diffusion tensor MRI measures in individuals with major depressive disorder. *Psychiatry Res.: Neuroimaging*, 264, 1–9, 2017.

55. Reece, A.G. and Danforth, C.M., Instagram photos reveal predictive markers of depression. *EPJ Data Sci.*, 6, 1, 1–2, 2017.
56. Wager, T.D. and Woo, C.-W., Imaging biomarkers and biotypes for depression. *Nat. Med.*, 23, 1, 16–17, 2017.
57. Walsh, C.G., Ribeiro, J.D., Franklin, J.C., Predicting risk of suicide attempts over time through machine learning. *Clin. Psychol. Sci.*, 5, 3, 457–469, 2017.
58. Franklin, J.C., Ribeiro, J.D., Fox, K.R. *et al.*, Risk factors for suicidal thoughts and behaviors: A meta-analysis of 50 years of research. *Psychol. Bull.*, 143, 2, 187–232, 2017.
59. Just, M.A., Pan, L., Cherkassky, V.L. *et al.*, Machine learning of neural representations of suicide and emotion concepts identifies suicidal youth. *Nat. Hum. Behav.*, 1, 12, 911–919, 2017.
60. Chekroud, A.M., Zotti, R.J., Shehzad, Z. *et al.*, Cross-trial prediction of treatment outcome in depression: A machine learning approach. *Lancet Psychiatry*, 3, 3, 243–250, 2016.
61. Chung, Y., Addington, J., Bearden, C.E. *et al.*, Use of machine learning to determine deviance in neuroanatomical maturity associated with future psychosis in youths at clinically high risk. *JAMA Psychiatry*, 75, 9, 960–968, 2018.
62. Petrone, J., FDA approves stroke-detecting AI software. *Nat. Biotechnol.*, 36, 4, 290–290, 2018.
63. Lundberg, S.M., Nair, B., Vavilala, M.S. *et al.*, Explainable machine-learning predictions for the prevention of hypoxaemia during surgery. *Nat. Biomed. Eng.*, 2, 10, 749–760, 2018.
64. Patel, N.M., Michelini, V.V., Snell, J.M. *et al.*, Enhancing next-generation sequencing-guided cancer care through cognitive computing. *Oncologist*, 23, 2, 179–185, 2018.
65. Bahl, M., Barzilay, R., Yedidia, A.B., Locascio, N.J., Yu, L., Lehman, C.D., High-risk breast lesions: A machine learning model to predict pathologic upgrade and reduce unnecessary surgical excision. *Radiology*, 286, 3, 810–818, 2018.
66. Gurovich, Y., Hanani, Y., Bar, O. *et al.*, Identifying facial phenotypes of genetic disorders using deep learning. *Nat. Med.*, 25, 1, 60–64, 2019.
67. Goodfellow, I., Bengio, Y., Courville, A., Bengio, Y., *Deep learning*, MIT Press Cambridge, Cambridge, 2016.
68. Mintz, Y. and Brodie, R., Introduction to artificial intelligence in medicine. *Minim. Invasive Ther. Allied Technol.*, 28, 2, 73–81, 2019.
69. Buhr, S., FDA clears AliveCor's Kardiaband as the first medical device accessory for the Apple Watch, 2017. https://www.mpo-mag.com/contents/view_breaking-news/2017-11-30/fda-clears-first-apple-watch-medical-device-accessory
70. Victory, J., What did journalists overlook about the Apple Watch 'heart monitor' feature?, HealthNewsReview, 2018. https://www.apple.com/in/healthcare/apple-watch/],

71. Fingas, R., Apple Watch Series 4 EKG tech got FDA clearance less than 24hours before reveal, AppleInsider, 2018. https://appleinsider.com/articles/18/09/18/apple-watch-series-4-ekg-tech-got-fda-clearance-less-than-24-hours-before-reveal
72. Levine, B. and Brown, A., Onduo delivers diabetes clinic and coaching to your smartphone, Diatribe, 2018. https://diatribe.org/onduo-delivers-diabetes-clinic-and-coaching-your-smartphone
73. Han, Q., Ji, M., de Rituerto de Troya, I.M., Gaur, M., Zejnilovic, L., A hybrid recommender system for patient-doctor matchmaking in primary care, in: *IEEE 5th International Conference on Data Science and Advanced Analytics (DSAA)*, 481–490, 2018, arXiv.
74. Matheny, M., Israni, S.T., Ahmed, M., Whicher, D., Artificial intelligence in healthcare: The hope, the hype, the promise, the peril. *Natl. Acad. Med.*, 94–97, 2020.
75. Richardson, J.P., Smith, C., Curtis, S. *et al.*, Patient apprehensions about the use of artificial intelligence in healthcare. *NPJ Digit. Med.*, 4, 1, 140, 2021.
76. He, J., Baxter, S.L., Xu, J., Xu, J., Zhou, X., Zhang, K., The practical implementation of artificial intelligence technologies in medicine. *Nat. Med.*, 25, 1, 30–36, 2019.
77. Commission, E., Centre, J.R., Gómez-González, E., Gómez, E., *Artificial intelligence in medicine and healthcare : Applications, availability and societal impact*, Publications Office, 2020. 978-92-76-18454-6 (online), 10.2760/047666.
78. Kondo, I., Ozaki, K., Osawa, A., Support for patients and their family using artificial intelligence. *Brain Nerve*, 71, 7, 759–764, 2019.
79. Ellahham, S., Artificial intelligence: The future for diabetes care. *Am. J. Med.*, 133, 8, 895–900, 2020.
80. Fast, E. and Horvitz, E., Long-term trends in the public perception of artificial intelligence, in: *Proceedings of the Thirty-First AAAI Conference on Artificial Intelligence*, AAAI Press, San Francisco, California, USA, pp. 963–969, 2017.
81. Concannon, T.W., Fuster, M., Saunders, T. *et al.*, A systematic review of stakeholder engagement in comparative effectiveness and patient-centered outcomes research. *J. Gen. Intern. Med.*, 29, 12, 1692–1701, 2014.
82. Holzer, J.K., Ellis, L., Merritt, M.W., Why we need community engagement in medical research. *J. Investig. Med.*, 62, 6, 851–855, 2014.
83. Muthukrishnan, N., Maleki, F., Ovens, K., Reinhold, C., Forghani, B., Forghani, R., Brief history of artificial intelligence. *Neuroimaging Clin. N. Am.*, 30, 4, 393–399, 2020.
84. Yarborough, M., Edwards, K., Espinoza, P. *et al.*, Relationships hold the key to trustworthy and productive translational science: Recommendations for expanding community engagement in biomedical research. *Clin. Transl. Sci.*, 6, 4, 310–313, 2013.

85. Borry, P., Schotsmans, P., Dierickx, K., What is the role of empirical research in bioethical reflection and decision-making? An ethical analysis. *Med. Healthcare Philos.*, 7, 1, 41–53, 2004.
86. Morley, J., Machado, C.C.V., Burr, C. *et al.*, The ethics of AI in healthcare: A mapping review. *Soc. Sci. Med.*, 260, 113172, 2020.
87. Juravle, G., Boudouraki, A., Terziyska, M., Rezlescu, C., Trust in artificial intelligence for medical diagnoses, in: *Real-World Applications in Cognitive Neuroscience*, pp. 263–282, 2020.
88. Rowe, J., How AI will help healthcare administrators streamline operations?, AI Powered Healthcare, 2020. https://www.healthcareitnews.com/ai-powered-healthcare/how-ai-will-help-healthcare-administrators-streamline-operations
89. Anonymous, How artificial intelligence can make hospital administration more efficient, eviCore Healthcare, 2020. https://www.evicore.com/insights/how-artificial-intelligence-can-make-hospital-administration-more-efficient
90. Daley, S., 35 Examples of AI in healthcare that will make you feel better about the future, builtin, 2022. https://dl.acm.org/doi/abs/10.1145/3433996.3434006#pill-authors__contentcon
91. Wolff, J., Pauling, J., Keck, A., Baumbach, J., Success factors of artificial intelligence implementation in healthcare. *Front. Digit. Health*, 3, 594971, 2021.
92. Wolff, J., Pauling, J., Keck, A., Baumbach, J., Systematic review of economic impact studies of artificial intelligence in healthcare. *J. Med. Internet Res.*, 22, 2, e16866, 2020.
93. Le, L.K.-D., Sanci, L., Chatterton, M.L., Kauer, S., Buhagiar, K., Mihalopoulos, C., The cost-effectiveness of an internet intervention to facilitate mental health help-seeking by young adults: Randomized controlled trial. *J. Med. Internet Res.*, 21, 7, e13065, 2019.
94. Li, J., Parrott, S., Sweeting, M. *et al.*, Cost-effectiveness of facilitated access to a self-management website, compared to usual care, for patients with type 2 diabetes (HeLP-Diabetes): Randomized controlled trial. *J. Med. Internet Res.*, 20, 6, e201, 2018.
95. Gomes, M., Murray, E., Raftery, J., Economic evaluation of digital health interventions: Methodological issues and recommendations for practice. *PharmacoEcon.*, 40, 4, 367–378, 2022.
96. Allen, D., Gillen, E., Rixson, L., The effectiveness of integrated care pathways for adults and children in healthcare settings: A systematic review. *JBI Database Syst. Rev. Implement. Rep.*, 7, 3, 80–129, 2009.
97. Boden, M.A., Creativity, in: *Artificial Intelligence*, pp. 267–291, 1996.
98. Lee, S.-I., Celik, S., Logsdon, B.A. *et al.*, A machine learning approach to integrate big data for precision medicine in acute myeloid leukemia. *Nat. Commun.*, 9, 1, 42, 2018.
99. Seh, A.H., Zarour, M., Alenezi, M. *et al.*, Healthcare data breaches: Insights and implications. *Healthcare*, 8, 2, 133, 2020.

100. Fernández-Alemán, J.L., Señor, I.C., Lozoya, PÁO, Toval, A., Security and privacy in electronic health records: A systematic literature review. *J. Biomed. Inf.*, 46, 3, 541–562, 2013.
101. Meskys, E., Kalpokiene, J., Jurcys, P., Liaudanskas, A., Regulating deep fakes: Legal and ethical considerations. *J. Intellect. Prop. Law Pract.*, 15, 1, 24–31, 2020.
102. Frank, M.R., Autor, D., Bessen, J.E. *et al.*, Toward understanding the impact of artificial intelligence on labor. *Proc. Natl. Acad. Sci.*, 116, 14, 6531–6539, 2019.
103. Nait Aicha, A., Englebienne, G., van Schooten, K., Pijnappels, M., Kröse, B., Deep learning to predict falls in older adults based on daily-life trunk accelerometry. *Sensors*, 18, 5, 1654, 2018.
104. Paul, D., Sanap, G., Shenoy, S., Kalyane, D., Kalia, K., Tekade, R.K., Artificial intelligence in drug discovery and development. *Drug Discovery Today*, 26, 1, 80–93, 2021.
105. Pu, L., Naderi, M., Liu, T., Wu, H.-C., Mukhopadhyay, S., Brylinski, M., eToxPred: A machine learning-based approach to estimate the toxicity of drug candidates. *BMC Pharmacol. Toxicol.*, 20, 1, 2, 2019.
106. Perc, M., Ozer, M., Hojnik, J., Social and juristic challenges of artificial intelligence. *Palgrave Commun.*, 5, 1, 61, 2019.
107. Coiera, E., Kocaballi, B., Halamka, J., Laranjo, L., The digital scribe. *NPJ Digit. Med.*, 1, 1, 58, 2018.
108. Kuziemsky, C., Maeder, A.J., John, O. *et al.*, Role of artificial intelligence within the telehealth domain. *Yearb. Med. Inform.*, 28, 01, 035–040, 2019.
109. Bhatt, A., Artificial intelligence in managing clinical trial design and conduct: Man and machine still on the learning curve? *Perspect. Clin. Res.*, 12, 1, 1–3, 2021.
110. Harrer, S., Shah, P., Antony, B., Hu, J., Artificial intelligence for clinical trial design. *Trends Pharmacol. Sci.*, 40, 8, 577–591, 2019.
111. Lin, W.-C., Chen, J.S., Chiang, M.F., Hribar, M.R., Applications of artificial intelligence to electronic health record data in ophthalmology. *Transl. Vis. Sci. Technol.*, 9, 2, 13, 2020.
112. Moglia, A., Georgiou, K., Georgiou, E., Satava, R.M., Cuschieri, A., A systematic review on artificial intelligence in robot-assisted surgery. *Int. J. Surg.*, 95, 106151, 2021.

14

Role of Artificial Intelligence in Machine Learning for Diagnosis and Radiotherapy

Sanket Chintawar[1], Vaishnavi Gattani[1], Shivanee Vyas[1] and Shilpa Dawre[1,2]*

[1]Department of Pharmaceutics School of Pharmacy & Technology Management, SVKMs, NMIMS Babulde Banks of Tapi River, Shirpur, Maharashtra, India
[2]Department of Pharmaceutics, School of Pharmacy, Vishwakarma University, Kondhwa, Pune, Maharashtra, India

Abstract
Currently there is a buzz about artificial intelligence (AI) and machine learning (ML) in every sector. The current chapter is focused on role of AI and ML in healthcare system especially diagnosis and radiotherapy. Different machine learning algorithm models such as supervised, unsupervised, semi-supervised, and reinforcement learning were also mentioned in this chapter. Herein authors also discusses role of AI in radiology and different types of radiation therapy with its mechanism of action. This chapter explores the ongoing research and implementation of AI and ML in diagnosis and radiotherapy. Successful application of AI and ML algorithms in radiotherapy has been discussed in detail. However, many challenges are there in clinical application of AI in diagnosis and radiotherapy at this time such as quality assurance, reproducibility, implementation, and interpretability.

Keywords: Artificial intelligence, machine learning, diagnosis, radiotherapy, machine learning models

**Corresponding author*: shilpadawre@gmail.com; Shilpa.dawre@nmims.edu;
ORCID: 0000-0003-2389-0002

Vivek Chavda, Krishnan Anand and Vasso Apostolopoulos (eds.) Bioinformatics Tools for Pharmaceutical Drug Product Development, (315–344) © 2023 Scrivener Publishing LLC

Abbreviations

PET	Positron emission tomography
AI	Artificial intelligence
ML	Machine learning
CT	Computed tomography
MR	Magnetic resonance
FDG	Fluorodeoxyglucose
CNN	Convolutional neural network
RL	Reinforcement learning
GAN	Generative adversarial network
DL	Deep learning
CAD	Computer aided detection
TPD	Total perfusion deficit
SPECT	Single Photon emission captured tomography
SGD	Stochastic gradient descent
DNN	Deep neural networks
ANN	Artificial neural networks
IMRT	Image-guided radiation therapy
ACS	American Cancer Society
VMAT	Volumetric modulated arc treatment
SBRT	Stereotactic body radiation therapy
IORT	Intraoperative radiation therapy
TSC	Trans sodium crocetin
LET	Linear energy transfer
SVM	Support vector machines
PCA	Principal component analysis
DSC	Dice similarity coefficient
MRGRT	MR guided radiotherapy
SLFNs	Single hidden layer feedforward neural networks
ELM	Extreme learning machine

ABS	Atlas-based segmentation
MBS	Lodel-based segmentation
QA	Quality assurance
PTV	Planning target volume
OAR	Organ at risk
AP	Auto Planning

14.1 Introduction

In recent times artificial intelligence (AI) has gained more attention both from academia and industry sector. It is one of the powerful modern tools which could 'think and act humanly without losing rationality'. Currently, AI has entered in every aspect of our lives including healthcare system. Artificial intelligence based on its application can be categorized into physical and virtual [1]. Physical element can be exemplified in sophisticated robots, medical devices, nanorobots, and limited mobility devices. The virtual element is implied by machine learning (study of algorithms). Often machine learning misleadingly arbitrated as AI. In current times patients request faster diagnosis and precision medication for treatment. Thus, physicians need to understand and analyze large amount of data in short span of time. Machine learning (ML) can assist in these circumstances in data analysis and providing more effective solutions. Enormous volume of data is available for computational process and algorithms. These algorithms can be utilized in healthcare system in risk management, imaging and diagnosis, drug discovery, personalized medicines, and hospital assistance [2]. Moreover, with the knowledge of deep learning and convolutional neural network (CNN), the ML competencies advanced considerably.

AI and ML in integration has been revolutionized the field of diagnosis and radiotherapy. Many pharma giant companies such as Roche, Pfizer, Johnson & Johnson, Novartis, etc. accepted and applying AI and ML in diagnosis of deadly diseases (Parkinson's disease, hepatitis virus, etc.) and in radiotherapy. These diseases are very complex in nature thus their treatment. Especially in the radiotherapy, AI has revolutionized the whole process. Due to rapid enhancement in AI based computational work several reviews has been published and focused on AI and ML in diagnosis and radiotherapy [3–5]. Moreover, many research findings discussed application of ML in quality assurance to avoid errors resulting delivery of right amount of prescribed drug [6]. This book chapter discusses about machine learning algorithms models, role of AI and ML in radiotherapy, and application for diagnosis of diseases.

14.2 Machine Learning Algorithm Models

It is a computer system based on a set of algorithms that employs many layers of analysis to analyze large amounts of data [7]. A computer can be taught to do a range of things such as make intelligent decisions or use specialized algorithms to accomplish a certain purpose. One of the most extensively used AI technologies for handling massive amounts of information is machine learning. It is a self-adjustable system that provides good analysis, organized as experience and fresh data accumulate. Machine learning strives to construct systems that automatically learn from their mistakes and evolve as a result of their experiences, which are stored in statistical models based on prior patterns of in-out data. These schemes are designed to mechanize the development of solutions depending on future inputs by displaying the essential arithmetical arrangements that appear in input-output data in order to build decision rules that require little to no human participation [8, 9]. There are several models that focus on technique development and improving the machine learning process. For the past three decades, machine learning has been a developing approach. It's now employed in a wide range of applications all around the world [10]. Controlling nanorobots so that they can discover their target region and navigate on their own, robotic surgery, data management, and other applications of machine learning in the real world are all examples of ML in action. Machine learning models include unsupervised, supervised, semi-supervised, and reinforcement learning [11].

14.2.1 Supervised Learning

Supervised learning is described by phrases like training data and desired labelled data. This consists of several training samples, each of which is combined with the required outputs. As a result, the first step in machine learning is to collect these training samples [12, 13]. Furthermore, each training sample must be expressed in a fashion that the computer program can understand, which can be done manually or automatically. Each letter, for example, represents a pixel block in imaging (typically rectangular). These raw pixels' intensities can be utilized to create a primitive feature representation. A feature vector is a collection of feature values that represents each input. Because real-world data is vast and non-manageable, thus significant amount of efforts are required to pre-process the data before creation of training data [14]. The efforts are required for the definition of an outcome values as well as a set of predictor values. If the model is optimized or trained to fit the input-output relationship, the model is categorized as supervised learning.

The two most important goals of supervised learning are classification and regression. The process of categorizing various inputs and procedures is referred to as "classification". The purpose of regression is to make predictions. The underlying premise and training/testing approaches in regression are similar to those used in classification. As a result, we'll concentrate on the categorization problem in the following section. With only two classes, binary categorization is the most fundamental method of classification [15]. For each sample, the supervised learner looks at the feature values and estimates which class it belongs. Depending on the purpose, the linear classifier is simple and applicable in separating the two classes. A quadratic classifier can subsequently be created using a more sophisticated decision boundary, such as a quadratic surface. Machine learning has presented a variety of models for constructing nonlinear decision boundaries.

14.2.2 Unsupervised Learning

Unsupervised learning refers to self-organizing algorithms that identify relationships without the use of previous samples. This model is ideal for discovering connections in a databank, but it doesn't predict the statistical significance of data. Unsupervised learning may identify inappropriate categories if the data has been developed [13]. Despite the fact that this model does not necessitate human intervention, it does necessitate a determination of the probability and relevance of the observed collections. Finally, deep learning systems acquire data connections via developmental testing, which can modify outcomes when more data is available. Deep learning is a unique approach to artificial intelligence [16]. It must be viewed from a variety of angles due to its ability to mix supervised and unsupervised approaches. It excels at handling large datasets with several dimensions and input sources. The output, on the other hand, is sometime incomprehensible because of its complicated arrangement. Thus, operates as a black box for operators, causing a serious threat to patients' wellbeing networks and convolutional neural networks [12].

14.2.3 Semi-Supervised Learning

The advantages of both supervised and unsupervised ML are combined in semi-supervised learning model. Moreover, it eludes the complication related to noticing enormous labelled data [17]. It uses a little amount of labelled data and a huge amount of unlabeled data. By grouping comparable data together and maintaining each group different from the others, cluster analysis organizes a dataset into homogeneous groupings. Clustering algorithms that are not supervised are frequently employed. No prior knowledge of the data's linkages is necessary because the goal is to detect similarities and contrasts between data items [13]. However, there are situations when certain details about cluster labels, outcome variables, or data connection information are available. In this circumstance, semi-supervised clustering is advantageous. Semi-supervised clustering categorizes unlabeled input using known cluster information [18]. A semi-supervised learning application such as a text document classifier is a common example. Due to the impossibility of finding a large amount of marked text documents in this condition, semi-supervised learning is the best alternative. Thus, semi-supervised learning allows the system to acquire from a lesser amount of labelled texts although categorizing a huge amount of unlabeled texts in the training set.

14.2.4 Reinforcement Learning (RL)

It is a deep learning technology that allows consumers to study in an interactive way through experiments while receiving advice from their activities and proficiencies. Unlike supervised learning, which educates the agent on how to do a task [19], reinforcement learning communicates good and negative behavior through incentives and penalties. In terms of objectives, reinforcement learning is distinct from unsupervised learning. Unsupervised learning seeks to find connections and variances amongst data elements, however RL is based on to find the best active model that maximizes the consumers' collective return [20].

SARSA (State-Action-Reward-State-Action) and Q-learning are RL approaches without model which have been extensively used [21]. Their methods of exploration differ, but their exploitation strategies are the same. Q-learning is a technique in which the user chooses the significance value. RL is used in cybernetics and industrial mechanization to allow a machine to create a self-regulated method that comprehends from its individual experiences and behavior. A good example is DeepMind's work on robotic manipulation using asynchronous policy updates and deep reinforcement learning [22]. Conversation bots (text, audio) that learn from user interactions and improve over time, abstractive text summarization algorithms, and learning best treatment plans in healthcare.

14.3 Artificial Learning in Radiology

Artificial intelligence is improving diagnostic imaging accuracy in radiology. Directly obtain a digital image of a patient for central archival and soft copy viewing. Similarly, AI has been successfully implemented in radiology [23, 24]. Due to the well digital imaging infrastructure, AI has been smoothly integrated into the radiology process. Large amount of data can be evaluated and sent in minutes. Deep learning AI could be used to automate the detection of regions of interest and diagnosis in patient images obtained by computed tomography, ultrasound (CT), X-ray, mammography, and magnetic resonance imaging (MRI) among other imaging modalities. Image recognition using AI and deep learning with CNNs has greatly improved, and it is now being used more frequently for diagnostic imaging [9, 11].

Radiation therapy is a technique for tumor treatment which uses radiation with excessive power to kill cancerous cells and decrease tumors. More than half of cancer patients, according to the American Cancer Society (ACS) receive radiation treatment [25]. Inside cancer cells, radiation has an impact on the genetic material known as DNA. A cancer cell which is unable to replace its DNA will eventually die due to its inability to create new cells. According to the American Cancer Society, noncancerous cells may be harmed by radiation, but most will recover. Radiation therapy will be carefully conducted according to clinical practitioner team to minimize injury to normal tissues and organs. The two most prevalent types of cancer radiation therapies are external and internal radiation treatment [26, 27]. The types of radiation treatments have been discussed in the following section. Radiation guidelines are influenced by location of tumor, mass of tumor, kind of cancer, and the patient's situation. Radiotherapy can be used to accomplish a few different treatment goals. For instance, enhance the efficiency of surgery, reduce the risk of tumor spreading, or ease the indications of progressive disease.

14.3.1 Types of Radiation Therapy

The radiation therapy can be classified into external and internal beam radiation.

14.3.1.1 External Radiation Therapy

This kind of radiotherapy is the most prevalent method of cancer management. External energy beams suggest that they are generated by a mechanism that is external to the body. The rays can infiltrate the body and reach the tumor site that can be accurately controlled by a medical practitioner. Teletherapy is alternative name for external beam radiation [28]. Brachytherapy and external beam radiation treatment work in a similar way. Both therapies use high-energy lasers to target and destroy cancer cells on a local level. The source of radiation in the two therapies, however, is different. Brachytherapy uses radiation from an implant and put it inside a tumor by a doctor [27]. The following are the several types of external beam radiation.

3D conformal radiation therapy: A three-dimensional computational model of the treatment area is created using computed tomography (CT) scans and sophisticated computer software. Treatments are focused more precisely to the tumor, sparing normal tissue in the area surrounding [29].
Intensity-modulated radiotherapy (IMRT)/volumetric modulated arc treatment (VMAT): This multi-beam technique changes the radiation strength and focuses it on the ill cells. This is accomplished using VMAT over an arc, which is more efficient [30].
Image-guided radiation (IGRT): It is a 3D imaging technique which assists in the best orientation to the aimed cells before starting the treatment. A CT scan is usually conducted before each therapy. Additional imaging techniques are ultrasound, X-rays, cameras that can trail the surface movement, and sensors that can trail inside cells [31].
Gamma Knife radiosurgery or Stereotactic radiosurgery: It is the "gold standard" for treatment of brain tumors and injuries with radiation. In many circumstances, the gamma knife can produce results that are analogous to or improved than traditional operation, devoid of the invasive cut or a lengthy hospital stay. Radiosurgery is usually a single treatment; however, it can also be divided into multiple treatments over several days [32].
Stereotactic body radiation therapy: It focuses on huge doses of high-intensity radiation. This form of treatment usually necessitates a series of one to five sessions. To reduce radiation to the healthy parts of body, advanced technologies are required which can regulate the breathing also [33].
Intraoperative radiation: Intraoperative radiation treatment (IORT) allows the delivery of radiation during surgery, potentially decreasing the requirement for later external radiation. Radiation is better targeted at areas where tumor development is still present [34].

14.3.1.2 Internal Radiation Therapy

It is the second most prevalent type of radiotherapy, also called as brachytherapy. At the time of therapy, a clinician allocates a radioactive material implant in or nearby the tumor. Implants exhibit a variety of shapes and sizes, including tubes, wires, capsules, seeds, and pellets. During brachytherapy, a person's treatment team injects the radioactive implant using a catheter or a larger instrument called an applicator [28]. Once the catheter has been put by the doctor, the radiation source will be implanted. Before removing the implant, the doctor might leave it in place for few days. In some circumstances, the implant could be inserted for short span of time (10-20 mins) and then repetitively for few weeks [35]. When the therapy is finished, the clinical practitioner will take out the applicator. Even though an implant can reside inside the body forever and ultimately discontinue the production of radiation.

14.3.1.3 Systemic Radiation Therapy

Additional category of internal radiotherapy is systemic radiation therapy. It entails eating a radioactive material that searches and eliminates malignant cells throughout the body. The radioactive chemical could potentially be injected into a person's vein by a healthcare practitioner [36].

14.3.2 Mechanism of Action

Radiation therapy works by destroying cancer cells' DNA. Photons or charged particles are the two energy sources that induce DNA damage [5]. Ionization of the atoms that forms DNA chain is responsible for damage, either directly or indirectly. When water is ionized, it generates free radicals, particularly hydroxyl radicals which can harm DNA. Free radicals are responsible for the majority of the radiation in photon therapy. Generally, biological system can repair damage to single-stranded and double-stranded DNA. However, double-stranded DNA breaks are difficult to repair resulting chromosomal abnormalities and genetic deletions. Cell death is more likely when double-stranded breaks are targeted. Cancer cells are stem like and fewer segregated cells as compared to normal discriminated cells, reproducing more often, and having a lower ability to repair sub-lethal injury. Cancer cells with ssDNA damage leads to cell death or proliferate at a slower rate [37].

The creation of oxygen deficit in solid tumor cells is one of the most serious side effects of photon radiation therapy. When a solid tumor's blood supply is reduced, hypoxia, or a lack of oxygen in the body can occur. By creating DNA-damaging free radicals, oxygen functions as a radiosensitizer, increasing the efficacy of a given dosage of radiation, tumor cells can be exposed to hypoxia may be twice than normal radiotherapy. Hypoxia can be overcome by various methods such as heat therapy that widens blood vessels to the cancerous cells, hypoxic cytotoxins (tissue poisons) like tirapazamine, blood substitutes that transfer additional oxygen, high-pressure oxygen tanks, and hypoxic cell radiosensitizer drugs such as misonidazole and metronidazole [37]. The use of chemical trans sodium crocetin (TSC) which increases the diffusion of oxygen as a radiosensitizer has been recently studied in preclinical and clinical trials.

Charged particles like neon ions, boron, protons, and carbon can directly destruct the DNA of cancerous cells through extraordinary-LET (linear energy transfer). They exhibit antitumor effect that is not dependent on tumor oxygen amount. Since they act primarily through undeviating energy allocation, it results into damage of double-stranded DNA. Charged particles and protons exhibit low side scattering in cells because of their huge mass, the beam does not expand significantly and remains focused on the tumor form which has minimum dose side effects on nearby tissue [37]. The Bragg peak effect can also be used to more precisely target the tumor. In proton treatment, the differences between intensity-modulated radiation therapy (IMRT) and charged particle therapy can be observed clearly. This method minimizes vigorous tissue damage. In IMRT, on the other hand, the usage of uncharged particles permits the radiation to destroy vigorous cells as it departs the body. This injury is not beneficial, and it has the potential to exacerbate treatment-related side effects. It also increases the risk of future cancer induction [38]. In some cases, where ionization is very harmful due to the closeness of other organs, this distinction is crucial (e.g., head and neck malignancies). Children are particularly vulnerable to X-ray radiation due to their growing bodies, and after 5 years, they have a 30% probability of relapse of cancer [36].

14.4 Application of Artificial Intelligence and Machine Learning in Radiotherapy

14.4.1 Delineation of the Target

It is an intricate, time consuming, and labor intensive process to contour organ at risk (OARs) and tumor volumes manually when radiotherapy targets are delineated. ML has been investigated as a solution by means of auto-detection or auto-contouring of normal structures or tumors in this process. Several commercially available software segmentation and packages have been available over the years, the most common is segmentation based on an Atlas or a Model (MBS) [7]. Images derived from computed tomography (CT) are applied in order to incorporate organ segmentation data. In recent years, clinicians have been able to obtain the best representation of patient anatomy by combining algorithms with body models. Radiation therapy planning has been automated using ML and DL techniques [8].

The Dice similarity coefficient (DCE) or Sorensen-Disc coefficient was invented to qualify the similarity between two contours. It is a statistical tool that compares the contours of a product and the performance of auto-segmentation software. This tool is constantly being refined and improved. Using deep learning, a team of researchers in the United Kingdom has investigated how to better define the OAR in patients with head and neck cancer. In this study, 663 patient images were analyzed to compare the results of ML and manual contouring. Comparing the results of ML with manual contouring on all OAR structures except the brainstem and right lens, clinically acceptable contours were achieved [9]. On the basis of MR images, deep learning-based tumor contouring to identify high-risk cardiothoracic vascular surgery CTVs has been shown to be closely related to contours drawn by clinicians [10]. Their multi-atlas-based-segmentation method further saves clinicians time with 50% of the auto-contour used clinically without any modification [8]. When compared to manually contouring, auto-contouring that has been improved by doctors can save 112 minutes per plan in the treatment of head and neck cancer [11]. Studies have investigated similar treatments for cancers such as prostate, lung, and breast [12]. Although we are making progress with machine learning and deep learning to save physicians time and generate high-quality outlines, we still have ways to go, we're still not at a point where these algorithms can completely replace clinicians. While machine learning (ML) can save clinicians time and increase their productivity, it can also offer significant potential benefits in radiotherapy target definition. This is particularly true for responsibilities such as contouring easily replicable organs at risk and deriving radiotherapy contours, which are repetitive and take a lot of time.

14.4.2 Radiotherapy Delivery

United Kingdom National Health Service is working on developing a strategy for adapting and implementing AI to enhance patient care and optimize it. Radiology have been interested in the potential applications of AI [13].

In the United Kingdom, the Royal College of Radiologists (RCR) named AI as one of the advanced high-tech developments in healthcare. As part of its effort to identify challenges in implementing AI in patient care, the RCR has actively reached out to a wide range of stakeholders. Before such technology can be applied to clinical practice, it is imperative that it should be supported by comprehensive evidence-based cost-benefit evaluations that investigate the legal framework, governance, quality assurance, and staff training concerns [8]. ML has been used to predict cancer survival in a variety of cancers, including breast cancer and lung cancer. ML can also be used to determine whether adaptive radiation will be needed if the anatomy changes during treatment [14]. ML has also been examined as a tool for improving the quality of radiotherapy. A prediction algorithm for IMRT plans has been created, which can detect variances of up to 3% while causing faults that are immediately recognizable [15]. A similar approach has also been investigated as part of the process of providing quality assurance for the VMAT radiotherapy programs used to treat prostate cancer. This model detects deviations and delivery errors in dose-volume histogram data received from the previous VMAT prostate plans [16]. In spite of the fact that it is capable of carrying out some tasks, such as identifying organ structures in radiological pictures, artificial intelligence is very different from the cognitive capacities of humans in terms of how it analyses information. Artificial intelligence may be able to recognize structures that are not seen by the human eye, but such capability may not be of clinical utility, and incorrect organ structures may be detected without the AI being aware of it [17]. It is often difficult to describe the exact algorithms used in AI and they are built without using clinical reasoning, but they are derived from intuition and empirical study [18]. Since these algorithms were developed by private initiatives, little information about them is available in the public domain. Machine learning is a process that detects links and uses a large pool of raw data to process. It is an iterative process with a number of computer models and algorithms. The radiation outlines, cancer images, and radiological data of patients are frequently saved on encrypted servers that are linked to other servers located in other locations. The absence of radiotherapy databases and diagnostic images of an adequate quality would be a significant threat to the development of machine methods in the field of radiotherapy [19]. In the past few years, ML algorithms have been used to predict cancer recurrences, most notably in breast and oral cancers, as well as cervical cancer. For the ML approach to training their models, large datasets are available in these cancer sites which facilitate progress in these cancer sites. Specifically, a breast cancer recurrence prediction model was able to provide high specificity and sensitivity [20]. The model even claims to be more effective than the routine models currently used in breast cancer screenings.

14.4.3 Image Guided Radiotherapy

In modern linear particle accelerators (Linac) these days, a CT scan using megavoltage X-rays can be performed daily as part of the treatment verification process [15]. Image-guided radiation can take advantage of patients' everyday anatomy to match treatment plans to them and prevent intra-fraction shifts, despite the lack of detail in the soft tissue structures. There may be a need to repeat a kilovoltage CT scan if the cone-beam megavoltage CT scans demonstrate major anatomical changes, such as weight loss or tumor displacement (for example, in head and neck radiation plans). Computed tomography pictures that use kilovoltage X-rays have enough contrast between soft tissue structures to help doctors design individualized radiation treatments for each unique patient [21]. It would require significant manual intervention for each of these steps, for the radiation dose to delivered, each cone-beam image must be evaluated by at least one or two experienced treatment radiographers on a regular basis. Senior radiologists, medical physicists, and clinical oncologists will discuss with each other when an anatomical mismatch is discovered. They will decide on whether to proceed or defer therapy and repeat the procedure using high-voltage X-ray CT scanning. These steps delay the treatment of patients and increase the department's workload. Moreover, linear accelerators coupled with magnetic resonance imaging technology are becoming increasingly common [22]. There will be a lot more training needed for radiographers, medical scientists, as well as consultants in clinical oncology in order to use the modern technology in a safe and effective manner. All of this paves the way for the development of a training program for medical and allied health professionals to occur concurrently with the growth of machine learning. The amount of human resources available is insufficient to satisfy the needs of an increasing amount of labor as well as to innovate and make use of contemporary technologies. Because the algorithm may "learn" alongside the personnel, the amount of time required to train employees will be reduced if machine learning is integrated with traditional training methods.

14.5 Implementation of Machine Learning Algorithms in Radiotherapy

Machine learning and other sophisticated models have become widely used to aid in prediction and decision-making across a broad variety of fields. Promising work has been done in tissue characterization, cancer staging, outcome prediction, automated segmentation, treatment planning, quality assurance, radiation oncology, and medical physics domains within the global diagnostic radiology (Figure 14.1). Machine learning can evaluate the performance of numerous components of a delivery system over time, such as the multileaf collimator (MLC), imaging system, mechanical, and dosimetric factors. Virtual Intensity-Modulated Radiation Therapy (IMRT) QA may forecast passing rates across many institutions that utilize different measurement techniques, treatment planning systems, and treatment delivery machines [23]. Prediction of QA passing rates and other metrics can have profound implications on the current IMRT process.

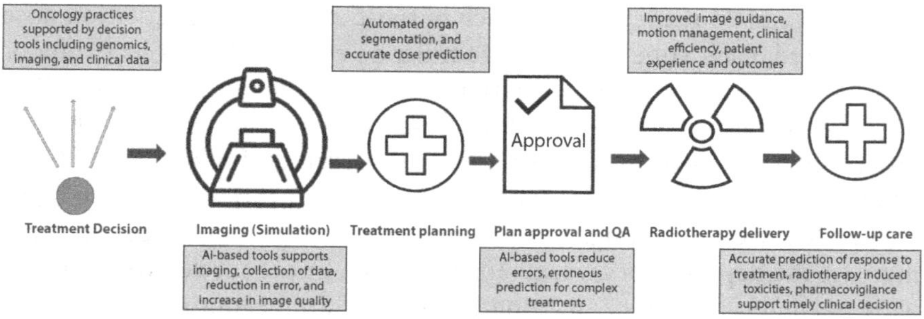

Figure 14.1 Application of artificial intelligence in radiotherapy.

14.5.1 Image Segmentation

Using multiple imaging modalities, AI algorithms were widely used for organ delineation and lesion segmentation. To achieve this goal, two diverse programs are often utilized: using the complete image or merely a subset of the image containing the required organ or lesion as inputs [24]. Organ segmentation is used to give clinically relevant characteristics or to narrow the search field for aims like software detection and radiation therapy planning. Due to the vast variation in shape and size of malignant lesions, lesion segmentation is more difficult than organ segmentation, despite their technical similarities. The treatment volume should be carefully calculated before beginning radiation planning. If conducted manually, this method is complex and time-consuming, as well as subject to considerable inter- and intra-observer variability. The feasibility of this technique (dice coefficient = 0.87) was determined using AI-based methods for automatic nasopharyngeal tumor cell segmentation from 18F-FDG PET/CT images and a U-Net architecture. Similar studies using convolutional neural networks for automatic tumor identification from PET/CT images for head and neck and lung cancers yielded promising results [25]. Despite this, totally automated lesion delineation from PET, CT, or MR imaging, or any combination of these images, remains a substantial issue due to the wide variation of lesion form and uptake associated with distinct cancers. To reflect actual overall population, sufficient huge amounts of the training sample must be collected, which may involve time-consuming image segmentation. Vendor-specific scanner performance, variances in positron emission tomography image collection, reformed methodologies, and standardization are all concerns in image segmentation.

14.5.2 Medical Image Registration

Deep learning image registration techniques are classified as training process (unsupervised, supervised, etc.), system designs (RL, CNN, etc.), productivity styles (thin alteration on regulator points, dense transformation, and parametric regression of change model, etc.), input image dimensions (entire image or segment-based,), and inference forms (one-shot prediction, iterative). DL-based medical image registration methods divided into seven categories, based on their methods, functions, and popularity: 1) Deep similarity-based methods; 2) generative adversarial networks (GAN) in medical image registration 3) RL-based methods, 4) unsupervised transformation prediction, 5) supervised transformation prediction, 6) registration validation using deep learning, and 7) other learning-based methods [26]. CNN was created to analyze highly structured information like pictures, which are often represented by grid-sampling data points. As a result, convolutional kernels were used in practically every specified methods of deep learning design.

14.5.3 Computer-Aided Detection (CAD) and Diagnosis System

Machine learning techniques were employed in the previous period to improve medical diagnosis and description of disorders using a method known as computer-aided diagnosis. Moreover, radiomic characteristics are commonly employed for prognosis, cancer subtyping, and lesion/tissue characterization [27]. Radiomic feature extraction can be done manually or automatically, while deep learning-based (automated) feature extraction has recently showed potential as a racist and discriminatory feature selection method [28]. To predict the risk of cancer growth, tumor aggressiveness, and the likelihood of malignancy, hand-crafted radiomic variables are usually fed into a classifier based on the imaging modalities' properties. Deep learning-based algorithms, on the other hand, use a sub-region of a picture as input and enhance result prediction accuracy by optimizing feature extraction (with minimal human participation) [29].

The primary purpose of AI-assisted lesion characterization is to describe a lesion's activity levels in order to detect false-positive diagnosis. Furthermore, lesion categorization is utilized in imaging genomics (the study of the architecture, utility, and progression of genomes) to investigate the correlation and interaction with histopathology employing radiomic parameters produced from the lesion as phenotypes. DL-based lesion analysis is not in-built as compared to manual structures, which are related to definite identified behaviors that are predictable during supervised training. Because they were chosen using a supervised learning technique, these attributes may be used in future genome discovery research.

When non-malignant tissue is the focus, such as parenchyma analysis to predict the risk of breast cancer, tissue characterization is sought in addition to malignant lesions to quantify the probability of disease development. Breast density and parenchymal patterns were linked to the risk of breast cancer using deep learning algorithms. Betancur *et al.* suggested a deep learning-based automated obstructive disease prediction model in myocardial perfusion SPECT imaging and compared the results to the TPD score, which is often used. A deep learning system was utilized to process a large cohort of patients (> 1600) in a multicenter trial to predict coronary artery disease by patient and vessel. Deep learning prediction beat TPD on average, according to the data [30].

Computer-aided diagnostic frameworks are used to characterize tissues or lesions in order to identify whether they are malignant or not. In breast cancer research, the advancement of AI-based approaches to discriminate among malignant and benign cancers is a major issue. Using deep learning-based feature fusion, successor radiomics-based computer-aided diagnostics improved diagnostic yield by a statistically significant margin [27]. While traditional radiomics-based approaches strive to provide favorable results, deep learning methods are increasingly being employed to provide additional decision support in the detection of various diseases such as lung cancer. According to Baek *et al.*, deep learning algorithms can provide superior prediction capability than manual radiomic features. To develop a U-net model for cancer identification, they solely used hand drawn outlines as underlying data. They discovered that combining deep learning-based feature fusion with successor radiomics-based computer-aided diagnosis enhanced diagnostic performance and had a statistically significant prediction value for picture features related to patient survival [31].

14.6 Deep Learning Models

Deep learning contains a lot of potential and has already inspired abundance of new research projects such as deep genomics, in recent years. Deep learning employs multiple processing layers to uncover trends in a large data set [32]. Deep learning is a type of artificial intelligence that consists of a collection of computer models that process data in several levels. The algorithm considers the disparities between actual and expected outputs throughout the training phase and modifies its internal weights to reduce the discrepancy. The system also generates a gradient vector for each weight, which depicts the error deviation as a function of weight change. The weight vector of the gradient vector is changed in the reverse way. A method known as stochastic gradient descent (SGD) is widely used to identify the best set of weights. In this approach, the system is given the input vector for a few examples and told to compute the output, error, and averaged gradient for those cases. Convolutional neural networks (CNNs) and deep neural networks (DNNs) are two deep learning-based networks that were recently developed and applied in complex radiotherapy calculations.

14.6.1 Deep Neural Networks

Unsupervised and supervised deep neural networks (DNNs) are the two forms of DNNs. It is common practice in machine learning to simplify the input and emphasize the most important pattern for the learning process. In most cases, the performance of the learning algorithm function reveals success rate of AI [33]. The sequential representation of the input data must be learned by many DNNs on their own. DNNs are multilayer artificial neural networks (ANNs) that combine many neural networks. DNNs use nodes to calculate data, with the output of the first layer becoming the input for the next layer, and so on, with the system's derived output being the final layer's output. Unsupervised deep learning models are preferred over supervised DNNs because they require less labelled data [34].

14.6.2 Convolutional Neural Networks

Convolutional neural networks (CNNs) excel at gathering and organizing enormous amount of data such as medical images. A pooling layer, convolutional layer, and an entire linked layer are different types of layers in CNN. The convolutional layer's work is to learn representations for the input by recognizing feature similarities from previous layers. The number of convolution layers corresponds to the number of convolution kernels used to compute feature maps. Each neuron in the feature map is linked to a concrete substrate neighboring neuron. The purpose of the pooling layer is to lessen the resolution of the feature map to achieve shift variance. A pooling layer is commonly placed between two convolutional layers, with each layer's and linked to future maps from the convolutional layer. The purpose of a completely linked layer is to perform high-level reasoning.

14.7 Clinical Implementation of AI in Radiotherapy

This section is the compilation of recent research findings of AI clinical implementation and application in various cancer diagnosis and radiotherapy (Table 14.1).

Chen *et al.* evaluated organs at risk (OAR) and superiority of planning target volume (PTV) developed by the auto-planning (AP) modules and the manual Pinnacle planning (manP). They studied applicability of AP in the field of radiotherapy for breast cancer imaging. In their study thirty subjects on breast-saving therapy were selected randomly. A physician used blind qualitative grading to compare the plans in terms of dosimetric characteristics and monitor units (MUs). The paired two-sided Wilcoxon signed-rank test was applied to evaluate statistical variances. When the D50 ($P = 0.04$) and conformal index ($P< 0.01$) of PTV in the manP and AP groups were compared, the conformal index ($P< 0.01$) and D50 ($P = 0.04$) of PTV in the AP group were lesser, whereas D1 was higher ($P = 0.03$). In terms of OAR dosimetry, the AP group's ipsilateral lung V20 Gy (P 0.01), V10 Gy (P 0.01), V5 Gy (P 0.05), and Dmean (P 0.01) were superior to the manP group's. In the AP group all subjects had lesser heart V40 Gy and Dmean compared to the manP group (P 0.01). Furthermore, twelve subjects breast cancer in left showed similar outcomes ($P \leq 0.01$). Although there was no statistical significance, the MU number of the IMRT module constructed by means of 2 dissimilar approaches was found greater in the AP group as compared to manP group (P = 0.32). The PTV and dosage distribution of the AP module were nearly identical to those of the manP module, and its OAR was less irradiated [35].

Jihong *et al.* showed that a commercially available AP module could be used to plan radiation therapy treatment for locally advanced nasopharyngeal cancer. This study comprised 22 patients with locally advanced NPC. VMAT schemes were created physically by a skilled physicist and robotically by the AP module for each patient. Automatic plans and manual plans were evaluated in terms of dose distribution, dosimetric characteristics, monitor units (MPs), and planning time. Meanwhile, the overall stage of the sickness was considered. The distribution of the decided dose by APs was equivalent to the MPs. Except for the spinal cord, the dosage factors of APs were greater than those of MPs for the OARs. The V50 and Dmax of the brainstem were significantly lower by 1.32 % and 1.0 Gy, respectively, in the APs, as were the Dmax of the optic nerves and chiasm ($p < 0.05$). In most cases, the APs were as good as or better than MPs, with the exception of a few patients with stage IV illness. Most OAR dosage variations were comparable in the two different schemes irrespective of phase, whereas APs offered superior brainstem sparing for stage III patients and enhanced parotid gland sparing for stage IV patients [36].

Spaek *et al.* observed at a combination of doxorubicin-ifosfamide chemotherapy and presurgical hypofractionated radiation therapy in slightly resectable soft tissue malignances. In the study 46 patients were included. At the beginning of the study, three of the patients had resectable lung metastases. The protocol treatment was given to forty-two people. Because of the toxicity of chemotherapy, the treatment was abruptly halted in two patients. After the second AI cycle, one patient died of infection because of bone marrow dysfunction; a second death had nothing to do with STS treatment. Amputations were carried out on three patients. They performed en bloc R0 resections in 72% of patients with the plan-to-treat analysis. In 15 patients, a dose decrease or treatment stoppage was required because of a 4.03 chemotherapeutic toxicity. Incidents related to injury happened in 18 patients, however only 6 of them were serious [37].

Sibolt *et al* studied clinical application of AI based cone-beam CT scan radiation therapy in the pelvic region. When compared automatically pre-treatment plans are comparable to PTV coverage and OAR doses. During simulated oART, more than 75% of AI fractions do not need minor adjustment and the improved scheme was best in 88% of instances. AI-segmentation flaws were linked to circumstances where training model of AI was not developed properly. The five patients who were provided with treatment first did fine with the intermediate process time of 17.6 minutes. When compared to non-ART bladder patients, treatment provided bladder patients had a 42% PTV decline indicating a 24-30% drop in V45Gy to the intestine cavity [38].

Fodor and colleagues evaluated toxicity of hypofractionated entire breast radiation therapy deprived of enhancement and the period of skin responses in a huge cohort of rarely-stage breast cancer patients. The average period of supplement was 72.4 months (IQR: 44.6-104.1). Acute RTOG toxicity was graded as follows: 69.8% Grade 1 (G1), 14.3% Grade 2 (G2), and 1.7% Grade 3 (G3). Edema-hyperpigmentation (E-H): G3 0.15, G2 4.41%G1 28.67%, fibrosis-atrophy-telangiectasia-pain (F-A-T-P): G1 14.6%, G2 3.2%, G3 0.8%, G4 0.1%. The intermediate period between the first incidence and the second occurrence was 6 months and 18 months, respectively. After surgery, 28.7% of patients had outstanding results, 41.5% had fair results, 20.3% had acceptable results, and 9.5% had bad results. After radiotherapy, 6.9% of patients had a modest change in breast appearance, 2.3% had a moderate change, and 1.3% had a notable change. Simultaneous chemotherapy, bolus administration, smoking, PTV planning, and obesity were all related with an increase severe toxicity. Acute toxicity was less common in patients under the age of 55. G2 E-H was linked to PTV and acute G2 poisoning. Increased risk of F-A-T-P was linked to PTV, concurrent chemotherapy, hypertension, and G2 acute toxicity. In a large cohort of patients, hypofractionated whole-breast radiation without boost showed mild acute and late damage. Between 18 and 42 months, 3.6% of individuals experienced moderate to significant changes in breast appearance [39].

Chao *et al.* analyzed patients with intracranial tumors using deep learning models to study the image division and standard outcomes by clinical depiction difficulties of cerebral edema post radiotherapy. They included patients with intracranial tumors receiving computer knife (CyberKnife M6) stereotactic radiosurgery followed by the treatment planning system (MultiPlan 5.1.3) to achieve previous to treatment and next four-month pictures of patients. They utilized tensor flow platform for the design of neural networks (Figure 14.2). For development of cerebral edema databank, they applied supervised learning model such as mask region-based convolutional neural networks (R-CNN) and region growing algorithms. The assessment coefficients such as Jaccard (intersection over union, IoU), volumetric overlap error (VOE), and DICE to analyze and study the processes in the image assembly for cerebral edema image subdivision and the standard as mentioned by the oncologists. When the VOE index was 0 and DICE and IoU indices were 1, the results were same to those designated by the clinician. Their study revealed the IoU index was 0.79, DICE index was 0.88, and the VOE index was 2.0. The Mask R-CNN model and the evaluated index, had the superlative effect on segmentation. This technique can be applied in the clinical practice in the future to attain good complex separation and offer clinical assessment as well as regulation plans [40].

Table 14.1 List of application of AI based technology applied, type of cancer or diseases, and their major findings.

Technology used	Disease	Major findings	References
AI-based algorithms in image-guided radiotherapy (IGRT)	Cancer	Tumor movement can be tracked, indecision in treatment can be minimized, and better precision.	[41]
ANN algorithms	Prostate Cancer	Understanding of cancer improvised. An improved conclusion for patients can be attained via genomics, histopathology, imaging, and treatment.	[42]
AI tools	Prostate Cancer	AI tools supported effective risk stratification and warrants further assessment for improving disease management.	[43]
Deep-learning heart segmentation on CT images	Breast cancer	Deep-learning algorithms can be used effectively in all areas of medicine and make clinical care better.	[44]

(Continued)

Table 14.1 List of application of AI based technology applied, type of cancer or diseases, and their major findings. (*Continued*)

Technology used	Disease	Major findings	References
Self-attention neural networks	Head and neck cancer	The ANN combines the volumetric data of patients and structured clinical data to produce a predictive model for multi-site, multi-modal tumor analysis.	[45]
Supervised machine-learning algorithm	Basal cell carcinoma	ML helps predict MDT decisions for MMS vs traditional surgery or radiotherapy for a large population of patients.	[46]
Computed tomography (CT)-based deep learning	Lung cancer	Transportability and validity of the CT-based deep learning prediction model for radiotherapy candidates.	[46]
CNNs	Breast cancer	Model demonstrated excessive potential to fasten the treatment preparation process while continuing consistent plan quality.	[47]

(*Continued*)

Table 14.1 List of application of AI based technology applied, type of cancer or diseases, and their major findings. (*Continued*)

Technology used	Disease	Major findings	References
Volumetric modulated arc treatment (VMAT) decision assistance system based on artificial intelligence (DST)	Head and neck cancer	DST-AI tools facilitated a significantly improved treatment directive across all OARs for this generalized H&N patient cohort, according to a study.	[48]
Logistic regression, decision tree model	Preeclampsia	Study suggested that AI based tools ease collection of laboratory data in second and third trimester and helped early detection of preeclampsia. These strategies help enhance maternal and fetal preeclampsia outcomes in normal prenatal treatment.	[49]
The average similarity coefficient for dice (DSC)	Breast cancer	Artificial intelligence-generated models have shown that the developed models are superior to human-generated ones.	[50]

(*Continued*)

Table 14.1 List of application of AI based technology applied, type of cancer or diseases, and their major findings. (*Continued*)

Technology used	Disease	Major findings	References
MR guided radiotherapy	Lung cancer	Stereotactic body radiation therapy (SBRT) incorporating MR guided radiotherapy (MRgRT) for the treatment of (ultra-) central tumors.	[51]
Robust segmentation method	Nasopharyngeal Carcinoma	Deep learning CNN and CE-MRI approach showed a robust method of segmenting NPC tumors with accuracy has been developed and segmentation can be done within seconds.	[52]
SPE-CT scans of dopamine transporters with ioflupane-123	Parkinson's disease	Study is the proof of concept that CNN can pretrain nonmedical images and assist the analysis of ^{123}I SPECT scans.	[53]
AI based chest x-ray images	COVID-19 pneumonia	In comparison to other pneumonia classes, COVID-19 pneumonia could be distinguished by its AUC of 0.98 and micro-average of 0.99.	[54]

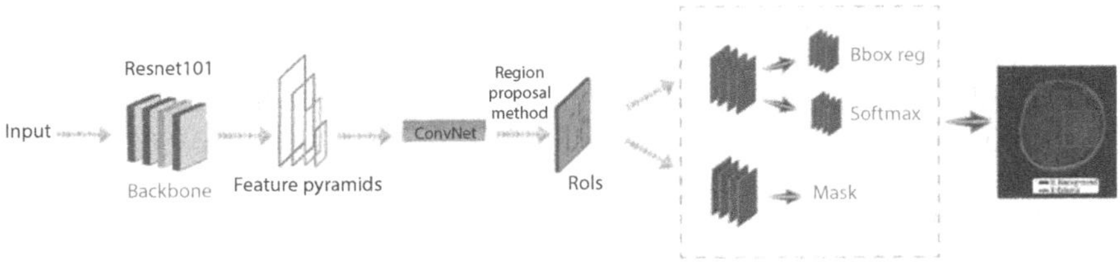

Figure 14.2 Mask R-CNN network architecture diagram. RoI generates a region of interest [40].

14.8 Current Challenges and Future Directions

Artificial intelligence and machine learning are modern tools and have proven very effective specifically for diagnosis and radiotherapy. However, it was observed that it has few limitations, and due to lack of clinician inputs and data bottleneck this technology is less supportive than claimed. Developers and researchers need to collect a large amount of imaging data to feed in AI models and apply it. Even after application, continuous monitoring is required for the performance of these technologies. Furthermore, validation, reproducibility, and quality assurance are required to translate these AI and ML-based approaches in clinical practice. Another challenge in AI-based approaches is performance and interpretability (decision tree). Technical groups are developing "explainable AI," which can improve performance and interpretable models. However, to date not been achieved successfully. In addition to that deep learning, models are not easily transportable across diverse hospitals. In advancement for these approaches, radiologists and researchers play an important role in labeling training datasets and developing new knowledge from image data. In summary, with the advancement and high performance of AI and ML approaches in diagnosis and radiotherapy, its use is progressively increasing and in the future also it could be used as an effective tool for the diagnosis and radiotherapy.

References

1. Amisha, Malik, P., Pathania, M., Rathaur, V., Overview of artificial intelligence in medicine. *J. Fam. Med. Prim. Care*, 8, 7, 2328, 2019. [Internet] Available from: https://journals.lww.com/10.4103/jfmpc.jfmpc_440_19.
2. Nayyar, A., Gadhavi, L., Zaman, N., Machine learning in healthcare: Review, opportunities and challenges, in: *Machine Learning and the Internet of Medical*

Things in Healthcare, pp. 23–45, Elsevier, Amsterdam, 2021, [Internet] Available from: https://linkinghub.elsevier.com/retrieve/pii/B9780128212295000112.
3. Hardy, M. and Harvey, H., Artificial intelligence in diagnostic imaging: Impact on the radiography profession. *Br. J. Radiol.*, 93, 1108, 20190840, 2020. [Internet] Available from: https://www.birpublications.org/doi/10.1259/bjr.20190840.
4. Elemento, O., Leslie, C., Lundin, J., Tourassi, G., Artificial intelligence in cancer research, diagnosis and therapy. *Nat. Rev. Cancer*, 21, 12, 747–752, 2021. [Internet] Available from: https://www.nature.com/articles/s41568-021-00399-1.
5. Hosny, A., Parmar, C., Quackenbush, J., Schwartz, L.H., Aerts, H.J.W.L., Artificial intelligence in radiology. *Nat. Rev. Cancer*, 18, 8, 500–510, 2018. [Internet] Available from: http://www.nature.com/articles/s41568-018-0016-5.
6. Segal, G., Segev, A., Brom, A., Lifshitz, Y., Wasserstrum, Y., Zimlichman, E., Reducing drug prescription errors and adverse drug events by application of a probabilistic, machine-learning based clinical decision support system in an inpatient setting. *J. Am. Med. Inform. Assoc.*, 26, 12, 1560–1565, 2019. [Internet] Available from: https://academic.oup.com/jamia/article/26/12/1560/5544737.
7. Tătaru, O.S., Vartolomei, M.D., Rassweiler, J.J. *et al.*, Artificial intelligence and machine learning in prostate cancer patient management—Current trends and future perspectives. *Diagnostics*, 11, 2, 354, 2021. [Internet] Available from: https://www.mdpi.com/2075-4418/11/2/354.
8. Boon, I., Au Yong, T., Boon, C., Assessing the role of artificial intelligence (AI) in clinical oncology: Utility of machine learning in radiotherapy target volume delineation. *Medicines*, 5, 4, 131, 2018. [Internet] Available from: http://www.mdpi.com/2305-6320/5/4/131.
9. Nikolov, S., Blackwell, S., Zverovitch, A. *et al.*, Deep learning to achieve clinically applicable segmentation of head and neck anatomy for radiotherapy. *arXiv*, 2021, 1–10, 2018. [Internet] Available from: http://arxiv.org/abs/1809.04430.
10. Li, Q., Xu, Y., Chen, Z. *et al.*, Tumor segmentation in contrast-enhanced magnetic resonance imaging for nasopharyngeal carcinoma: Deep learning with convolutional neural network. *Biomed. Res. Int.*, 2018, 1–7, 2018. [Internet] Available from: https://www.hindawi.com/journals/bmri/2018/9128527/.
11. Speight, R., Karakaya, E., Prestwich, R. *et al.*, Evaluation of atlas based auto-segmentation for head and neck target volume delineation in adaptive/replan IMRT. *J. Phys. Conf. Ser.*, 489, 012060, 2014. [Internet] Available from: https://iopscience.iop.org/article/10.1088/1742-6596/489/1/012060.
12. Bell, L.R., Dowling, J.A., Pogson, E.M., Metcalfe, P., Holloway, L., Atlas-based segmentation technique incorporating inter-observer delineation uncertainty for whole breast. *J. Phys. Conf. Ser.*, 777, 012002, 2017. [Internet] Available from: https://iopscience.iop.org/article/10.1088/1742-6596/777/1/012002.
13. Kortesniemi, M., Tsapaki, V., Trianni, A. *et al.*, The European Federation of Organisations for Medical Physics (EFOMP) white paper: Big data and deep learning in medical imaging and in relation to medical physics profession.

Phys. Med., 56, 90–93, 2018. [Internet] Available from: https://linkinghub.elsevier.com/retrieve/pii/S1120179718313152.
14. Zhao, W., Shen, L., Islam, M.T. *et al.*, Artificial intelligence in image-guided radiotherapy: A review of treatment target localization. *Quant. Imaging Med. Surg.*, 11, 12, 4881–4894, 2021. [Internet] Available from: https://qims.amegroups.com/article/view/76804/html.
15. Valdes, G., Chan, M.F., Lim, S.B., Scheuermann, R., Deasy, J.O., Solberg, T.D., IMRT QA using machine learning: A multi-institutional validation. *J. Appl. Clin. Med. Phys.*, 18, 5, 279–284, 2017. [Internet] Available from: https://onlinelibrary.wiley.com/doi/10.1002/acm2.12161.
16. Liu, Z., Liu, F., Chen, W. *et al.*, Automatic segmentation of clinical target volumes for post-modified radical mastectomy radiotherapy using convolutional neural networks. *Front. Oncol.*, 10, 581347, 2021. [Internet] Available from: https://www.frontiersin.org/articles/10.3389/fonc.2020.581347/full.
17. Diaz-Escobar, J. and Kober, V., Natural scene text detection and segmentation usingphase-basedregionsandcharacterretrieval. *Math. Probl. Eng.*, 2020, 1–17, 2020. [Internet] Available from: https://www.hindawi.com/journals/mpe/2020/7067251/.
18. Siddique, S. and Chow, J.C.L., Artificial intelligence in radiotherapy. *Rep. Pract. Oncol. Radiother.*, 25, 4, 656–666, 2020. [Internet] Availablefrom: https://linkinghub.elsevier.com/retrieve/pii/S1507136720300444.
19. Iqbal, M.J., Javed, Z., Sadia, H. *et al.*, Clinical applications of artificial intelligence and machine learning in cancer diagnosis: Looking into the future. *Cancer Cell Int.*, 21, 1, 270, 2021. [Internet] Available from: https://cancerci.biomedcentral.com/articles/10.1186/s12935-021-01981-1.
20. Jhee, J.H., Lee, S., Park, Y. *et al.*, Prediction model development of late-onset preeclampsia using machine learning-based methods. *PloS One*, 14, 8, e0221202, 2019. [Internet] Available from: https://dx.plos.org/10.1371/journal.pone.0221202.
21. Goldman, L.W., Principles of CT: Radiation dose and image quality. *J. Nucl. Med. Technol.*, 35, 4, 213–225, 2007. [Internet] Available from: http://tech.snmjournals.org/cgi/doi/10.2967/jnmt.106.037846.
22. Crockett, C.B., Samson, P., Chuter, R. *et al.*, Initial clinical experience of MR-guided radiotherapy for non-small cell lung cancer. *Front. Oncol.*, 11, 2021. [Internet] Available from: https://www.frontiersin.org/articles/10.3389/fonc.2021.617681/full.
23. Palareti, G., Legnani, C., Cosmi, B. *et al.*, Comparison between different D-Dimer cutoff values to assess the individual risk of recurrent venous thromboembolism: Analysis of results obtained in the DULCIS study. *Int. J. Lab. Hematol.*, 38, 1, 42–49, 2016.
24. Liu, X., Song, L., Liu, S., Zhang, Y., A review of deep-learning-based medical image segmentation methods. *Sustainability*, 13, 3, 1224, 2021. [Internet] Available from: https://www.mdpi.com/2071-1050/13/3/1224.

25. Wei, L. and El Naqa, I., Artificial intelligence for response evaluation with PET/CT. *Semin. Nucl. Med.*, 51, 2, 157–169, 2021. [Internet] Available from: https://linkinghub.elsevier.com/retrieve/pii/S0001299820301136.
26. Fu, Y., Lei, Y., Wang, T., Curran, W.J., Liu, T., Yang, X., Deep learning in medical image registration: A review. *Phys. Med. Biol.*, 65, 20, 20TR01, 2020. [Internet] Available from: https://iopscience.iop.org/article/10.1088/1361-6560/ab843e.
27. Chan, H., Hadjiiski, L.M., Samala, R.K., Computer-aided diagnosis in the era of deep learning. *Med. Phys.*, 47, 5, e218–e227, 2020. [Internet] Available from: https://onlinelibrary.wiley.com/doi/10.1002/mp.13764.
28. Preuss, K., Thach, N., Liang, X. *et al.*, Using quantitative imaging for personalized medicine in pancreatic cancer: A review of radiomics and deep learning applications. *Cancers (Basel)*, 14, 7, 1654, 2022. [Internet] Available from: https://www.mdpi.com/2072-6694/14/7/1654.
29. Sharma, N., Sharma, R., Jindal, N., Machine learning and deep learning applications-A vision. *Global Transitions Proc.*, 2, 1, 24–28, 2021. [Internet] Available from: https://linkinghub.elsevier.com/retrieve/pii/S2666285X21000042.
30. Betancur, J., Commandeur, F., Motlagh, M. *et al.*, Deep learning for prediction of obstructive disease from fast myocardial perfusion SPECT. *JACC Cardiovasc. Imaging*, 11, 11, 1654–1663, 2018. [Internet] Available from: https://linkinghub.elsevier.com/retrieve/pii/S1936878X18301311.
31. Suh, C.H., Lee, K.H., Choi, Y.J. *et al.*, Oropharyngeal squamous cell carcinoma: Radiomic machine-learning classifiers from multiparametric MR images for determination of HPV infection status. *Sci. Rep.*, 10, 1, 17525, 2020. [Internet] Available from: https://www.nature.com/articles/s41598-020-74479-x.
32. Hesamian, M.H., Jia, W., He, X., Kennedy, P., Deep learning techniques for medical image segmentation: Achievements and challenges. *J. Digit. Imaging*, 32, 4, 582–596, 2019.
33. Huang, D., Bai, H., Wang, L. *et al.*, The application and development of deep learning in radiotherapy: A systematic review. *Technol. Cancer Res. Treat.*, 20, 153303382110163, 2021. [Internet] Available from: http://journals.sagepub.com/doi/10.1177/15330338211016386.
34. Bao, W., Lianju, N., Yue, K., Integration of unsupervised and supervised machine learning algorithms for credit risk assessment. *Expert Syst. Appl.*, 128, 301–315, 2019. [Internet] Available from: https://linkinghub.elsevier.com/retrieve/pii/S0957417419301472.
35. Chen, K., Wei, J., Ge, C. *et al.*, Application of auto-planning in radiotherapy for breast cancer after breast-conserving surgery. *Sci. Rep.*, 10, 1, 10927, 2020. [Internet] Available from: http://www.nature.com/articles/s41598-020-68035-w.
36. Jihong, C., Kaiqiang, C., Yitao, D., Xiuchun, Z., Yanyu, C., Penggang, B., Evaluation of auto-planning in VMAT for locally advanced nasopharyngeal carcinoma. *Sci. Rep.*, 12, 1, 4167, 2022. [Internet] Available from: https://www.nature.com/articles/s41598-022-07519-3.
37. Spałek, M.J., Koseła-Paterczyk, H., Borkowska, A. *et al.*, Combined preoperative hypofractionated radiotherapy with doxorubicin-ifosfamide chemotherapy in

marginally resectable soft tissue sarcomas: Results of a phase 2 clinical trial. *Int. J. Radiat. Oncol.*, 110, 4, 1053–1063, 2021. [Internet] Available from: https://linkinghub.elsevier.com/retrieve/pii/S0360301621001942.

38. Sibolt, P., Andersson, L.M., Calmels, L. *et al.*, Clinical implementation of artificial intelligence-driven cone-beam computed tomography-guided online adaptive radiotherapy in the pelvic region. *Phys. Imaging Radiat. Oncol.*, 17, 1–7, 2021. [Internet] Available from: https://linkinghub.elsevier.com/retrieve/pii/S2405631620300816.
39. Fodor, A., Brombin, C., Mangili, P. *et al.*, Toxicity of hypofractionated whole breast radiotherapy without boost and timescale of late skin responses in a large cohort of early-stage breast cancer patients. *Clin. Breast Cancer*, 7, 363–370, 2021. [Internet] Available from: https://linkinghub.elsevier.com/retrieve/pii/S1526820921003451.
40. Chao, P.-J., Chang, L., Kang, C.-L. *et al.*, Using deep learning models to analyze the cerebral edema complication caused by radiotherapy in patients with intracranial tumor. *Sci. Rep.*, 12, 1, 1555, 2022. [Internet] Available from: https://www.nature.com/articles/s41598-022-05455-w.
41. Vandewinckele, L., Claessens, M., Dinkla, A. *et al.*, Overview of artificial intelligence-based applications in radiotherapy: Recommendations for implementation and quality assurance. *Radiother. Oncol.*, 153, 55–66, 2020.
42. Tătaru, O.S., Vartolomei, M.D., Rassweiler, J.J. *et al.*, Artificial intelligence and machine learning in prostate cancer patient management—Current trends and future perspectives. *Diagnostics*, 11, 2, 1–20, 2021.
43. Wulczyn, E., Nagpal, K., Symonds, M. *et al.*, Predicting prostate cancer specific-mortality with artificial intelligence-based Gleason grading. *Commun. Med.*, 1, 1, 10, 2021. [Internet] Available from: http://www.nature.com/articles/s43856-021-00005-3.
44. Zeleznik, R., Weiss, J., Taron, J. *et al.*, Deep-learning system to improve the quality and efficiency of volumetric heart segmentation for breast cancer. *NPJ Digit. Med.*, 4, 1, 43, 2021. [Internet] Available from: http://www.nature.com/articles/s41746-021-00416-5.
45. Le, W.T., Vorontsov, E., Romero, F.P. *et al.*, Cross-institutional outcome prediction for head and neck cancer patients using self-attention neural networks. *Sci. Rep.*, 12, 1, 3183, 2022. [Internet] Available from: https://www.nature.com/articles/s41598-022-07034-5.
46. Andrew, T.W., Hamnett, N., Roy, I., Garioch, J., Nobes, J., Moncrieff, M.D., Machine-learning algorithm to predict multidisciplinary team treatment recommendations in the management of basal cell carcinoma. *Br. J. Cancer*, 126, 4, 562–568, 2022. [Internet] Available from: https://www.nature.com/articles/s41416-021-01506-7.
47. Van de Sande, D., Sharabiani, M., Bluemink, H. *et al.*, Artificial intelligence based treatment planning of radiotherapy for locally advanced breast cancer. *Phys. Imaging Radiat. Oncol.*, 20, 111–116, 2021. [Internet] Available from: https://linkinghub.elsevier.com/retrieve/pii/S2405631621000713.

48. Sher, D.J., Godley, A., Park, Y. *et al.*, Prospective study of artificial intelligence-based decision support to improve head and neck radiotherapy plan quality. *Clin. Transl. Radiat. Oncol.*, 29, 65–70, 2021. [Internet] Available from: https://linkinghub.elsevier.com/retrieve/pii/S2405630821000501.
49. Jhee, J.H., Lee, S., Park, Y. *et al.*, Prediction model development of late-onset preeclampsia using machine learning-based methods. *PloS One*, 14, 8, 1–12, 2019.
50. Liu, Z., Liu, F., Chen, W. *et al.*, Automatic segmentation of clinical target volumes for post-modified radical mastectomy radiotherapy using convolutional neural networks. *Front. Oncol.*, 10, 1–8, 2021.
51. Crockett, C.B., Samson, P., Chuter, R. *et al.*, Initial clinical experience of MR-guided radiotherapy for non-small cell lung cancer. *Front. Oncol.*, 11, 1–10, March 2021.
52. Li, Q., Xu, Y., Chen, Z. *et al.*, Tumor segmentation in contrast-enhanced magnetic resonance imaging for nasopharyngeal carcinoma: Deep learning with convolutional neural network. *BioMed. Res. Int.*, 2018, 2018.
53. Kim, D.H., Wit, H., Thurston, M., Artificial intelligence in the diagnosis of Parkinson's disease from ioflupane-123 single-photon emission computed tomography dopamine transporter scans using transfer learning. *Nucl. Med. Commun.*, 39, 10, 887–893, 2018.
54. Baltazar, L.R., Manzanillo, M.G., Gaudillo, J. *et al.*, Artificial intelligence on COVID-19 pneumonia detection using chest xray images. *PloS One*, 16, 10, e0257884, 2021. [Internet] Available from: https://dx.plos.org/10.1371/journal.pone.0257884.

15

Role of AI and ML in Epidemics and Pandemics

Rajashri Bezbaruah, Mainak Ghosh, Shuby Kumari, Lawandashisha Nongrang, Sheikh Rezzak Ali, Monali Lahiri, Hasmi Waris and Bibhuti Bhushan Kakoti*

Department of Pharmaceutical Sciences, Faculty of Science and Engineering, Dibrugarh University, Dibrugarh, Assam, India

Abstract

The healthcare industry, as well as business and society, have been revolutionized by Artificial Intelligence (AI) and Machine Learning (ML). Currently, microbiology, biochemistry, genetics, structural biology, and immunological concepts have all seen significant advances. In contrast, the fields of bioinformatics have seen considerable expansion in order to handle this massive data influx. The field of bioinformatics, which tries to use computational methods for a better understanding of biological sciences, sits at the crossroads of data science and wet lab. Several innovative databases and computational techniques have been proposed in this sector to advance immunology research, with many of them relying on artificial intelligence and machine learning to anticipate complicated immune system activities, such as epitope identification for lymphocytes. Models based on machine learning skilled on specific proteins have provided inexpensive and quick-to-implement strategies for the discovery of effective viral treatments in the recent decade. Given a target biomolecule, these models can predict inhibitor candidates using structural data. The emergence of the coronavirus COVID-19 has resulted in significant network data traffic and resource optimization demands, rendering standard network designs incapable of dealing calmly with COVID-19's consequences. Researchers are encouraged by the use of Machine Learning (ML) and Artificial Intelligence (AI) in previous epidemics, which offers a novel strategy to combating the latest COVID-19 pandemic.

***Keywords*:** Artificial intelligence, machine learning, COVID-19, vaccine, Ebola

**Corresponding author*: bibhutikakoti@dibru.ac.in; ORCID id: 0000-0003-4492-9439

Vivek Chavda, Krishnan Anand and Vasso Apostolopoulos (eds.) Bioinformatics Tools for Pharmaceutical Drug Product Development, (345–370) © 2023 Scrivener Publishing LLC

15.1 Introduction

Artificial Intelligence (AI) and Machine Learning (ML) have transformed the healthcare industry and even businesses and the society that we live in. As days go by new modern innovations have come up making our lives so much easier. In the field of medicine, these logical techniques have resulted in labor, time, and even cost savings in the development of novel drugs and agents [1]. Artificial Intelligence (AI) may be defined as the study of, "intelligent agents", whereby it can identify our potentiality and maximize it for optimal activity. AI mainly mimics the human mind making our work so much easier especially in solving problems [2]. Machine Learning (ML) is also related to AI. It mainly collects data from previous studies and interprets this data for use in an ongoing study by creating protocols for that said study [3]. Figure 15.1 depicts how AI and ML has helped millions of people digitally for pandemic preparedness and response through several ways.

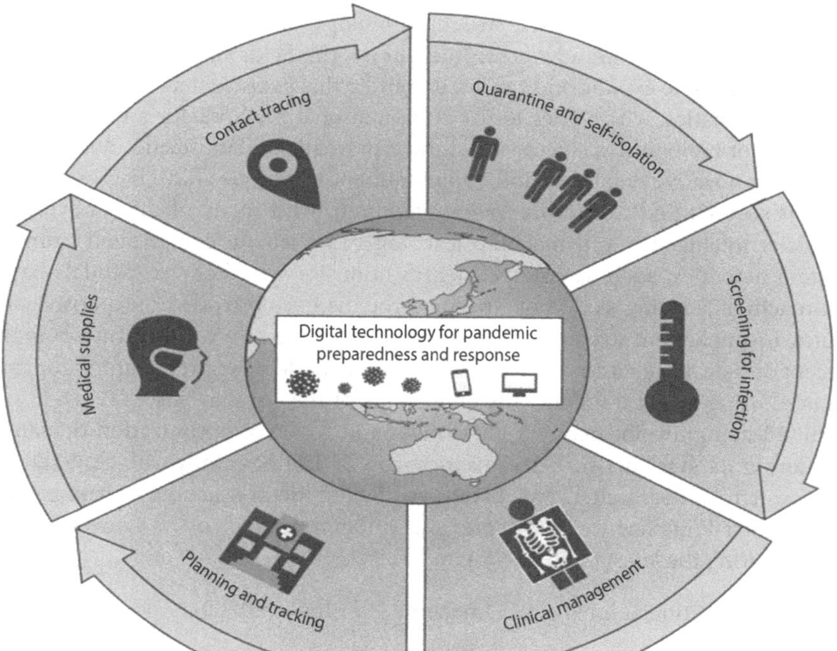

Figure 15.1 Pandemic preparedness and response using digital technology. (Adopted from [10] under CC BY 4.0 License).

The use of Artificial Learning Deep Learning is the main aspect of COVID-19 detection and management [4]. There are several numbers of algorithms that have been used in healthcare, viz. Glucometer in Diabetes, Angiography, and ECG in cardiac-related problems, etc. [5]. The following literature review talks about the importance of AI and ML in the field of medicine, mainly focusing on vaccine development during any epidemic or pandemic particularly the Ebola Virus and Coronavirus outbreak which has affected millions of people in the last decade. Several AI algorithms have been used in healthcare during an epidemic and pandemics like Random Forest (RF), Decision Tree (DT), Support Vector Machine (SVM), Convolutional Neural Network (CNN), etc. [6]. Furthermore, a combination of AI, ML, and systems biology is said to reduce any failures that may be related to the efficacy of vaccine development [7]. The use of AI has minimized the problem in all aspects humans are facing on social, cultural, economic, and political levels globally [8]. Randomized Controlled Trials (RCTs) have been stated to be the most appropriate model based on ethics, to be followed in clinical trials during an outbreak [9].

15.2 History of Artificial Intelligence (AI) in Medicine

In 1950, the concept of intelligence, using computers was first explained by Alan Turning. He mentioned a simple test later on named as "Turning Test" in the book "Computer and Intelligence" to test the capability of computers to determine human intelligence [11, 12]. In 1956, Jon McCarthy coined the name "Artificial Intelligence". Initially, AI's main focus was the development of machines that involve the functions of humans. Based on this, for the first time in 1961 first industrial robot arm "Unimate" involved the assembly line and worked as an automated die casting. In 1964, great scientist Joseph Weizenbaum developed Eliza, which was used as Chatterbots for the future to mimic conversation [13]. The first mobile robot was created to interact with complex instructions a name as "First Electronic person". In 1971 MYCIN was formed which mainly provides to trial pathogenesis of bacteria and provides antibiotic treatment based on a person's body weight. Whereas EMYCIN (1976) and INTERNIST-1 (1972) were later developed as a source of medical knowledge for physicians which is used in primary care in diagnosis [14]. To enhance communication between the biochemical and clinical research, in 1973, "The Stanford University Medical Experimental – Artificial Intelligence in

Medicine", a computer system was formed. In 1976, the CASNET model (it is one work of model building, consultation, and database) was used for the consultation of Glaucoma treatment, this model could also be applicable to gather information along with providing advice to the physicians to maintain patients' health.

In 1986, The University of Massachusetts introduced a support system, namely DXplain, used to diagnose diseases based on symptoms and is also used as an electronic medical textbook that provides information regarding the disease. In the 1990s reintroduce Machine learning (ML) technology and set up a new era called the modern era of AIM [15]. In 2000, "deep learning" became famous [6]. In 2007 a technique was developed called Deep QA, which mainly analyse unstructured content using natural language and different types of searches to create a possible answer. Deep QA is also applicable to provide medicine based on patients' electronic medical reports and opens a new era to clinical decision-making, which is evidence-based. To create meaningful conversation "Eliza" technology was applied in the year 2011 in "SIRI" (Apple's virtual assistant) and Alexa (virtual assistant of Amazon) in 2014. In 2015, the chatbot was created as "Pharmabot" which is work to assist pediatric patients along with their parents by giving medication education, whereas Mandy was initiated in the year 2017 for primary care of patients. Between 2018 to 2020 Al trials were done in Gastroenterology [16, 17]. In 2018, a medical device "Dx-DR" was approved by FDA that was mainly for patient care without physicians. In 2020, declared the first reimbursement to the hospitals regarding the use of AI Technologies [5].

15.3 AI and MI Usage in Pandemic and Epidemic (COVID-19)

AI refers to the capacity of computer systems to complete tasks and approximate human intelligence. Machine learning is one of the subcategories of artificial intelligence. Patients' personal health data is summarized using AI-based technology, which is then used to construct an information regarding dataset that aids physicians in making conclusions and monitoring a personalized routine for the treatment of patients thus AI-based skills are frequently used to inspect the effects of disease prevention, therapies, and patient consequences. Several approaches based on machine learning (ML), coevolutionary as well as deep neural networks, and Bayesian networks have been created to aid with healthcare advancements using intelligent computing systems [18]. The amount of data acquired by public health monitoring systems has increased dramatically as information and communication technologies have advanced. When AI-based methodologies are paired with solid disease management platforms, a road for complete analysis opens up, allowing stakeholders to properly respond to an epidemic or pandemic [19].

Infectious disease epidemiology, like Middle East respiratory syndrome (MERS), Kyasanur forest disease, Chikungunya, Zika, and Ebola, COVID-19. AI-based technologies have been successfully used in all of these diseases [20–35]. The deadly tick-borne viral infectious disease Kyasanur Forest Illness (KFD) is endemic to South Asia that has claimed the lives of thousands of people every year for the past decade. A new cloud computing-based e-Healthcare framework has been designed to monitor KFD-affected patients in the early stages of infection and reduce the outbreak. A site warning system has also been built in order to provide GPS-based location data of each KFD afflicted user and risk-prone zones as quickly as possible in order to avert the outbreak [36].

MERS-CoV is an airborne virus that is rapidly disseminated and has a high mortality rate. An effective cloud computing system is developed that uses a Bayesian belief network to anticipate MERS-CoV-infected patients and gives a geographic-based risk valuation to regulate the epidemic. The system provided high classification accuracy as well as an acceptable geographic-based risk assessment [37].

Chikungunya is a mosquito-borne infection that is transmitted quickly throughout infected areas. Its outbreak produces acute illness, which can develop into a chronic condition. An IoT and fog-based healthcare strategy is developed to identify and manage the CHV outbreak. The fog layer is being used to evaluate possibly infected individuals and give diagnostic and preventive alerts to them using fuzzy-C means (FCM). Moreover, on the cloud server, social network analysis (SNA) is employed to represent the current stage of the CHV outbreak [38]. The Zika virus is a mosquito-borne disease that is rapidly spreading across the globe. A system that integrates cloud computing, mobile phones, fog computing, as well as Internet of things (IoT)-based sensor devices to avert and regulate the spread of Zika virus disease [39].

15.3.1 SARS-CoV-2 Detection and Therapy Using Machine Learning and Artificial Intelligence

Early identification and screenings can help prevent pandemic infections like SARS-CoV-2 from spreading, also save time and money throughout the diagnostic procedure. By being cheaper than the old system, the development of an expertise tool for healthcare supports in the new order of detection, screening, and treatment of SARS-CoV-2 carriers. ML and AI are utilized to improve the assessment and screening technique of the recognized patient using radio imaging technology such as X-Ray, computed tomography (CT), and clinical blood sample data [40].

15.3.2 SARS-Cov-2 Contact Tracing Using Machine Learning and Artificial Intelligence

If a person has been identified with COVID-19 and the diagnosis has been verified, contact tracing is the next essential step in preventing the transmission of pathogens further. The virus is communicated from person to person mostly through nasal discharges, saliva, or, droplets according to the World Health Organization. Many Countries employed fruitfully digital contact tracing apps like COVIDSafe (Australia), Stopp Corona (Austria), conjunction with Alipay (China), Aarogya Setu (India), UAE (TraceCovid), NHS COVID-19 App (UK) were planned to diminish the exertion and supplement the efficiency of the traditional healthcare diagnosis procedures [41].

15.3.3 SARS-CoV-2 Prediction and Forecasting Using Machine Learning and Artificial Intelligence

On clinical and mammographic factor datasets, new studies revealed a novel model utilizing a controlled multi-layered recursive classifier named XGBoost. After the use of the model, researchers revealed that three key characteristics "high-sensitivity C-reactive protein", "lymphocyte", and "lactic dehydrogenase (LDH)" of the 75 features clinical as well as blood samples showed in the highest rank of 90% accuracy in predicting and assessing COVID-19 patient into general, severe, and mortality rate [42].

15.3.4 SARS-CoV-2 Medicines and Vaccine Using Machine Learning and Artificial Intelligence

AutoDock Vina is a virtual screening and molecular docking program with a proposed model that uses a deep learning algorithm using COVID-19's 3C-like proteinase and FDA-approved 3,410 existing pharmaceuticals on the market. Figure 15.2 states that ML and AI has found out many ways to diagnose COVID-19, and also treatment of it in a stepwise manner. Antazanavir, a common antiretroviral drug used to treat HIV, was found to

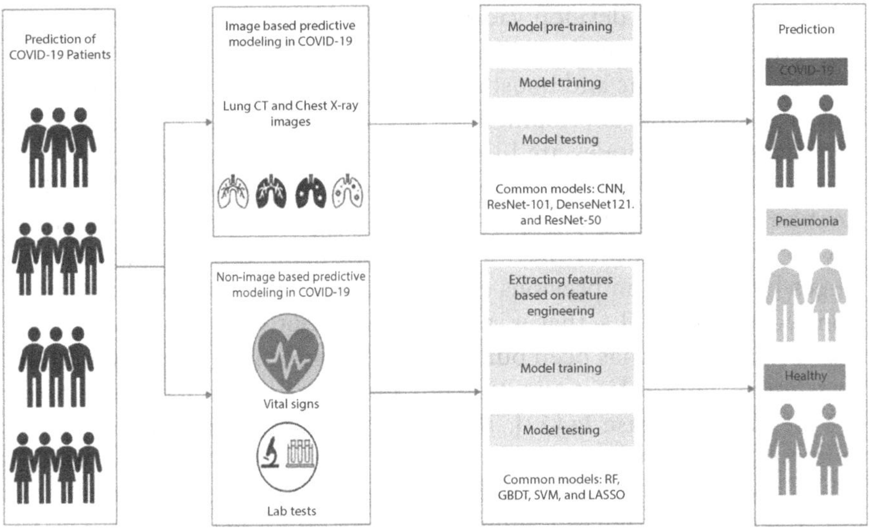

Figure 15.2 A schematic diagram of using ML (Machine Learning) and DL (Deep Learning) techniques in COVID-19 diagnostic and treatment.

be the best drug for COVID-19 treatment, after Remdisivir. Furthermore, some drugs, such as lopinavir, darunavir and ritonavir were recommended to combat viral proteinases, according to the findings. It was also discovered that antiviral medicines like as Kaletra could be used to treat COVID-19 human patients. Malaria is commonly treated with the amodiaquine and chloroquine compounds. A merger of computational screening method with docking techniques and machine learning for choosing supplementary medication to explore on SARS-CoV-2 was also proposed after a decade of drug development based on ML and AI technology was discovered [43, 44].

15.4 Cost Optimization for Research and Development Using AI and ML

Cost optimization of simulation based method is a process of optimization that integrates various optimization techniques regarding simulation modeling and its analysis. This method has several steps including problem definition, system definition, model formulation, project planning, model translation, input data collection, experimentation, verification and validation [45, 46]. Simulation modeling is very expensive and time consuming to develop vaccines during pandemic situation against the pathological agents [47]. This has limited contribution to reduce the severity of pandemic and boost up the research and development of vaccine. Research and development of vaccine is not safe [48], stochastic optimization techniques are likely to be accurate representations of the unpredictable outcomes of Drug research and development [49]. Various stochastic modelling techniques have been applied in drug research and development process to meet a variety of portfolio optimization challenges [50]. Based on previous evidence, a two step stochastic optimization techniques [51] – that is, a step-by-step optimization of objectives with uncertainty – has been built to find optimal research portfolios and costs for moving at least one vaccine candidate per pandemic infectious disease through phase 2a [52]. The minimum number of ideal candidates required to achieve at least one phase 2b–3 ready candidate for an epidemic infectious disease has been calculated in stage 1 from nonclinical research to clinical phase 1 and phase 2 [53]. Using such data on accessible lines per pandemic and epidemic infectious disease the range number of vaccine required by the research and development stage to proceed at least one of them through to the ending of phase 2a have been estimated [54]. Stage 2 builds on stage 1's results to determine the minimum and maximum boundaries of vaccine candidates per research and development stage from which minimum expenditure of developing at least one phase 2b–3 ready candidate per epidemic infectious disease may be computed [55]. To optimize the cost of vaccine development with the aid of advanced technologies, such as the Internet of Things, with a focus on ev commended to l to phase 2a may cost $31–68 million ($14–159 million range), assuming no risk of failure [56]. The entire cost of moving an epidemic viral disease vaccine via clinical phase 2a, and on other hand, is determined by the likelihood of success and the vaccine research and development pipeline structure [57]. No effective vaccine potent substance exist for a specific pandemic viral disease, 11 to 21 non clinical candidates would be needed to complete phase 2a, costing $319–469 million ($137 million–11 billion) [58].

15.5 AI and ML in COVID 19 Vaccine Development

Artificial intelligence (AI) has played a significant role into scientific consciousness, with new discoveries being published at an incredible rate. Artificial intelligence (AI) is a discipline of computer science that can help patients in different ways. It is frequently instantiated and can be used to develop intelligent systems as a piece of software [59]. The emerging application of AI in disease diagnosis has expanded the AI horizon (refer to Figure 15.3). The fields of medicine and science are one of the most promising applications in healthcare, locations, which could be tracked past to the mid-twentieth century. Several health-related decision-support systems have been proposed and successfully developed by researchers [60]. Disease diagnosis by utilizing the AI system based on rules was successful in the late 1970s [61] and has proven to be beneficial in illness detection [62], analyzing ECG images [63], deciding on the best treatment, etc., as well as generating hypothesis for doctors. Modern AI, unlike this first-generation knowledge-based AI system, which depends on experts' past medical knowledge and formulation-based principles, uses machine learning techniques to obtain answers, data patterns and connections [64–66]. The return of AI has sparked speculation over whether AI-doctors will soon be able to take the role of human doctors. While this is the case, researchers anticipate that AI-driven intelligent systems will become more prevalent in the future and can substantially assist human physicians with making better and more accurate diagnosis, faster decisions, and in some cases, removing the need of human decisions. The current success of AI in healthcare [40] can be linked to

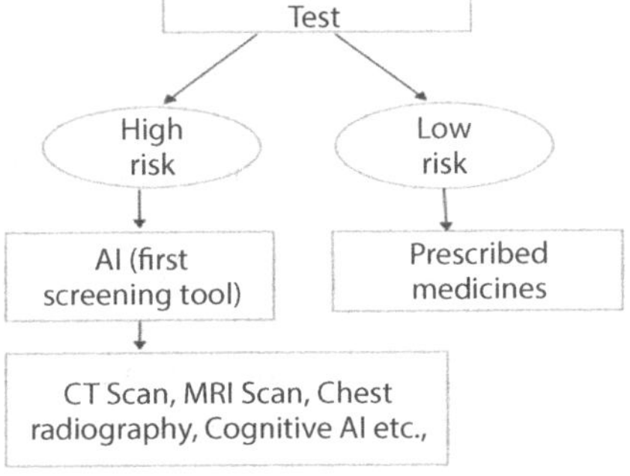

Figure 15.3 Process of disease diagnosis using AI.

greater usage of advancement of digital technology and development of big data analytics in healthcare. Increasing widespread use of digital apparatus has made it useful to gather and obtain these purposes [68]. Data via mobile applications nonetheless, AI research in healthcare is still in its infancy, the majority of technology focuses on three areas: malignancy, neurobiology, and cardiovascular diseases. Evidence-based decision-making insights into medical data can be revealed by a powerful AI and can be utilized for decision-making and forecasting in the future [69–71]. Researchers argue that because AI has proven effective in healthcare, it should be used in other fields as well. They debated that since AI has potential impact in the medicinal field, it should be used in other fields as well. It's also possible that it could help in the fight against viral disease from pandemic forecasting to anti-viral-replication discovery AI has shifted the way we think about health system. Current SARS-CoV AI research suggests that it may be beneficial whereby, viral infection and infected populations can be detected, the next epidemic can be predicted, the attack pattern can be discovered, and even the future outbreak may be predicted in search of a remedy [72–74]. Several recent studies have demonstrated the ramifications of AI where machine learning (ML) algorithm are used (Table 15.1 shows the most frequently used AI algorithms), *viz.*, biological data mining in detection, diagnosis, and treatment, in COVID-19 categorization and vaccine development [75]. The AI algorithms utilized were analyzed and compared by the authors who analyzed the information and gave a series of recommendations for the future Metrics for evaluation of research. On the other hand, it focuses on the research on a larger scale, not limited to the incorporation of diagnosis, detection, epidemic forecasting, and performance evaluation since these are all applications of AI. It is recommended for the future scientists in AI and machine learning applications with COVID-19 as an example whereby the present AI-based research has been carried out in order to combat the COVID-19 epidemic.

During the past few years due to COVID-19, the awareness among people has been going on increasing due to the loss of millions of lives, affecting large number of people and causing the death of greater than 1 million people globally as of October 2020 [76]. WHO then declared COVID-19 as a Global Pandemic on March 11, 2020. Early detection, isolation, and treatment of this pandemic can avoid other people to come in contact with the affected one [77]. Many people worldwide are affected by this virus due to the continuous mutation in their genomic sequence and more losses is expected to be felt for years to come [78]. Due to this, new several

Table 15.1 The most frequently used AI algorithm.

Random Forest (RF)	It is a machine learning (ML). It helps in the Prediction of mortality rate of COVID-19 Patients with high accuracy. It is analyses by the cohort study method [85].
Prophet Forecasting Model (PFM)	It is basically outlined by Facebook for analyzing the time series of time analysis. It is best method for prediction of active rate, cured rate, death rate [86].
Support Vector Machines (SVM)	It applies on labelled set of data, produces series of labelled input-output mapping function. It is used as regression method and classification method [87].
Convolutional Neural Networks (CNN)	It is highly used deep learning models in image classification. CNN is used with a quantum circuit are used in COVID-19 detection. Utilizing CNN in combined with chest X-ray helps in detection of COVID-19 [6].
Decision Trees (DT)	It helps in recognition and prediction of COVID-19 disease with the help of blood-gas data using the Chi-squared Automatic Interaction Detector (CHAID) with decision tree model. In clinical trials they include individuals greater than 18 years and firstly their blood values are measured and at completion of trials they measure the presence of carboxyhemoglobin [88].
XG-Boost (XGB)	XG-Boost in combination with LR-model can accurately predict COVID-19 patients and night monitoring by applying radar monitoring data, as it measures the heart rate, respiratory rate, body motion etc., and it is uploaded in real time via WI-FI [89].

(*Continued*)

Table 15.1 The most frequently used AI algorithm. (*Continued*)

Extra Trees (ET)	It is a group of learning model, as it boosts the prediction accuracy by constructing several randomized decision trees. It is different from random forest classifier due to construction of decision trees [90].
Gradient Boosting Machine Light	It depends on the decision of tree algorithm and then it produces tree in leaf-wise. It can handle large amount of data with less usage of memories. It uses a histogram-based algorithm [91].
Adaptive Boost	In modified version of dataset it includes small decision trees. It leads to increase in the weight of wrongly classified training sample and also decreases the weight for correctly classified [92].
Assay Bayesian Machine Learning model (for EBOV)	This is an FDA-approved screening model for discovering agents to use against Ebola Virus (EBOV). Three active compounds were identified *in vitro* as a result of these models: pyronaridine, quinacrine and tilorone. A further investigation found that when given intraperitoneally to mice infected with mouse-adapted EBOV at 30 mg/kg/day, tilorone has 100% effective *in vivo*. This implies that the data on inhibiting EBOV can be used to detect and test new drugs for their effectiveness *in vivo* [93].
Susceptible Exposed Infectious Recovered (SEIR)	This is the most common type of mechanical modelling technique in predicting the extent to which COVID-19 will spread through the population. Other aspects of the pandemic, such as the accuracy of testing methods, under-reporting of cases and intervention effectiveness, can also be determined using these models [94].

discoveries has been announced at a remarkable rate, Artificial intelligence come into existence since the late 1970s and helpful in analyzing several diseases [79]. It is explained as the use of medical software for the diagnosis of disease with minimal human intervention [80]. Artificial intelligence (AI) and machine learning (ML) have been widely used to fight against covid-19 pandemic [81]. There are many advancements in relation to AI which can represent an effective measure to face major challenges [82]. There are several methods available in IT, and the continued increase in computational power in AI has the ability to find patterns and relationships from data and this has emerged as an alluring area [83]. There are several applications that are included in AI Deep Learning, Machine learning, Robotics, and nanorobots. All these outcomes mainly focus on global research on AI, and it is also considered as an equipment to fight with COVID-19 pandemic [8].

Main application of AI in the COVID-19 pandemic:

- Early identification and diagnosis of the infection and prevention [84].
- Analyze the detection level of infection by the virus [50].
- Automatic treatment for the treatment [49].
- Tracking and forecasting the nature of the virus [50].
- Reducing the workload of health workers [55].
- Development of drugs and vaccines [49].

15.6 Efficacy of AI and ML in Vaccine Development

Since the outbreak of the coronavirus, researchers and healthcare providers have been working to find a cure. Experts from all around the world have encouraged the establishment of a viable option to deal with the production of substances likes vaccine for the disease [95, 96]. For disease like COVID 19 machine learning/artificial intelligence (ML/AI) technologies are both potential solutions. The trip is intriguing. As per choice of drug concerned towards the regimen for infected patients' urgent evaluation on current old remarkable drugs for a novel viral carrier in a human being is possible is necessary [96]. Taiwanese scientists are developing a new model to aid in the development of a revolutionary medicine. Following the application of the two datasets, a model based of ML and AI technology was developed. The study found that eight drugs such as vismodegib, gemcitabine, clofazimine, brequinar, conivaptan, bedaquiline, and tolcapone, celecoxib are virtually efficacious for SARS-CoV treatment by utilizing the two models based on the above two theories on two datasets (one using the 3C-like protease constraint and other data-holding records of infected SARS-CoV, SARS-CoV-2 [95]. In order to emphasize the requirement for an antiviral drug, several scientists from all over the world designed an appropriate and particular drug-target model. The open-source molecular docking software namely autodock using appropriate predefined model which incorporate a core learning assay using COVID-19's 3C-like proteinase and about 3410 currently available drugs are approved by FDA. Beside the rampant use of Remdesivir, another drug namely Antanazavir appeared to be one of the mostly used anti-HIV drug . Furthermore, the findings demonstrated that certain drugs aren't as effective as other [2]. To combat viral proteinases, drugs such as darunavir, ritonavir, and lopinavir have been proposed [2, 97]. Antiviral chemicals were also discovered to be effective. Kaletra, for example, could be used to treat COVID-19 humans' patients. A group of scientists from America came up with the drug for treating another viral disease like Ebola. They started their work using a group of Ebola virus carrier in an vitro in 2014 [12]. The study advocated a combination of amodiaquine and chloroquine, which is commonly used to treat malaria. Furthermore, combination of computational screening techniques with molecular docking application and machine learning for choosing supplementary treatment to research on SARS-CoV-2 was proposed after uncovering a decade of drug development based on ML and AI technology [98]. The chosen review paper used a variety of approaches and technologies, ranging from a traditional statistical classification method to a cutting-edge AI and machine learning algorithm [99]. The use of computational tools in combination with docking applications was found to be more active in predicting the reusability of an existing old drug on COVID-19 medication and dramatically reduce the level of a risk factor in the development of a more cost-effective medicine development process [100]. During this time of urgency, the use of machine learning and artificial intelligence can amplify the discovery program help by reducing the time it takes to find a new treatment or medication for the carrier [101, 102].

15.7 Artificial Intelligence and Machine Learning in Vaccine Development: Clinical Trials During an Epidemic and Pandemic

Many recent advances in the development of effective vaccines during an epidemic or a pandemic are with the help of AI and ML. These two computational tools are the most useful since they reduce the cost, time and labor in the development of any vaccine. For speeding up the development process of a vaccine when in dire need, a joint venture between Machine Learning (ML), Artificial Intelligence (AI) and Systems Biology rational approaches can reduce the failures in enhancing the efficacy of the vaccine developed [7] (Figure 15.4).

Furthermore, each potential vaccine candidate must always be assessed in people for protective effectiveness, immunogenicity and safety, prior to getting licensed for use [103, 104]. After such safety assessment, each vaccine candidate follows a unique development path, based on the availability of a pre-existing vaccine, the kind of vaccine, targeted population and disease epidemiology. The standard pharmaceutical Research and Development (R&D) pipeline consisting of preclinical (*in vivo* and *in vitro*) and clinical trials has to be followed in every drug development process [105–107]. On conducting clinical trials on the vaccines developed, on the other hand, have additional protocols to be followed. Unlike other medications which are administered to the diseased patient, preventive vaccines are first given to healthy people; as a result, their safety after receiving the drug should be considered and it should be to a maximal degree. A more

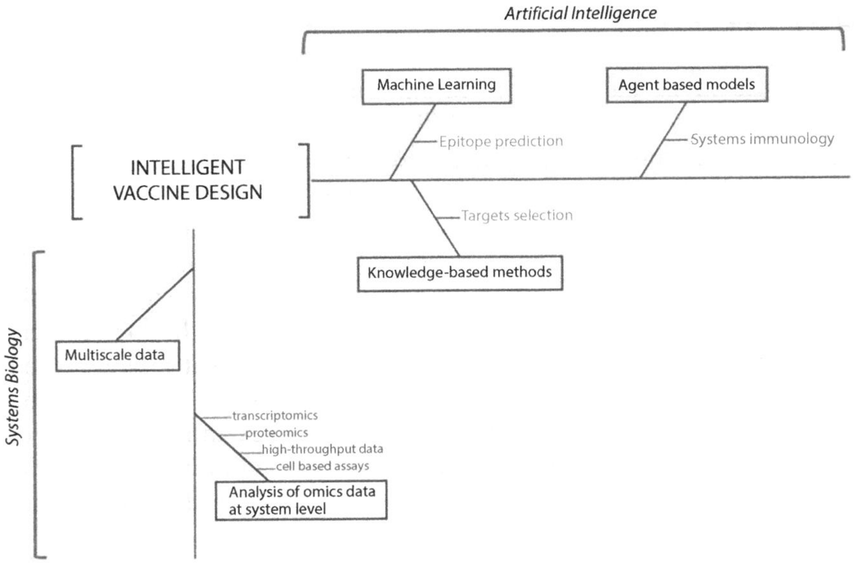

Figure 15.4 The combination of artificial intelligence and systems biology for intelligent vaccine.

targeted immunization approach is required particularly for susceptible populations (e.g., pregnant women, elderly people, patients with a low immunity, and healthcare workers), [108, 109].

As newly developed vaccines reach human trials, Machine Learning (ML) increases the success and efficiency of trials during the initial phases by applying simulation techniques (for an improved treatment) from the data that was collected from previous trials to develop protocols to follow during the trials. Artificial Intelligence (AI) lets investigators upload the protocols and uses algorithms to identify the barriers and overcome them to make the trial a successful one [3].

During an outbreak of disease i.e., an epidemic (E.g. Ebola virus) or a pandemic (E.g. COVID-19), clinical trials are greatly affected due to the limited access to manpower, healthcare and medical facilities resources. In such cases, a strict protocol has to be followed but this can be affected by the delayed or missed conducting and recording of the study report, assessment of safety and efficacy and reporting adverse events. Medical administration and oversight may be severely strained if study participants are unable to visit healthcare institutions.

15.8 Clinical Trials During an Epidemic

15.8.1 Ebola Virus

During the Ebola pandemic, planning and executing clinical research involved dealing with many ethical difficulties. At first, the stakeholders argued whether conducting clinical studies during an outbreak was even ethical [110]. They stated that clinical research must be well-designed to answer questions about the disease and to assess the efficacy and safety of prospective agents. Due to the high mortality rate of Ebola, it was important to identify an effective therapeutic at the earliest to tackle the outbreak. There was a difference in opinion among the researchers on how the clinical trials should be designed but in the end, they found out that a Randomized controlled trials (RCTs) were the most ethical and a proper design to be used in the epidemic since they allow researchers to examine the results of similar groups of persons who has or has not been administered with the investigational agent. Therefore, every effort should be made to implement them in case of an epidemic [111].

Currently, a specific treatment or vaccine for Ebola has not been licensed for use but several agents have been developed in the last decade.

15.8.2 SARS-CoV-2

COVID-19 has no approved treatments or vaccines at this time. With the number of cases expected to increase dramatically, this represents a massive unmet medical need. A Press Release was made mentioning that Chloroquine, Remdesivir, Umifenovir, Favipiravir, and Ribavarin are chosen by DeepVir, a deep learning AI model for repurposing to tackle the virus and all of them are under COVID-19 clinical trials in various locations throughout the world [20, 112–114]. Another ongoing clinical trial against COVID-19 is by using machine learning and artificial intelligence, whereby, the algorithm seeks to investigate a novel method for diagnosis of COVID-19 infection in the peripheral blood [115].

15.9 Conclusion

Artificial Intelligence (AI) is an emerging and promising technology for detecting early coronavirus infections and tracking the state of affected individuals. By building helpful procedures, it can effectively enhance therapeutic uniformity and selection. This chapter focuses on measuring the value of deep learning, machine learning, and other artificial intelligence methodologies in the fight against COVID-19, a global epidemic. Several studies have shown that AI and machine learning can reliably distinguish between Ebola, seasonal flu, and COVID-19 illnesses. AI and machine learning put a strong emphasis on diagnosis and detection. Methods ranging from disease detection to pandemic forecasting were presented as state-of-the-art. On a range of levels, these were compared and contrasted, with a focus on the data used, input properties, AI and ML technology, and their various field goals. We have provided a range of informative information throughout the text, including the nature of the application, the use of AI and ML, and the corresponding assessment conducted for each research. Our study has several limitations, but at the same path, it gives some avenues for future research in the identified track. To begin, we searched for relevant information citing a few specified key terms. Although our search key terms yielded fruitful outcomes for achieving our study's purpose, there's a chance we missed any important origin that didn't present in our searches. Then, we believe that the important parameters that we have found, investigated, and reported in this article are contemporary and recent materials linked to the pandemic and AI approaches. Therefore, future work is required to collect and evaluate more relevant origins.

References

1. Santoshi, S. and Sengupta, D., Artificial intelligence in precision medicine: A perspective in biomarker and drug discovery, in: *Artificial Intelligence and Machine Learning in Healthcare* [Internet], A. Saxena and S. Chandra (Eds.), pp. 71–88, Springer Singapore, Singapore, 2021, Available from: https://doi.org/10.1007/978-981-16-0811-7_4.
2. Rong, G., Mendez, A., Bou Assi, E., Zhao, B., Sawan, M., Artificial intelligence in healthcare: Review and prediction case studies. *Engineering*, 6, 3, 291–301, 2020.
3. Weissler, E.H., Naumann, T., Andersson, T. *et al.*, Correction to: The role of machine learning in clinical research: Transforming the future of evidence generation. *Trials*, 22, 1, 1–15, 2021. 10.1186/s13063-021-05489-x
4. Sarosh, P., Parah, S.A., Mansur, R.F., Bhat, G.M., Artificial intelligence for COVID-19 detection - A state-of-the-art review, 2 November 2020.
5. Thomas, B., Artificial intelligence: Review of current and future applications in medicine. *Fed. Pract.*, 38, 11, 527–538, 2021.
6. Loey, M., El-Sappagh, S., Mirjalili, S., Bayesian-based optimized deep learning model to detect COVID-19 patients using chest X-ray image data. *Comput. Biol. Med.*, 142, 105213, 2022.
7. Russo, G., Reche, P., Pennisi, M., Pappalardo, F., The combination of artificial intelligence and systems biology for intelligent vaccine design. *Expert Opin. Drug Discov.*, 15, 11, 1267–1281, 2020.
8. Nayak, J. and Naik, B., Intelligent system for COVID-19 prognosis: A state-of-the-art survey. *Appl. Intell.*, 51, 5, 2908–2938, 2021.
9. National Academies of Sciences, Engineering, and Medicine. Integrating Clinical Research into Epidemic Response: The Ebola Experience. Washington, DC: *The National Academies Press.* 2017. Available on: https://doi.org/10.17226/24739.
10. Whitelaw, S., Mamas, M.A., Topol, E., Van Spall, H.G.C., Applications of digital technology in COVID-19 pandemic planning and response. *Lancet Digit. Health*, 2, 8, e435–e440, 2020.
11. Chahal, D. and Byrne, M.F., A primer on artificial intelligence and its application to endoscopy. *Gastrointest. Endosc.*, 92, 4, 813–820.e4, 2020.
12. Ramesh, A.N., Kambhampati, C., Monson, J.R.T., Drew, P.J., Artificial intelligence in medicine. *Ann. R. Coll. Surg. Engl.*, 86, 5, 334–338, 2004.
13. Kaul, V., Enslin, S., Gross, S.A., History of artificial intelligence in medicine. *Gastrointest. Endosc.*, 92, 4, 807–812, 2020.
14. Kulikowski, C.A., Beginnings of artificial intelligence in medicine (AIM): Computational artifice assisting scientific inquiry and clinical art - with reflections on present AIM challenges. *Yearb. Med. Inform.*, 28, 1, 249–256, 2019.
15. Ford, J., Software review. *Bioinformatics*, 11, 5, 575–576, 1995.

16. Comendador, B.E.V., Francisco, B.M.B., Medenilla, J.S., Nacion, S.M.T., Serac, T.B.E., Pharmabot: A pediatric generic medicine consultant chatbot. *J. Autom. Control Eng.*, 3, 2, 137–140, 2015.
17. Ni, L., Lu, C., Liu, N., Liu, J., MANDY: Towards a smart primary care chatbot application. *Commun. Comput. Inf. Sci.*, 780, 38–52, 2017.
18. Khan, R., Srivastava, A.K., Gupta, M., Kumari, P., Kumar, S., Medicolite-machine learning-based patient care model. *Comput. Intell. Neurosci.* [Internet], 2022, 8109147, 2022, Available from: https://pubmed.ncbi.nlm.nih.gov/35126501.
19. Wong, Z.S.Y., Zhou, J., Zhang, Q., Artificial intelligence for infectious disease big data analytics. *Infect. Dis. Health*, 24, 1, 44–48, 2019.
20. Chavda VP, Kapadia C, Soni S, Prajapati R, Chauhan SC, Yallapu MM, Apostolopoulos V. A global picture: therapeutic perspectives for COVID-19. *Immunotherapy*. 14, 5, 351–371, 2022.
21. Chavda, V.P. and Apostolopoulos, V., Global impact of delta plus variant and vaccination. *Expert Rev. Vaccines*, 21, 5, 597–600, 2022, Available from: https://doi.org/10.1080/14760584.2022.2044800.
22. Chavda, V.P., Patel, A.B., Vaghasiya, D.D., SARS-CoV-2 variants and vulnerability at the global level. *J. Med. Virol.*, 97, 7, 2986–3005, 2022, Available from: https://doi.org/10.1002/jmv.27717.
23. Chavda, V.P., Pandya, A., Pulakkat, S., Soniwala, M., Patravale, V., Lymphatic filariasis vaccine development: Neglected for how long? *Expert Rev. Vaccines*, 20, 11, 1471–1482, 2021.
24. Chavda, V.P., Gajjar, N., Shah, N., Dave, D.J., Darunavir ethanolate: Repurposing an anti-HIV drug in COVID-19 treatment. *Eur. J. Med. Chem. Rep.* [Internet], 3, 100013, 2021, Available from: https://www.sciencedirect.com/science/article/pii/S2772417421000133.
25. Chavda, V.P., Feehan, J., Apostolopoulos, V., A veterinary vaccine for SARS-CoV-2: The first COVID-19 vaccine for animals. *Vaccines*, 9, 6, 631, 2021.
26. Chavda, V.P., Bezbaruah, R., Athalye, M. *et al.*, Replicating viral vector-based vaccines for COVID-19: Potential avenue in vaccination arena. *Viruses*, 14, 4, 759, 2022.
27. Chavda, V.P., Hossain, M.K., Beladiya, J., Apostolopoulos, V., Nucleic acid vaccines for COVID-19: A paradigm shift in the vaccine development arena. *Biologics*, 1, 3, 337–356, 2021.
28. Basu, D., Chavda, V.P., Mehta, A.A., Therapeutics for COVID-19 and post COVID-19 complications: An update. *Curr. Res. Pharmacol. Drug Discovery* 3, 100086, 2022, Available from: https://www.sciencedirect.com/science/article/pii/S2590257122000062.
29. Chavda, V.P., Pandya, R., Apostolopoulos, V., DNA vaccines for SARS-CoV-2: Towards third generation vaccination era. *Expert Rev. Vaccines*, 20, 12, 1549–1560, 2021.
30. Chavda, V.P., Vora, L.K., Vihol, D.R., COVAX-19® vaccine: Completely blocks virus transmission to non-immune individuals. *Clin. Complement.*

Med. Pharmacol. [Internet], 1, 1, 100004, 2021, Available from: https://www.sciencedirect.com/science/article/pii/S2772371221000048.

31. Chavda, V.P., Kumar, A., Banerjee, R., Das, N., Ayurvedic and other herbal remedies for dengue: An update. *Clin. Complement. Med. Pharmacol.*, 2, 3, 100024, 2022.
32. Chavda, V.P., Ertas, Y.N., Walhekar, V. *et al.*, Advanced computational methodologies used in the discovery of new natural anticancer compounds. *Front. Pharmacol.*, 12, 702611, 2021.
33. Chavda, V.P., Vora, L.K., Pandya, A.K., Patravale, V.B., Intranasal vaccines for SARS-CoV-2: From challenges to potential in COVID-19 management. *Drug Discovery Today* [Internet], 26, 11, 2619–2636, 2021, Available from: https://www.sciencedirect.com/science/article/pii/S1359644621003317.
34. Chavda, V.P., Patel, A.B., Vihol, D. *et al.*, Herbal remedies, nutraceuticals, and dietary supplements for COVID-19 management: An update. *Clin. Complement. Med. Pharmacol.* 2, 1, 100021, 2022, Available from: https://www.sciencedirect.com/science/article/pii/S2772371222000031.
35. Chavda, V.P., Pandya, R., Apostolopoulos, V., DNA vaccines for SARS-CoV-2: Toward third-generation vaccination era. *Expert Rev. Vaccines*, 20, 12, 1549–1560, 2021.
36. Majumdar, A., Debnath, T., Sood, S.K., Baishnab, K.L., Kyasanur forest disease classification framework using novel extremal optimization tuned neural network in fog computing environment. *J. Med. Syst.*, 42, 10, 1–6, 2018.
37. Sandhu, R., Sood, S.K., Kaur, G., An intelligent system for predicting and preventing MERS-CoV infection outbreak. *J. Supercomput.*, 72, 8, 3033–3056, 2016.
38. Sood, S.K. and Mahajan, I., Wearable IoT sensor based healthcare system for identifying and controlling chikungunya virus. *Comput. Ind.*, 91, 33–44, 2017.
39. Sareen, S., Gupta, S.K., Sood, S.K., An intelligent and secure system for predicting and preventing Zika virus outbreak using Fog computing. *Enterp. Inf. Syst.*, 11, 9, 1436–1456, 2017.
40. Lalmuanawma, S., Hussain, J., Chhakchhuak, L., Applications of machine learning and artificial intelligence for COVID-19 (SARS-CoV-2) pandemic: A review. *Chaos Solitons Fractals* [Internet], 139, 110059, 2020, Available from: https://www.sciencedirect.com/science/article/pii/S0960077920304562.
41. Vaishya, R., Javaid, M., Khan, I.H., Haleem, A., Artificial Intelligence (AI) applications for COVID-19 pandemic. *Diabetes Metab. Syndr.* [Internet], 14, 4, 337–339, 2020, Available from: https://pubmed.ncbi.nlm.nih.gov/32305024.
42. Yan, L., Zhang, H.-T., Goncalves, J. *et al.*, An interpretable mortality prediction model for COVID-19 patients. *Nat. Mach. Intell.*, 2, 5, 283–288, 2020.
43. Vickers, N.J., Animal communication: When i'm calling you, will you answer too? *Curr. Biol.*, 27, 14, R713–R715, 2017.

44. Xu, Z., Su, C., Xiao, Y., Wang, F., Artificial intelligence for COVID-19: Battling the pandemic with computational intelligence. *Intell. Med.*, 2, 1, 13–29, 2022.
45. Kuster, A.C. and Overgaard, H.J., A novel comprehensive metric to assess effectiveness of COVID-19 testing: Inter-country comparison and association with geography, government, and policy response. *PLoS One*, 16, 3, 1–21, 2021.
46. Lai, S., Ruktanonchai, N.W., Zhou, L. *et al.*, Effect of non-pharmaceutical interventions to contain COVID-19 in China. *Nature*, 585, 7825, 410–413, 2020.
47. Wooldridge, M. and Jennings, N., Intelligent agents: Theory and practice. *Knowl. Eng. Rev.*, 10, 2, 115–152, 1995.
48. Grams, R.R., Zhang, D., Yue, B., Medical diagnostic decision support systems-past, present and future: A threaded biblibography and brief commentary. *J. Med. Syst.*, 20, 3, 129–140, 1996.
49. Haleem, A., Vaishya, R., Javaid, M., Khan, I.H., Artificial Intelligence (AI) applications in orthopaedics: An innovative technology to embrace. *J. Clin. Orthop. Trauma*, 11, S80–S81, 2020.
50. Biswas, K. and Sen, P., Space-time dependence of corona virus (COVID-19) outbreak. *arXiv*, 1, 1, 5–7, 2020.
51. Stebbing, J., Phelan, A., Griffin, I. *et al.*, COVID-19: Combining antiviral and anti-inflammatory treatments. *Lancet Infect. Dis.*, 20, 4, 400–402, 2020.
52. Sohrabi, C., Alsafi, Z., O'Neill, N. *et al.*, World Health Organization declares global emergency: A review of the 2019 novel coronavirus (COVID-19). *Int. J. Surg.*, 76, 71–76, 2020.
53. Tian, H., Liu, Y., Li, Y. *et al.*, An investigation of transmission control measures during the first 50 days of the COVID-19 epidemic in China. *Sci. (80-.)*, 368, 6491, 638–642, 2020.
54. Bobdey, S. and Ray, S., Going viral – COVID-19 impact assessment: A perspective beyond clinical practice. *J. Mar. Med. Soc.*, 22, 1, 9, 2020.
55. Gozes, O., Frid-Adar, M., Greenspan, H. *et al.*, Rapid AI development cycle for the coronavirus (COVID-19) pandemic: Initial results for automated detection & patient monitoring using deep learning CT image analysis. *Radiol. Artif. Intell.*, 3, 5–8, 2020.
56. Pirouz, B., Haghshenas, S.S., Haghshenas, S.S., Piro, P., Investigating a serious challenge in the sustainable development process: Analysis of confirmed cases of COVID-19 (new type of Coronavirus) through a binary classification using artificial intelligence and regression analysis. *Sustain (United States)*, 12, 6, 5–8, 2020.
57. Ting, D.S.W., Carin, L., Dzau, V., Wong, T.Y., Digital technology and COVID-19. *Nat. Med.*, 26, 4, 459–461, 2020.
58. Wan, K.H., Huang, S.S., Young, A.L., Lam, D.S.C., Precautionary measures needed for ophthalmologists during pandemic of the coronavirus disease 2019 (COVID-19). *Acta Ophthalmol.*, 98, 3, 221–222, 2020.

59. Li, L., Qin, L., Xu, Z. *et al.*, Using artificial intelligence to detect COVID-19 and community-acquired pneumonia based on pulmonary CT: Evaluation of the diagnostic accuracy. *Radiology*, 296, 2, E65–E71, 2020.
60. Das, S., Mishra, A., Roy, P., Automatic diabetes prediction using tree based ensemble learners. *Proc. Int. Conf.*, 2, 2, 21–29, 2018.
61. Syed, A.H. and Khan, T., Machine learning-based application for predicting risk of type 2 diabetes mellitus (T2DM) in Saudi Arabia: A retrospective cross-sectional study. *IEEE Access*, 8, 199539–199561, 2020.
62. Joshi, A., Joshi, B.C., A ul Mannan, M., Kaushik, V., Epitope based vaccine prediction for SARS-COV-2 by deploying immuno-informatics approach. *Inform. Med. Unlocked*, 19, March, 100338, 2020.
63. Littrup, P.J., Freeman-Gibb, L., Andea, A. *et al.*, Cryotherapy for breast fibroadenomas. *Radiology*, 234, 1, 63–72, 2005.
64. Ardakani, A.A., Kanafi, A.R., Acharya, U.R., Khadem, N., Mohammadi, A., Application of deep learning technique to manage COVID-19 in routine clinical practice using CT images: Results of 10 convolutional neural networks. *Comput. Biol. Med.*, 121, March, 103795, 2020.
65. Mahmud, T., Rahman, M.A., Fattah, S.A., CovXNet: A multi-dilation convolutional neural network for automatic COVID-19 and other pneumonia detection from chest X-ray images with transferable multi-receptive feature optimization. *Comput. Biol. Med.*, 122, May, 103869, 2020.
66. Kohmer, N., Westhaus, S., Rühl, C., Ciesek, S., Rabenau, H.F., Brief clinical evaluation of six high-throughput SARS-CoV-2 IgG antibody assays. *J. Clin. Virol.*, 129, May, 104480, 2020.
67. Wu, J., Zhang, P., Zhang, L. *et al.*, Rapid and accurate identification of COVID-19 infection through machine learning based on clinical available blood test results. *medRxiv*, 2020, Available from: https://doi.org/10.1101/2020.04.02.20051136
68. Sarraf, D.P., Gupta, P.P., Keshwar, S., Public's Knowledge and beliefs towards universal safety precautions during. *J. Drug Deliv. Ther.*, 10, 133–141, 2020.
69. Mor, S., Saini, P., Wangnoo, S.K., Bawa, T., Worldwide spread of COVID-19 pandemic and risk factors among co-morbid conditions especially diabetes mellitus in India. *Res. J. Pharm. Technol.*, 13, 5, 2530–2532, 2020.
70. Arora, G., Joshi, J., Mandal, R.S., Shrivastava, N., Virmani, R., Sethi, T., Artificial intelligence in surveillance, diagnosis, drug discovery and vaccine development against COVID-19. *Pathogens*, 10, 8, 1048, 2021.
71. Marcus, J.L., Sewell, W.C., Balzer, L.B., Krakower, D.S., Artificial intelligence and machine learning for HIV prevention: Emerging approaches to ending the epidemic. *Curr. HIV/AIDS Rep.*, 17, 3, 171–179, 2020.
72. Feng, S., Feng, Z., Ling, C., Chang, C., Feng, Z., Prediction of the COVID-19 epidemic trends based on SEIR and AI models. *PLoS One*, 16, 1 January, 1–15, 2021.

73. Malik, Y.S., Sircar, S., Bhat, S. *et al.*, How artificial intelligence may help the COVID-19 pandemic: Pitfalls and lessons for the future. *Rev. Med. Virol.*, 31, 5, 1–11, 2021.
74. Khemasuwan, D. and Colt, H.G., Applications and challenges of AI-based algorithms in the COVID-19 pandemic. *BMJ Innov.* [Internet], 7, 2, 387 LP–398, 2021, Available from: http://innovations.bmj.com/content/7/2/387.abstract.
75. Ghimire, A., Thapa, S., Jha, A.K., Kumar, A., Kumar, A., Adhikari, S., AI and IoT solutions for tackling COVID-19 pandemic, in: *Proceedings of the 4th International Conference on Electronics, Communication and Aerospace Technology, ICECA 2020*, IEEE, pp. 1083–1092, 2020. Available from: https://doi.org/10.1109/ICECA49313.2020.9297454
76. Garibaldi, B.T., Chisolm, M.S., Berkenblit, G.V. *et al.*, Review of the published literature to characterise clinical excellence in COVID-19 care. *Postgrad. Med. J.*, 1–7, 2021.
77. Islam, M.N., Inan, T.T., Rafi, S., Akter, S.S., Sarker, I.H., Islam, A.K.M.N., A systematic review on the use of AI and ML for fighting the COVID-19 pandemic. *IEEE Trans. Artif. Intell.*, 1, 3, 258–270, 2021.
78. Garg, S., Kim, L., Whitaker, M. *et al.*, Hospitalization rates and characteristics of patients hospitalized with. *Morb. Mortal. Wkly. Rep., US Dep. Heal. Hum. Serv. Dis. Control Prev.*, 69, 15, 458–464, 2020.
79. de Dombal, F.T., Computer-aided diagnosis of acute abdominal pain. The British experience. *Rev. Epidemiol. Sante Publique*, 32, 1, 50–56, 1984.
80. Haleem, A., Javaid, M., Vaisha, R., Since January 2020 Elsevier has created a COVID-19 resource centre with free information in English and Mandarin on the novel coronavirus COVID-19. The COVID-19 resource centre is hosted on Elsevier Connect, the company's public news and information. *Curr. Med. Res. Pract.*, 10, January, 78–79, 2020.
81. Sarker, I.H. and Kayes, A.S.M., ABC-RuleMiner: User behavioral rule-based machine learning method for context-aware intelligent services. *J. Netw. Comput. Appl.*, 168, June, 102762, 2020.
82. Piccialli, F., di Cola, V.S., Giampaolo, F., Cuomo, S., The role of artificial intelligence in fighting the COVID-19 pandemic. *Inf. Syst. Front.*, 23, 6, 1467–1497, 2021.
83. Shorten, C., Khoshgoftaar, T.M., Furht, B., Deep learning applications for COVID-19. *J. Big Data*, 8, 1, 1–54, 2021.
84. Aminian, A., Safari, S., Razeghian-Jahromi, A., Ghorbani, M., Delaney, C.P., COVID-19 Outbreak and surgical practice: Unexpected fatality in perioperative period. *Ann. Surg.*, 272, 1, e27–e29, 2020.
85. Wang, J., Yu, H., Hua, Q. *et al.*, A descriptive study of random forest algorithm for predicting COVID-19 patients outcome. *PeerJ*, 8, 1–19, 2020.
86. Li, Q., Feng, W., Quan, Y.H., Trend and forecasting of the COVID-19 outbreak in China. *J. Infect.*, 80, 4, 469–496, 2020.

87. Farhat, N.H., Photonit neural networks and learning mathines the role of electron-trapping materials. *IEEE Expert. Syst. Appl.*, 7, 5, 63–72, 1992.
88. Huyut, M. and Üstündağ, H., Prediction of diagnosis and prognosis of COVID-19 disease by blood gas parameters using decision trees machine learning model: A retrospective observational study. *Med. Gas Res.*, 12, 2, 60–66, 2022.
89. Dong, C., Qiao, Y., Shang, C. *et al.*, Non-contact screening system based for COVID-19 on XGBoost and logistic regression. *Comput. Biol. Med.*, 141, 28, 105003, 2022.
90. Rustam, F., Ashraf, I., Mehmood, A., Ullah, S., Choi, G.S., Tweets classification on the base of sentiments for US airline companies. *Entropy*, 21, 11, 1–22, 2019.
91. Debjit, K., Islam, S., Rahman, A., Pinki, F.T., Nath, R.D., An improved machine-learning approach for COVID-19 prediction using Harris Hawks optimization and feature analysis using SHAP. December 2019, 1–19, 2022.
92. Shahi, T.B., Sitaula, C., Paudel, N., A hybrid feature extraction method for nepali COVID-19-related tweets classification. *Comput. Intell. Neurosci.*, 2022, 2022. Available from: https://doi.org/10.1155/2022/5681574
93. Anantpadma, M., Lane, T., Zorn, K.M. *et al.*, Ebola virus bayesian machine learning models enable new in vitro leads. *ACS Omega*, 4, 1, 2353–2361, 2019.
94. Bansal, A., Padappayil, R.P., Garg, C., Singal, A., Gupta, M., Klein, A., Utility of artificial intelligence amidst the COVID 19 pandemic: A review. *J. Med. Syst.*, 44, 9, 156, 2020.
95. Kwekha-Rashid, A.S., Abduljabbar, H.N., Alhayani, B., Coronavirus disease (COVID-19) cases analysis using machine-learning applications. *Appl. Nanosci.*, 2021. 0123456789.
96. Jiang, F., Jiang, Y., Zhi, H. *et al.*, Artificial intelligence in healthcare: Past, present and future. *Stroke Vasc. Neurol.*, 2, 4, 230–243, 2017.
97. Ahmad, M.A., Eckert, C., Teredesai, A., Interpretable machine learning in healthcare, in: *Proceedings of the 2018 ACM International Conference on Bioinformatics, Computational Biology, and Health Informatics*, ACM, New York, NY, USA, pp. 559–560, 2018.
98. Naseem, M., Akhund, R., Arshad, H., Ibrahim, M.T., Exploring the potential of artificial intelligence and machine learning to combat COVID-19 and existing opportunities for LMIC: A scoping review. *J. Prim. Care Community Health*, 11, 2020.
99. Holzinger, A., Langs, G., Denk, H., Zatloukal, K., Müller, H., Causability and explainability of artificial intelligence in medicine. *Wiley Interdiscip. Rev. Data Min. Knowl. Discovery*, 9, 4, 1–13, 2019.
100. Esteva, A., Robicquet, A., Ramsundar, B. *et al.*, A guide to deep learning in healthcare. *Nat. Med.*, 25, 1, 24–29, 2019.

101. Fanioudakis, E., Geismar, M., Potamitis, I., Mosquito wingbeat analysis and classification using deep learning. *Eur. Signal Process. Conf.*, 2018-Sept., pp. 2410–2414, 2018.
102. Fong, S.J., Li, G., Dey, N., Gonzalez-Crespo, R., Herrera-Viedma, E., Finding an accurate early forecasting model from small dataset: A case of 2019-nCoV novel coronavirus outbreak. *Int. J. Interact. Multimedia Artif. Intell.*, 6, 1, 132, 2020.
103. Gomez, P. L., Robinson, J. M., Rogalewicz, J. A. Vaccine manufacturing. *Vaccines Sixth Ed.*, 44–57, 2012, doi:10.1016/B978-1-4557-0090-5.00019-7.
104. WHO Expert Committe on Biological Standardization, *Guidelines on clinical evaluation of vaccines: Regulatory expectations*; TRS 1004, Annex 9. *WHO Tech. Rep. Ser.*, 67, 1004(924), 503–575, 2017. Available on: https://www.who.int/publications/m/item/clinical-evaluation-of-vaccines-annex-9-trs-no-1004
105. Rolling, K.E. and Hayney, M.S., The vaccine development process. *J. Am. Pharm. Assoc.*, 56, 6, 687–689, 2016.
106. Han, S., Clinical vaccine development. *Clin. Exp. Vaccine Res.*, 4, 1, 46, 2015.
107. Regulators MTHE. European Medicines Agency, CAT Secretariat & US Food and Drug Administration. *Regen. Med.*, 6, 6 SUPPL., 90–96, 2011.
108. Miller, M.A. and Rathore, M.H., Immunization in special populations. *Adv. Pediatr.*, 59, 1, 95–136, 2012.
109. Cagigi, A., Rinaldi, S., Di Martino, A. *et al.*, Premature immune senescence during HIV-1 vertical infection relates with response to influenza vaccination. *J. Allergy Clin. Immunol.*, 133, 2, 592–594.e1, 2014.
110. Edwards, K.M. and Kochhar, S., Ethics of conducting clinical research in an outbreak setting. *Annu. Rev. Virol.* [Internet], 7, 1, 475–494, 2020, Available from: https://doi.org/10.1146/annurev-virology-013120-013123.
111. Spieth, P.M., Kubasch, A.S., Penzlin, A.I., Illigens, B.M.-W., Barlinn, K., Siepmann, T., Randomized controlled trials - a matter of design. *Neuropsychiatr. Dis. Treat.* [Internet], 12, 1341–1349, 2016, Available from: https://pubmed.ncbi.nlm.nih.gov/27354804.
112. Mongia A, Jain S, Chouzenoux E, Majumdar A. DeepVir: Graphical deep matrix factorization for *in silico* antiviral repositioning—Application to COVID-19. *J. Comput. Biol.*, 29, 5, 441–452, 2022.
113. Chavda, V. P., Chapter 4 Nanobased nano drug delivery: A comprehensive review. *Applications of Targeted Nano Drugs and Delivery Systems: Nanoscience and Nanotechnology in Drug Delivery*, Elsevier Inc., 2018. Available from: doi:10.1016/B978-0-12-814029-1.00004-1.
114. Chavda, V.P., Nanotherapeutics and nanobiotechnology, in: *Applications of Targeted Nano Drugs and Delivery Systems*, pp. 1–13, Elsevier, 2019. Available from: https://doi.org/10.1016/B978-0-12-814029-1.00001-6
115. Wang, L., Zhang, Y., Wang, D. *et al.*, Artificial intelligence for COVID-19: A systematic review [Internet]. *Front. Med.*, 8, 1–15, 2021, Available from: https://www.frontiersin.org/article/10.3389/fmed.2021.704256.

16

AI and ML for Development of Cell and Gene Therapy for Personalized Treatment

Susmit Mhatre[1], Somanshi Shukla[2], Vivek P. Chavda[3], Lakshmikanth Gandikota[4] and Vandana Patravale[2*]

[1]Department of Pharmacy Sciences, School of Pharmacy and Health Professions, Creighton University, Omaha, Nebraska, USA
[2]Department of Pharmaceutical Sciences and Technology, Institute of Chemical Technology, Mumbai, India
[3]Department of Pharmaceutic and Pharmaceutical Technology, L. M. College of Pharmacy, Ahmedabad, India
[4]Cell and Gene Therapy Products, Research and Development, Intas Pharmaceutical Ltd. (Biopharma Division), Ahmedabad, India

Abstract
Artificial Intelligence (AI) has the potential to revolutionize several aspects of human life, and medicine is one of them. For cell and gene-based therapies, the application of AI is still in its preliminary stages but holds tremendous potential. Personalized medicine demands an exhaustive understanding of genomic composition of individuals and the risk factors associated with them. The identification of suitable genes needs meticulous screening and characterization so that an individual has the highest compatibility and hence avails maximum therapeutic benefits. Machine learning (ML) based algorithms, a subset of AI, can help in the screening process. ML based models have successfully predicted stem cell differentiation, cell fate, and gene expression using algorithms trained with information already available from different individuals and pre-clinical and clinical studies. Based on the available datasets of genomic information and drug responses, several models have been able to predict the potency of cell therapies. Indeed, the potential of ML in personalized medicine through cell and gene therapies is worth investigating. This chapter discusses the fundamentals and applications of ML and other AI based techniques in developing predictive models for different aspects of cell and gene therapies.

**Corresponding author*: vb.patravale@ictmumbai.edu.in

Vivek Chavda, Krishnan Anand and Vasso Apostolopoulos (eds.) Bioinformatics Tools for Pharmaceutical Drug Product Development, (371–400) © 2023 Scrivener Publishing LLC

Keywords: Artificial intelligence, machine learning, predictive model, artificial neural networks, cell therapy, gene therapy, stem cell fate

16.1 Fundamentals of Cell Therapy

Cellular therapies have their roots from the 19th century and continue to expand their horizon for research and investment reasons. In 1889, the first cell therapy procedure was done by Charles Édouard Brown-Séquard, he was the first to develop hormone replacement therapy during his era. He also tried to reduce the effects of aging with the aid of animal injections. Cell therapy is stated as the transfer of allogeneic or autologous cellular components to the sufferer for therapeutic applications. It encompasses the stem cell (SC) and non-SC-based therapy, single-celled and multi-celled therapy, and various immune-phenotypes, isolation strategies, and control levels. As of today, cell therapy continues to grow in each aspect such as research, clinical safety and efficacy. According to the global market trends the cell therapy market is supposed to reach USD 23.0 billion by 2028. It usually makes use of allogeneic or autologous cells; it may include genetic engineering or gene alterations; and could also be used topically or in forms of injections, infusions, bio-scaffolds, or non-scaffold systems. It covers a wide range of therapies, such as rejuvenation, immunotherapy, and cancer treatment. Many cell-based therapies are currently being experimented, with a few exceptions such as the transfusion of hematopoietic SC (HSC) which is already a well-established treatment for blood-related diseases [1].

Therapies for many degenerative diseases can be developed because of the ability to convert SCs into differentiated cell types, such as brain cells, pancreas, or eyes. For instance, to cure or reduce the symptoms of Parkinson's disease which is caused by the loss of dopamine producing brain cells, there are a lot of clinical trials being performed using pluripotent SC-derived brain cells [2]. The loss of these dopamine producing cells in the brain from substantia nigra results in disruption of movement, muscle stiffness, and tremors [3]. To replace these lost cells, scientists have discovered dopamine-producing brain cells in human pluripotent SCs. SC-derived brain cells are currently being explored to see if they reduce the symptoms. Similar studies are being taken up to explore the advantages of SCs in the treatment of eye diseases that affect eyesight or can even cause blindness [4].

It is essential that one has a well-documented procedure to create the required cell types in a cost-effective manner, for cell therapy to be successful. The proliferation of the transplanted cells once implanted and integrated with the host cells to perform their function is also critical for the success. Additionally, one should also ensure that the regenerated cells don't show tumor-like growth in the host. Therefore, rigorous testing should be done before cell therapy is made available to patients. Translational Bioinformatics (TBI) studies will need to keep addressing implementation difficulties throughout the spectrum of disease in order to achieve the potential of customized medicine. The goal of this chapter is to assess the growing topic of TBI as it applies to therapeutic applications, as well as to identify recurring characteristics and present gaps in order to spur more investigation (Figure 16.1) [5, 6].

Cell therapy is used in many diseases for many organs and there are several delivery methods currently in use [7–11]. Therefore, the mechanism of the therapies involved in various treatments is broad. However, the main principles by which the therapeutic action is performed by the cells can be classified into two. The first is that the SC themselves when implanted into the site of injury (by systemic or local management) replace the damaged cells and start dividing to form new cells. In this way, the normal operation of the damaged organ is restored. An example of this is the use of cells to replace cardiomyocytes after myocardial infarction [12], to aid angiogenesis in ischemic stroke [13], or to produce cartilage matrix degeneration intervertebral disc [14]. The second is that cells produce soluble factors like chemokines, cytokines, and hormones. These factors make it easier

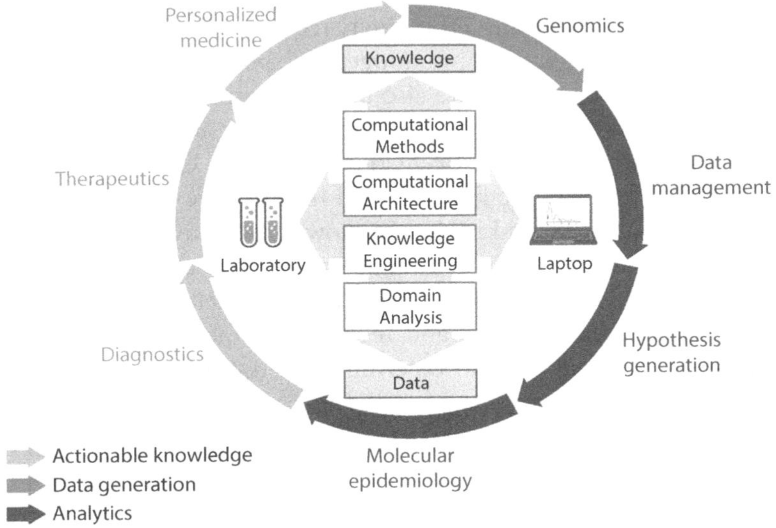

Figure 16.1 The clinical applications of translational bioinformatics. (Figure created with Biorender.com.)

for the body to heal itself by introducing local cells (stem) or attracting cells to move into transplanted regions. The cells with a smaller number of passages have shown to be much more effective in performing paracrine function than the cells with more number of passages [15]. The life of transported cells either through systemic or local administration is relatively small (days-weeks). This also comprises the naturally produced cells with the right therapeutic agents or that have undergone epigenetic mutations or are genetically engineered to release large amounts of substances that aid in angiogenesis, anti-apoptosis, and anti-inflammation [16].

There are many ways to classify cell therapies. The classification is based on their therapeutic application according to which they can be classified as neurological, cardiovascular, ophthalmic, regenerative, cancer therapy or immunotherapy. Another method of differentiation is based on whether the donor and recipient of the cells is the same individual (autologous), or different individuals (allogeneic), or even different species (xenogenic) [17].

16.1.1 Stem Cell Therapies

Several types of cells are tested for cell therapies. Embryonic SCs (ESCs) isolated from interior cellular part of blastocyst [18] show totipotency, giving a great opportunity for the discovery of new therapies. The main challenges for the lucrative use of ESCs are the designing of vigorous and repetitive systems of differentiation for determining the pure population density of isolated cells. Along with this, other safety requisites involve preventing the formation of teratoma and an immunogenic response during implantation. Behavioral considerations should also be taken into account. Induced pluripotent SC (iPSCs) isolated from somatic cells, are conditioned to produce pluripotent cells. The fibroblast cells on exposure to Oct3/4, Sox2, c-Myc and Klf4 [18] produced the first reported iPSCs. They show excellent differentiation capabilities, and in theory allow for the advancement towards curated treatment on the basis of an automated source (reprogramming) [19]. If iPSCs can be created from human somatic cells, this might lead to key therapeutic breakthroughs and regenerative medicine advancements [20]. However, we still need to determine the tumorigenic potential and long-term genetic stability for these therapies. Adult and infant SCs are divided into bone marrow, placenta, peripheral blood, umbilical blood, adipose and other differentiated tissues, to deliver as a progenitor for tissue-specific SC [21]. Detailed studies are needed to evaluate if certain cellular sources are of additional benefit during the treatment of certain diseases. Some of the important SCs used in clinical practices [21, 22].

16.1.1.1 Mesenchymal Stem Cells (MSCs)

These are high-strength cells, and are derived from bone marrow, peripheral blood, placenta, umbilical cord, and adipose. MSCs produce a broad range of cytokines, growth factors, chemokines, angiogenic substances and anti-inflammatory substances, and also perform immune functions. In addition, MSCs can promote the amplification of chronic SC, involving their use in tissue repair. They have also been thoroughly evaluated during pre-clinical and clinical studies and showed favorable results in the treatment of many grave diseases. However, many late-stage clinical trials have not met the basic requisites and thus the application of MSCs in systemic delivery is less well known [23].

16.1.1.2 Hematopoietic Stem Cells (HSCs)

These are isolated from bone marrow, peripheral blood, and umbilical cord. When transplanted, they migrate to bone marrow, where they regenerate themselves and rebuild the hematopoietic system. The first ones to be explored in the field of stem cells were the HSCs and till date, total bone marrow or HSC therapies are the sole SC-based treatments that got approval for the management of specific leukemia. HSCs for the management of autoimmune diseases have given good results when used in combination with transplantation [24].

16.1.1.3 Mononuclear Cells (MNCs)

MNCs are derived from peripheral blood and bone marrow. They also include hematopoietic immunoglobulins, lymphoid cells, macrophages, and monocytes. MNCs are widely researched during clinical trials for management of cardiovascular disease, neurological disorders, and acute ischemia of the organs [24].

16.1.1.4 Endothelial Progenitor Cells (EPCs)

These are derived from bone marrow, peripheral blood, and umbilical cord. They account for almost 1% of the whole MNC peripheral population and are distinguished by the expression of VEGFR2 endothelial-specific markers and the HSC markers (e.g., CD34 and CD133). Till now, no cell surface markers have been distinguished as specific to all EPCs, and therefore, search for SC unique markers is still going on [25]. EPCs play a vital role in formation of new blood vessels that is the targeted therapeutic effect with reference to ischemic diseases.

16.1.1.5 Neural Stem Cells (NSCs) or Neural Progenitor Cells (NPCs)

NSCs are highly differentiated cells derived from the tissues of the fetal or adult nervous system. In the adult brain, NSCs are present in the sub ventricular zone (SVZ) of lateral ventricles and the sub granular zone of the hippocampal dentate gyrus. Isolation from epithelium and spinal cord could also be done. Due to their capabilities to form functional neurons and glia, NSCs are also regarded for the development of an effective treatment of neurological disorders [26].

16.1.2 Adoptive Cell Therapy

Adoptive cell therapy is also known as cellular immunotherapy. It is a therapy that uses immune cells to fight diseases. A few of the processes include directly isolating and expanding immune cells, while others involve genetic modification of the immune cells (genetically modified cells) to improve their ability to fight diseases [27]. In the case of cancer, killer T cells are prominent players, due to their property to bind antigen to the surface of cancer cells [28]. Adoptive cell therapies utilize this natural ability and can be used in a variety of ways.

16.1.2.1 Tumor-Infiltrating Lymphocyte (TIL) Therapy

The presence of the lethal T cells is not always sufficient to ensure that the job of destroying the tumor will be done. A possible setback is that these T cells must first be activated by exposure to the antigen before they can effectively perform their function of killing cancer cells, and they must also be able to retain that function long enough to support an effective immune response [29, 30]. One more possible setback could be that the T cells are present in insufficient quantities.

A form of diagnostic treatment that attempts to solve these problems is TIL therapy. The method regenerates the naturally occurring T-cell population that has already invaded diseased cells, then activates and expands them [31]. Later, a sufficient amount of these activated T cell populations is reintroduced into patients, where they perform their normal function [32].

16.1.2.2 *Engineered T-Cell Receptor (TCR) Therapy*

It is not always necessary that the T-cells have recognized the tumor. And in some cases, the T-cells may not be activated and expanded into sufficient quantities to function properly. In these cases, physicians might use a technique known as engineered T-cell receptor (TCR) therapy [33].

This method also includes capturing T-cells in patients, but in place of simply activating and amplifying the available tumor-resistant T-cells, they could be implanted with a novel T-cell receptor that enhances its ability to target specific cancer antigens [34].

16.1.2.3 *Chimeric Antigen Receptor (CAR) T Cell Therapy*

The aforementioned therapies of TIL and TCR can only target the antigen when it is complexed with antigen presenting cells such as the major histocompatibility complex (MHC). But the recent developments in adoptive cell therapies have allowed physicians to overcome this barrier [35]. Scientists arm the patient's T cells with an artificial receptor known as chimeric antigen receptor (CAR).

A major benefit of these receptors is their ability to bind to antigens that have not been processed or are bound to MHCs. However, CAR T cells can only detect the immunogens themselves that are naturally expressed in the cell environment, so the range of potent antigens is smaller than TCRs. CARs potential is being evaluated in a variety of ways for different types of cancers. A method currently in clinical research is using SCs to create an unlimited source of off-shelf CAR T cells [36].

16.1.2.4 *Natural Killer (NK) Cell Therapy*

It is a very recent approach in adoptive cell therapy to use other body cells, such as natural killer (NK) cells. An application considered in the clinic includes arming these NK cells with cancer-targeting CARs [37]. The NK cell is a kind of immune effector cell that is capable of responding quickly and effectively against tumors. Adoptive NK cell cancer immunotherapy was first shown in clinical trials against hematological malignancies a decade ago. The challenge of obtaining large quantities of NK cells, scaling up *ex vivo* to therapeutic size, and maintaining *in vivo* survival and function of injected NK cells has slowed development. It is time to re-explore the therapeutic potentials of NK cells using new tools such as iPSC-NK and genetic engineering approaches, as well as fresh understandings of NK cell biology. Despite the obstacles, existing licensed NK cell-based therapeutics and forthcoming pre-clinical and clinical trials remain enticing.

16.2 Fundamentals of Gene Therapy

Genetic therapy is a way to treat genetic/chronic disorders by modifying, down regulating, or replacing the genes of an individual. It can be performed *in-vitro* or *in-vivo*. During the *in-vivo* process, the therapeutic genes are delivered directly into the patient's cells, whereas in *ex-vivo* delivery, the therapeutic gene is incorporated into foreign cells before they are induced into the body. For this, the therapeutic modified genes are placed in an inactivated virus such as retroviruses, lentiviruses or adeno-associated viruses. Cell therapy is a form of *ex-vivo* gene therapy [38].

Despite the flexible therapeutic approach, the success of it lies in guaranteeing that gene therapy is specifically targeted at the right cells and tissues [39]. Along with molecular guidance, other hurdles faced by geneticists consist of the unintentional inclusion of genes from the delivery vehicle, and accurate testing of the natural immune response of the body in response to the viral vectors that carry the gene modified DNA payloads. A prominent solution to all the before-mentioned hurdles is understanding the human genome, a method that fragments and sequences the different parts of DNA for better understanding of their function [40]. However, the human genome comprises more than 3 billion elements and the analysis of this amount of data using common statistical methods can be tedious, resource-intensive, and complex. In such situations, ML proves to be a useful tool. It is one of the methods used in AI to generate automated intelligent behavior using mathematical data. It provides an opportunity to learn from statistical data and perform learning-based actions. Through ML, large and complicated data analysis can be done in a fast and efficient way.

The two main applications of AI in genetics are: 1) Identification of the therapeutic target genes and 2) the off target effects.

16.2.1 Identification

For humans, it is a very difficult and time-taking procedure to understand the enormous information contained in an individual's DNA. This process can be made more systematic and precise by using machines for its main purpose. ML speeds up the analysis of sequential data and successfully predicts genetic mutations coupled to a specific disorder [41, 42]. Algorithms are designed based on motifs identified in large datasets, which are then translated into human models to evaluate their impact.

ML algorithms can be used for comparing the difference in the level of genetic expression of the malignant and normal tissue samples taken from a host, and predictions can be made as to which genes are associated with the disease [43]. Programs can be trained to perform these predictions depending on the overexpression or under-expression of the targeted gene in the malignant sample when compared with the normal sample, accumulating more data for every progressive batch of fed data. The capacity of machine learning technologies to find essential traits in complicated datasets demonstrates their value. Artificial Neural Networks (ANNs), Bayesian Networks (BNs), Support Vector Machines (SVMs), and Decision Trees (DTs) are among the approaches that have been extensively used in cancer research to construct predictive analytics, leading to efficient and optimal strategic planning. Even though it is clear that the application of machine learning algorithms may increase our knowledge of cancer development, adequate validation is required before these technologies can be used in clinical practice [44].

AI along with 3D imaging also helps in identifying genetic mutations that cause tumors. For example, one can detect the presence of glioma using a patient's brain scans with an accuracy of around 97%. Using techniques of deep-learning and neural networks, devices can identify the presence of mutations so that physicians can provide better treatment to patients without the use of biopsy and surgeries [45]. Through these processes, ML presents amazing opportunities for automatic diagnosis of diseases such as cancer [46].

16.2.2 Treatment

A considerable advantage that favors genetic engineering is its ability to slice out genes that cause disorders. Genetic engineering is an approach used to alter genetic sequences using nuclease. In genetic engineering, the nucleotide sequence is incorporated, replaced, retrieved, or altered in certain positions of the human genome to treat a specific disorder [47]. The cuts made by the nuclease are repaired using the ligase enzyme for the formation of a modified gene. The improvement of the current gene editing technologies, along with the development of new approaches such as CRISPR (clustered regularly interspaced short palindromic repeats) provides a more flexible route for gene modification. CRISPR is a targeted approach for DNA modification which has the potential to create multiple genetic mutations in one go. Alternative genetic engineering tools include, zinc finger nucleases (ZFNs) and transcription activator-like effector nucleases (TALEN) that creates a nick in specific DNA sequences [48].

Though technologies like CRISPR have seen a significant advancement, error chances are still significant in them, and safety should be considered a priority for genetic manipulation. ML algorithms are beneficial in sourcing out where mutations should be subjected and how DNA should be aligned later to reduce the chances of error in the process [49]. Mutagenic processes have a specific connection with surrounding bases that distinguishes them. Only a few basic examples, such as CpG hypermutability, provide direct evidence for this idea. For a more sophisticated scenario, we tested whether the molecular origin of a point mutation can be determined using just sequence context [50]. A logistic regression classifier performed well in distinguishing between the various mutation classes. The top classifier's feature set and information content analyses are in agreement, indicating that our findings may be applied to additional mutation classification issues [49].

AI holds lot of applications in the personal medicine field, the prerequisite for which is that the treatment should be specific to the requirement of one patient when compared with another. The fingerprint regions of human DNA has over three million differences when compared with other individuals, indicating there might be a very high probability that the mutations in the genome causing cancer in one individual may differ in location and level from another individual suffering from cancer [51]. Analogous to diagnosing a disease on a genomic basis, AI can help associate the harmful mutations in the genes to the target gene therapy [52]. To be able to anticipate from future datasets, artificial intelligence systems use learning methodologies based on categorization or pattern recognition to (multi-dimensional) input data. These massive digitization initiatives will substantially aid AI algorithms, which may help build genotype-phenotype relationships for genetic illnesses and have the capacity to infer a plethora of phenotypic relationships and linkages. Of course, gathering massive amounts of digital data will only be useful if the data contains important clinical data for AI systems to model (Figure 16.2) [53].

DNA repair post editing is another potential area for using AI. When changes are made in the DNA using Cas9 enzyme, a spontaneous alternation is made in the DNA strand depending on the guide RNA. In a publication of 2018 in Nature, Sherwood *et al.* explained how they directed a machine-readable algorithm called in Delphi to predict DNA-modifications made using Cas-9. They used experimental data from around 1,872 sequences which were cut, inserted and then ligated into the mouse and human cell lines. The program showed that 5-11% of the guide RNA used created single, predictable genetic alterations in the human genome

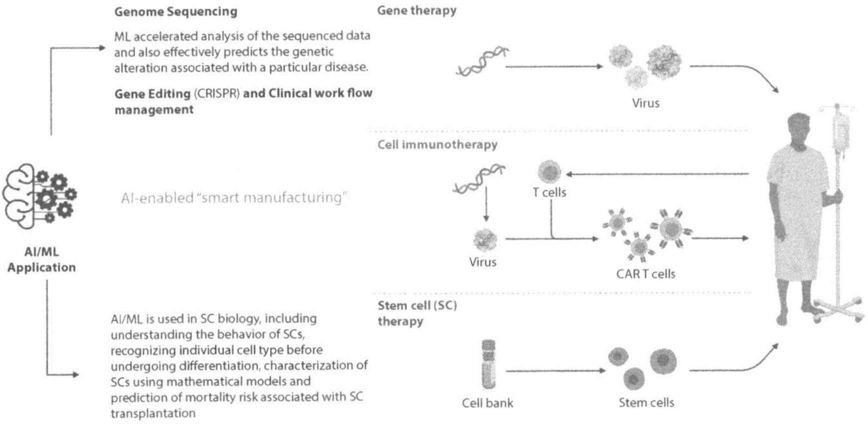

Figure 16.2 Overview of AI/ML application for cell and gene therapy development. (Figure created with Biorender.com.)

for over 50% of the edited results, suggesting that edits aren't random [54]. Algorithms used to predict changes that will be done based on modified sequences can enhance the accuracy of identifying which guide RNA is leading to which mutation.

16.3 Personalized Cell Therapy

Personal medicine is often referred to as providing "the right patient with the right treatment with the right dose at the right time". It incorporates methods such as "accurate medicine", "stratified medicine" and "pharmacogenomics", and is an alternative to the traditional method of treatment design based on "general patients" and "one size fits all". Autologous cell therapy is undoubtedly one of the most tailored treatments, using patient cells to produce a bespoke product that is returned to the original donor only. AI can also be utilized to develop human-specific predictive models for SCs, regenerated tissue and immune cells in children and adults [55]. These predictive models can cleave the entire genome and break down the immune profile of a patient in a matter of a short time and curate treatments based on the patient's genetic makeup and immune system. AI strategies can be used for development and enhancement of innovative SC clinical trials and gene therapy in pediatric patients through accurate treatment designing, predicting clinical results, interpreting patient recruitment and retention, learning data entry, and applying it to new data, thereby

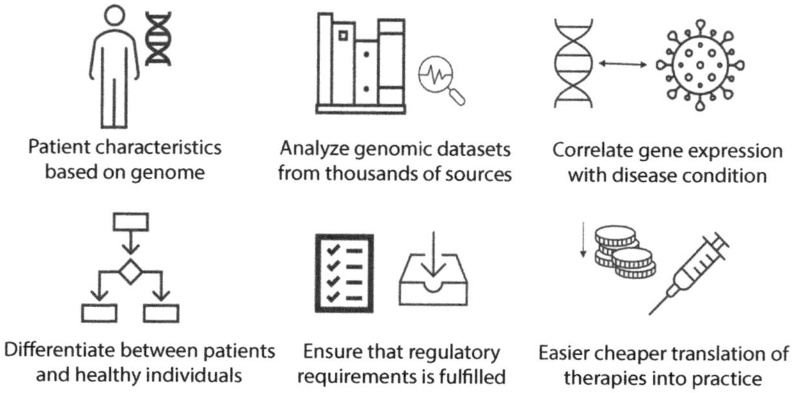

Figure 16.3 Goals of AI in precision medicine.

reducing complexity and cost. Recently, AI has been a part of a number of projects in the field of science, healthcare and medicine [56]. Figure 16.3 shows some of the goals to be achieved by AI.

16.4 Manufacturing of Cell and Gene-Based Therapies

The production of any cell and gene-based therapy requires a carefully controlled and meticulously planned process. Like any biologic's therapy, a major challenge in cell therapies is minimizing the batch-to-batch variation [57]. The starting material for cell therapy manufacturing is cells obtained from a donor. This makes it very important to have an improvised process for different cell types based on their application, storage conditions and shelf life, reagents and buffers requirements, etc. A minor alteration in the process parameters when culturing the cells can largely affect the quality of the final product. Similarly, to comply with the stringent regulatory requirements of cell therapy manufacturing, manufacturers need to employ good manufacturing practices. In general, the manufacturing process begins with the selection of media and reagents that meet the necessary qualifications of high quality, ease of handling, sterile processing, regulatory compliance, and minimal batch variations. Specific types of cells relevant to the therapy from the whole sample obtained from the donor are first isolated. A primary requirement is to have enough cell load in the isolated sample [58]. These specific cells then may be engineered to improve their therapeutic activity by adding targeting ligands or by conjugating with acting proteins [59]. The cells are then cultured in the media, a process that may take hours, days, or even weeks. At every stage of manufacturing, there must be a check on the number of cells in the sample, along with following the necessary temperature, aeration, and quality requirements. After the culture is done, the cells are extracted, purified, washed, filtered, harvested, concentrated, and formulated into an appropriate formulation [60]. This step may require addition of excipients, adjuvants and cryopreservants.

An essential element of cell therapy manufacturing is continuous and extensive monitoring of in-line parameters. Manual process monitoring can potentially lead to variations, especially depending on the experience and expertise of the operators and this can directly impact the final product quality. In such cases, automation becomes very useful in providing control over the manufacturing process. Using in-line sensors, robots that do precise compounding, and systems that accurately maintain incubation conditions, manual errors can be eliminated. Many large-scale manufacturers have adopted first and second-generation automation technologies that allow ease and flexibility in cell therapy manufacturing [61]. However, an aspect of large-scale manufacturing which needs further automation is the process of scaling up new therapies. For instance, clinical experiments make use of adherent cells to produce vectors like adeno-associated viruses and lentiviruses. These cell systems are unable to be replicated on a large scale as the cell lines require frequent manual handling [62]. There are more challenges to large scale production of cell therapies such as process complexity, final product characterization, lack of process monitoring capability, etc.

ML is a powerful tool that can be employed to overcome large-scale translation challenges. A prediction-based model can run an analysis based on data already available and return scale-up parameters and process specifications, which otherwise may require expensive experiments to be repeated [63]. Artificial neural networks are the most common ML based approaches in manufacturing of biopharmaceuticals and cell therapies [64]. A set of 'soft sensors' can estimate real-time critical process parameters and critical quality attributes on the basis of other on-line measurements [65]. A multivariate data analysis model can predict the implications of the change in donor cells and other raw materials on the final cell therapy product manufactured [66]. For example, Li *et al.* used Raman spectroscopy and chemometrics to rapidly identify, characterize and assess the quality of complex cell culture media components in a large-scale manufacturing of cells using principal component analysis and soft independent modeling of class analogy [67]. Schauba and colleagues presented [68] "a framework for advanced bioprocess data analysis consisting of multivariate data analysis (MVDA), metabolic flux analysis (MFA), and pathway analysis for mapping of large-scale gene expression data sets. This data analysis platform was applied in a process development project with an IgG-producing Chinese hamster ovary (CHO) cell line in which the maximal product titer could be increased from about 5 to 8 g/L. Principal component analysis (PCA), k-means clustering, and partial least-squares (PLS) models were applied to analyze the macroscopic bioprocess data. MFA and gene expression analysis revealed intracellular information on the characteristics of high-performance cell cultivations. By MVDA, for example, correlations between several essential amino acids and the product concentration were observed. Also, grouping into rather cell specific productivity-driven and process control-driven processes could be unraveled. By MFA, phenotypic characteristics in glycolysis, glutaminolysis, pentose phosphate pathway, citrate cycle, coupling of amino acid metabolism to citrate cycle, and in the energy yield could be identified. By gene expression analysis 247 deregulated metabolic genes were identified which are involved, inter alia, in amino acid metabolism, transport, and protein synthesis." The model has the potential to predict whether a particular culture media will produce a high-quality product, which makes it easier to design a process and its parameters. In another study, Grzesik *et al.* employed a design of experiments and ML based model to optimize T cell cultures in one experimental step as one-time optimization [69]. The model considered 12 major media components such as buffers, metabolically active compounds, proteins, trace elements, etc. Based on the prediction model, the formulations developed had a higher T cell expression. Moreover, the formulations had an expression precisely as predicted by the algorithm.

A Process Analytical Technology system, consisting of multivariate tools for design, data acquisition and analysis, process analyzers, process control tools and continuous improvement and knowledge management tools, can be used in biomanufacturing for controlling manufacturing processes (Figure 16.4). A combination of this system with RNA sequencing and multivariate data analysis can lead to new critical quality attributes, thus evaluating additional critical process parameters for a product with higher control on its manufacturing parameters [70]. RNA-Seq is now most often used to discover genes that are differentially expressed between two or more conditions. Despite the relevance of Gene Set Analysis (GSA) in interpreting RNA-Seq findings, the limits of GSA approaches established for microarrays in the context of RNA-Seq data remain unknown [71]. Numerous statistical and machine learning problems are involved in analyzing RNA-seq data at four distinct levels (samples, genes, transcripts, and exons), many of which are still difficult to answer [72]. Higher the

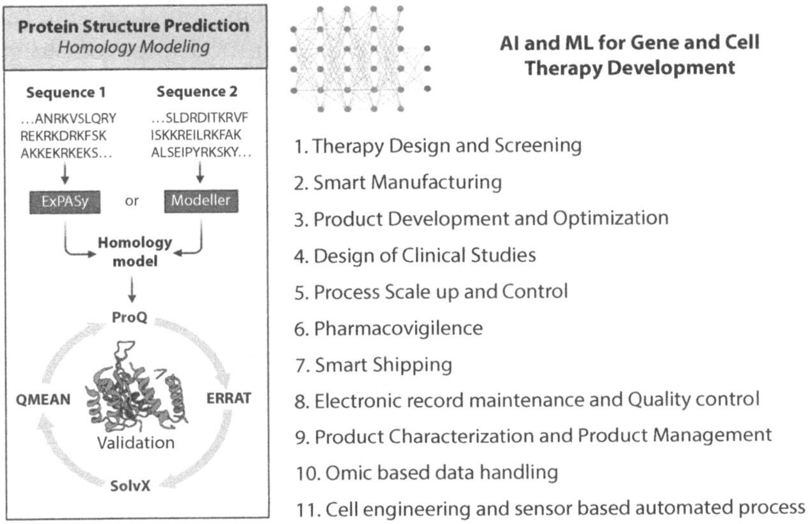

Figure 16.4 Possible involvement of AI and ML in cell and gene therapy product development. (Figure created with Biorender.com.)

process parameters and more frequently are they measured, higher will be understanding of the process and better will be the prediction of the model for better quality of the final product. In summary, ML based algorithms have prospective applications in predicting the selection of raw materials, process parameters and designing a manufacturing process when scaling up from a laboratory to an industry. Furthermore, even when operators and biopharma engineers use comparable production procedures, there are significant variances based on the exact vector operation to be used in each batch or patient. To double-check the uniqueness of the particularities connected with such production, ongoing monitoring is essential. As a result, each patient must be associated with a particular batch that is made and monitored using both singularities (specific objectives) and commonalities (universal specifications).

16.5 Development of an Omics Profile

The goal of an accurate diagnosis is to hypothesize the best treatment plan based on the individual's genetic profile. Drug responses combined with genomic, proteomic, epigenomic, metabolomics, transcriptomic data gives precise network prediction for disorders. Using multi-omics data, along with somatic mutations, methylomes, somatic exome mutations and transcriptomes of 1000 cell lines, ML can be used in modeling work to gain insight on genomic attributes of the process and reaction mechanism of drugs [73]. The most effective methods that utilize ML include multiple profiling datasets, and improve scoring with regression models to determine drug sensitivity [74]. Given the non-linear and convulsion relationship amongst the different types of omic functions, the future ML software can be responded to solve complex multi-omics patterns [75]. In biomedicine, multi-omics data is rich and complicated, allowing for data-driven insights and automated illness categorization. The knowledge gained from this data will help us better understand and define healthy baselines and disease markers. Digital image identification, single-cell clustering, and virtual drug screening are examples of cutting-edge deep neural network applications, showcasing the breadth and potential of machine learning in biomedicine. Significantly, AI and systems biology have embraced big data difficulties, and emerging biotechnology-derived medicines may be able to help with precision medicine deployment.

Support vector machine (SVM), a supervised learning-based platform, is one of the most extensively used methods of analyzing multi-omics data. Keeping the maximum distance feasible amongst the various categories of sample data points, it forms a linear hyperplane [76]. Along with being directed for a specific function, these ML algorithms can also search for appropriate properties for improved execution in the future. SVM-based methods are widely used to detect subtypes of cancer and to extract vital elements like biomolecules that play a role. The main purpose of doing so, is to re-classify cancer on the basis of cellular factors rather than tissue types [77]. Random forest algorithms are also seldom considered. They are made up of a number of decision trees, all of which are made using a training set and a random vector. The decision tree acts as a distributor. Each tree votes in favor of the most approved class, and then it is selected [78]. In addition to SVM-based learning algorithms, unregulated learning methods such as auto-encoders also help in decreasing the "large" size of multi-omics data. Auto-encoders include an encoder and a decoder. The encoder separates motifs from big input data, and decoder attempts to create output that is very similar to input using only extracted motifs. In this way, it does not include obsolete data [79].

Epigenomics of oncogenic networks can precisely predict regulome activity, disease progression and epigenomic-transcriptomic interactions [80]. Also, epigenetic mutations in the genetic material are complicated and often resource specific, making their mechanical comprehension a task. To manage the ultra-high dimensional regression, an elastic net is used in epigenomic data. This net is formed by combination of ridge reduction and lasso regularization (prevent over-equilibrium) [81]. Epigenomic and metabolic data helped to create biomarkers and predict clocks in aging, using these methods [82]. Improved by ML methodology, epigenetic markers including methylation of the promoter are used as a continuous readout of transcriptional accessibility and molecular processes that guide tissue maintenance, development, disease status, and ultimately aging. Following the advances in multiplex barcoding, interpretation of the new data will always be a challenge that the researchers will have to face [82].

16.6 ML in Stem Cell Identification, Differentiation, and Characterization

iPSCs are widely investigated tools of personalized therapy, cells that hold the potential to be differentiated into any kind of cell. An obvious critical step in developing therapies using the SCs is controlling the differentiation of the cells and identifying them at the stages of development and manufacturing. For example, SC that are originated from a particular tissue, have some residual memory and a chance of reverting back to their origin [83]. A minor variation in the culture conditions or manufacturing parameters can have an impact on the differentiation of the SC [84]. The manual way of checking the induction and differentiation of SC is by expert evaluation of the morphology changes, which allows a scope for person-to-person variation. For SC therapy manufacturing at an industrial level, an automation is important to ensure consistency in the characterization. ML algorithms based on data from several databases can make accurate predictions on the fate of SC, without having to evaluate the actual cell samples manually (Figure 16.5). One possible dataset could be of the microscopic images of different stages of SC differentiations, or a continuous trajectory of the same. These images can be then associated with the culture parameters and the final differentiation product. A ML algorithm can be trained to read such images and predict the differentiation fate of SC. Zhang *et al.* used a live cell imaging microscopic system 2 days after retroviruses infection expressing different genes [85]. They considered 11 morphological features of SC such as area, volume, sphericity, nucleo-cytoplasm ratio, ellipsoids prolate, ellipsoid oblate, etc. A model was then developed using XGBoost, an optimized distributed gradient library, using optimized features and timeframe. The model had an accuracy of 52% for the progenitor SC.

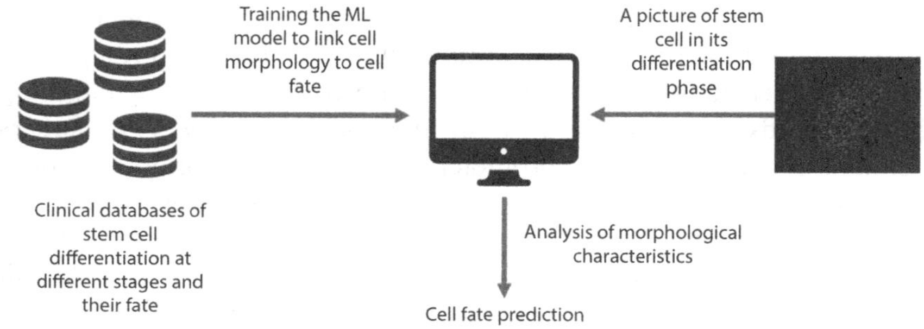

Figure 16.5 A brief overview of stem cell prediction using morphology recognition.

A subset of ML that has found various applications in cell and gene therapies is artificial neural networks. These are based on concept of a human neural network, but instead composed of node layers. The node is a representative of a neuron and connects to another node like neurons in the human brain. These nodes work on threshold signaling, where if a sufficient signal is generated, a communication between two nodes is established [86]. Artificial neural networks, similar to other ML algorithms discussed previously, can predict the types of SC by looking at their morphological features. A technique called semantic segmentation breaks down microscopic images of SC to pixels and assigns an object characteristic or class to the pixel [87]. Such a segmentation allows identification of cell location and classification [88]. In a study, an algorithm was trained with phase-contrast micrographs of MSCs [89]. Cell clusters were segmented, and the SC were characterized on the basis of their morphological and textural features. The algorithm had 86% precision in segmentation of low to moderately dense SC.

ML also finds potential applications in characterization of SC by identification of the differentiated cell types. The alteration in the morphology of SC during the differentiation phase can be detected and logically assigned to SC fate using ML algorithms. A model developed by Zhu *et al.* could predict the fate of SC on basis of the differentiation inducer used [90]. Such models can make predictions on the fate right at the beginning of the SC development [91]. A ML based approach to evaluate the biosafety and bioefficacy of SC therapy is another example of use of computational tools in therapy profiling and characterization [92].

Tumorigenesis is often a concern with SC when the cells lose their own identity and become tumor cells [93]. Combining cancer research and SC research datasets for various ML models can be explored as a method of better understanding SC fate. The proliferation ability, morphological features and cell surface markers for SC and cancer cells are different, and hence, using these parameters from datasets of both the type of cells, one can train a ML model to distinguish between the two cells [94]. Based on this information, the model can predict if a SC has risk of tumorigenesis by looking at the initial or intermittent morphological features. A model can be used to predict and evaluate the changes in SC behavior in a specific environment, with the goal of establishing the influence on biosafety for therapeutic usage. Thus, ML may be used to characterize SC using images, paving the way for future applications of ML in cell therapies.

16.7 Machine Learning in Gene Expression Imaging

Gene expression control is one of the most important biological challenges. Until recently well-planned control would not have been possible, especially for eukaryotes because of their complex genetic regulation. With the advancement of ML along with the increasing database size, models that predict the gene expression levels of a regulatory sequence is in today's time a successful vision. Such models are the base of algorithms that allow users to design regulatory sequences to achieve a certain level of genetic expression [95].

Today, a growing database of genomic and transcriptomic research is available for analysis. Such datasets provide an opportunity for the use of ML methods, such as using predictive sequence activity models when prior knowledge is not available. If adequate data were provided, these models could perform normal operations and predict the activity of an unseen sequence. Many relevant biological problems have already been resolved in this way on a regular basis, including gene structure prediction [96], protein function, location, and structure [97], and protein-protein interactions with DNA [98].

ML prepares speculative models by entering the criterions based on the huge input database and the subsequent results you want, the so-called training data. These training datasets are then employed to forecast results for new, unseen test data. A trained ML model can be used to prognosticate novel gene sequence function. This prediction can then be used as a factor for a design algorithm that searches sequences to achieve the targeted expression level by amplification of that expression, taking specific limitations (e.g., sequencing construction or homology) into account [99]. Two commonly used methods in design are: iterative guided mutations and element selection, but alternatives to it such as generative adversarial networks (GANs), adaptive sampling and paired deep learning models are also being looked upon.

Ashraf *et al.* used a machine learning model to identify genetic biomarkers to survive breast cancer. The study analyzed the genetic function of the live vs. deceased for each therapy for over a period of five years. The computational model forms a set of biomarkers for patients who were subjected to different treatments. This new approach can be optimized so that it can be applied to identify the appropriate biomarker genes (signature) for various types of cancer and even in cases in which patients need or have received multiple gene therapies [100].

16.8 AI in Gene Therapy Target and Potency Prediction

For any therapies including small molecules and biologics, it is critical that the active molecules have targeted action within the therapeutic window. The pharmacokinetics and pharmacodynamics of small molecules are relatively easy to study since a suitable animal model can be designed. The variation in individual response is not a large factor as much as the safety and efficacy of the drugs. However, for cell and gene therapies, since the goal is to develop a personalized treatment, individual responses to any therapy become important to be studied. Other than the safety and efficacy, the compatibility of a therapy with an individual becomes a crucial consideration. Several approaches can be adopted to understand cellular response with different experimental settings [101, 102]. ML algorithms can help in developing prediction models that use genomic information of individuals and datasets of responses of different drugs in other individuals [103]. The objective of such a model is to analyze the genomic data of thousands of individuals and train the ML model with drug responses of those patients. This can be done by assigning a special role to specific genes of interest and labelling the patients as those who exhibited a response and those who did not. Finally, the genomic profile of an individual seeking the cell therapy can be mapped and fed into the model [56, 104].

Franks *et al.* used gene expression data from peripheral blood cells of 63 participants of the 'Scleroderma: Cyclophosphamide or Transplantation' clinical trial [105] and identified treatments responses [106]. The participants were divided into groups based on their intrinsic gene expression before the trial. Only the participants who completed the clinical trial were considered. They were studied for event-free survival and for differentially expressed genes. A ML algorithm was used to assign to individuals from clinical trials to groups that showed a higher expression of a group of genes. The genes were earlier showed to be the biomarkers on intrinsic subsets. The algorithm mapped these data points using multinomial elastic net classification. It could predict these patterns in new datasets with 85% accuracy [107]. In another study, a supervised ML model identified targets and predicted the outcomes in diffuse large B-cell lymphoma [108]. The model was trained using a dataset of 6817 gene expressions in diagnostic tumor from patients who were administered chemotherapies on different drugs. The model firstly divided the patients two groups based on their 5-year survival rates. Then it accurately assigned the patients with a high-risk of lymphoma into either one of the groups of mortality. The model predicted the genes that govern B-cell receptor signaling, serine/threonine phosphorylation pathways, and apoptosis.

Any ML based model is a predictive pre-clinical approach to understand the extent of targeted activity and therapeutic efficacy. However, ML algorithms hold tremendous potential to accurately and quickly identify key genes from an individual's genome and make a prediction about the potency of cell-based therapy [109, 110]. The most important advantage of using a computational approach is cost-effectiveness and non-invasiveness. Unlike an experimental setting, a prospective analysis is possible with a predictive model.

16.9 Conclusion and Future Prospective

The advent of personalized medicine has made it possible to convincingly tackle diseases that were previously considered incurable. Cell and gene therapies, most well-known personalized medicines approaches, have been discussed in length in this chapter. The challenges to personalized medicine are many and need extensive screening before a therapy can make it to clinical practice. ML and other AI based techniques when paired with medicine can help overcome these challenges. In a nutshell, ML models use the information already available in different databases and use the data as points to create a correlation tree. These models can use different techniques such as multiple regression, principal component analysis, decision trees etc. This makes a prediction model which can assign any new datapoint to other factors that may have a cause-effect relation. With regards to cell and gene therapy, the application of prediction models is seen in predicting the SC differentiation fate, gene expressions, cell therapy potency, etc., which has been discussed in the chapter. The current procedures for the above-mentioned goals are incapable of achieving desirable timescales and efficiency. Undoubtedly, the integration of AI with medicine can overcome these challenges faster and non-invasively. The resources required for a prediction model over experimental evaluation are minimal. In the near future, there is potential of many biologics manufacturing companies and large medical centers adopting AI into practice, making it easier, faster and more convenient for the advantages of personalized medicine to be delivered to patients.

References

1. Mount, N.M., Ward, S.J., Kefalas, P., Hyllner, J., Cell-based therapy technology classifications and translational challenges. *Philos. Trans. R. Soc. Lond. B. Biol. Sci.* [Internet], 370, 1680, 20150017, 2015, Available from: https://pubmed.ncbi.nlm.nih.gov/26416686.
2. Liu, Z. and Cheung, H.-H., Stem cell-based therapies for parkinson disease. *Int. J. Mol. Sci.* [Internet], 21, 21, 8060, 2020, Available from: https://pubmed.ncbi.nlm.nih.gov/33137927.
3. Stoker, T.B., Stem cell treatments for parkinson's disease, in: *Parkinson's Disease: Pathogenesis and Clinical Aspects* [Internet], T.B. Stoker and J.C. Greenland (Eds.), Codon Publications, Brisbane (AU), 2018 Dec 21, Chapter 9, Available from: https://www.ncbi.n.
4. Singh, M.S., Park, S.S., Albini, T.A. *et al.*, Retinal stem cell transplantation: Balancing safety and potential. *Prog. Retin. Eye Res.* [Internet], 75, 100779, 2020, Available from: https://pubmed.ncbi.nlm.nih.gov/31494256.
5. Regan, K. and Payne, P.R.O., From molecules to patients: The clinical applications of translational bioinformatics. *Yearb. Med. Inform.* [Internet], 10, 1, 164–169, 2015, Available from: https://pubmed.ncbi.nlm.nih.gov/26293863.
6. Qazi, S. and Raza, K., Chapter 1 - Translational bioinformatics in healthcare: Past, present, and future [Internet], in: *Advances in Ubiquitous Sensing Applications for Healthcare*, K. Raza, N.B.T. Dey, TB in H and M (Eds.), pp. 1–12, Academic Press, Cambridge, Massachusetts, 2021, Available from: https://www.sciencedirect.com/science/article/pii/B978032389824900001X.
7. Mao, A.S. and Mooney, D.J., Regenerative medicine: Current therapies and future directions. *Proc. Natl. Acad. Sci. U. S. A.* [Internet], 112, 47, 14452–14459, 2015, Available from: https://pubmed.ncbi.nlm.nih.gov/26598661.
8. Zakrzewski, W., Dobrzyński, M., Szymonowicz, M., Rybak, Z., Stem cells: Past, present, and future. *Stem Cell Res. Ther.* [Internet], 10, 1, 68, 2019, Available from: https://doi.org/10.1186/s13287-019-1165-5.
9. Sterner, R.C. and Sterner, R.M., CAR-T cell therapy: Current limitations and potential strategies. *Blood Cancer J.* [Internet], 11, 4, 69, 2021, Available from: https://doi.org/10.1038/s41408-021-00459-7.

10. Oncology, T.L., CAR T-cell therapy for solid tumours. *Lancet Oncol.* [Internet], 22, 7, 893, 2021, Available from: https://doi.org/10.1016/S1470-2045(21)00353-3.
11. Maus, M.V., CD19 CAR T cells for adults with relapsed or refractory acute lymphoblastic leukaemia. *Lancet* [Internet], 398, 10299, 466–467, 2021, Available from: https://doi.org/10.1016/S0140-6736(21)01289-7.
12. Jackson, K.A., Majka, S.M., Wang, H. *et al.*, Regeneration of ischemic cardiac muscle and vascular endothelium by adult stem cells. *J. Clin. Invest.*, 107, 11, 1395–1402, 2001.
13. Kalka, C., Masuda, H., Takahashi, T. *et al.*, Transplantation of *ex vivo* expanded endothelial progenitor cells for therapeutic neovascularization. *Proc. Natl. Acad. Sci. U. S. A.*, 97, 7, 3422–3427, 2000.
14. Hiraishi, S., Schol, J., Sakai, D. *et al.*, Discogenic cell transplantation directly from a cryopreserved state in an induced intervertebral disc degeneration canine model. *JOR Spine* [Internet], 1, 2, e1013, 2018, Available from: https://doi.org/10.1002/jsp2.1013.
15. *2017 TERMIS - Americas Conference & Exhibition Charlotte*, NC December 3-6, 2017, vol. 23(S1), pp. S1–159, 2017 Dec, Tissue Eng Part A.
16. Yagi, H., Soto-Gutierrez, A., Parekkadan, B. *et al.*, Mesenchymal stem cells: Mechanisms of immunomodulation and homing. *Cell Transplant.*, 19, 6, 667–679, 2010.
17. Wang, L.L.-W., Janes, M.E., Kumbhojkar, N. *et al.*, Cell therapies in the clinic. *Bioeng. Transl. Med.* [Internet], 6, 2, e10214–e10214, 2021, Available from: https://pubmed.ncbi.nlm.nih.gov/34027097.
18. Takahashi, K. and Yamanaka, S., Induction of pluripotent stem cells from mouse embryonic and adult fibroblast cultures by defined factors. *Cell*, 126, 4, 663–676, 2006.
19. Ye, L., Swingen, C., Zhang, J., Induced pluripotent stem cells and their potential for basic and clinical sciences. *Curr. Cardiol. Rev.* [Internet], 9, 1, 63–72, 2013, Available from: https://pubmed.ncbi.nlm.nih.gov/22935022.
20. Yamanaka, S., Induction of pluripotent stem cells from mouse fibroblasts by four transcription factors. *Cell Prolif.* [Internet], 41 Suppl 1, Suppl 1, 51–56, 2008, Available from: https://pubmed.ncbi.nlm.nih.gov/18181945.
21. Buzhor, E., Leshansky, L., Blumenthal, J. *et al.*, Cell-based therapy approaches: The hope for incurable diseases. *Regen. Med.* [Internet], 9, 5, 649–672, 2014, Available from: https://doi.org/10.2217/rme.14.35.
22. Mousaei Ghasroldasht, M., Seok, J., Park, H.-S., Liakath Ali, F.B., Al-Hendy, A., Stem cell therapy: From idea to clinical practice. *Int. J. Mol. Sci.* [Internet], 23, 5, 2850, 2022, Available from: https://pubmed.ncbi.nlm.nih.gov/35269990.
23. Ankrum, J. and Karp, J.M., Mesenchymal stem cell therapy: Two steps forward, one step back. *Trends Mol. Med.*, 16, 5, 203–209, 2010.

24. Choi, E.W., Adult stem cell therapy for autoimmune disease. *Int. J. Stem Cells* [Internet], 2, 2, 122–128, 2009, Available from: https://pubmed.ncbi.nlm.nih.gov/24855531.
25. Raval, Z. and Losordo, D.W., Cell therapy of peripheral arterial disease: From experimental findings to clinical trials. *Circ. Res.*, 112, 9, 1288–1302, 2013.
26. Reynolds, B.A. and Weiss, S., Generation of neurons and astrocytes from isolated cells of the adult mammalian central nervous system. *Science*, 255, 5052, 1707–1710, 1992.
27. Roybal, K.T. and Lim, W.A., Synthetic immunology: Hacking immune cells to expand their therapeutic capabilities. *Annu. Rev. Immunol.* [Internet], 35, 229–253, 2017, Available from: https://pubmed.ncbi.nlm.nih.gov/28446063.
28. Varela-Rohena, A., Carpenito, C., Perez, E.E. *et al.*, Genetic engineering of T cells for adoptive immunotherapy. *Immunol. Res.* [Internet], 42, 1–3, 166–181, 2008, Available from: https://pubmed.ncbi.nlm.nih.gov/18841331.
29. Nurieva, R., Wang, J., Sahoo, A., T-cell tolerance in cancer. *Immunotherapy* [Internet], 5, 5, 513–531, 2013, Available from: https://pubmed.ncbi.nlm.nih.gov/23638746.
30. Houghton, A.N. and Guevara-Patiño, J.A., Immune recognition of self in immunity against cancer. *J. Clin. Invest.* [Internet], 114, 4, 468–471, 2004, Available from: https://pubmed.ncbi.nlm.nih.gov/15314682.
31. Lee, S. and Margolin, K., Tumor-infiltrating lymphocytes in melanoma. *Curr. Oncol. Rep.* [Internet], 14, 5, 468–474, 2012, Available from: https://pubmed.ncbi.nlm.nih.gov/22878966.
32. Wu, R., Forget, M.-A., Chacon, J. *et al.*, Adoptive T-cell therapy using autologous tumor-infiltrating lymphocytes for metastatic melanoma: Current status and future outlook. *Cancer J.* [Internet], 18, 2, 160–175, 2012, Available from: https://pubmed.ncbi.nlm.nih.gov/22453018.
33. Fesnak, A.D., June, C.H., Levine, B.L., Engineered T cells: The promise and challenges of cancer immunotherapy. *Nat. Rev. Cancer* [Internet], 16, 9, 566–581, 2016, Available from: https://pubmed.ncbi.nlm.nih.gov/27550819.
34. Zhao, L. and Cao, Y.J., Engineered T cell therapy for cancer in the clinic. *Front. Immunol.* [Internet], 10, 2250, 2019, Available from: https://pubmed.ncbi.nlm.nih.gov/31681259.
35. Chmielewski, M., Hombach, A.A., Abken, H., Antigen-specific T-cell activation independently of the MHC: Chimeric antigen receptor-redirected T cells. *Front. Immunol.* [Internet], 4, 371, 2013, Available from: https://pubmed.ncbi.nlm.nih.gov/24273543.
36. Dai, H., Wang, Y., Lu, X., Han, W., Chimeric antigen receptors modified T-cells for cancer therapy. *J. Natl. Cancer Inst.* [Internet], 108, 7, djv439, 2016, Available from: https://pubmed.ncbi.nlm.nih.gov/26819347.
37. Liu, S., Galat, V., Galat4, Y., Lee, Y.K.A., Wainwright, D., Wu, J., NK cell-based cancer immunotherapy: From basic biology to clinical development. *J. Hematol. Oncol.* [Internet], 14, 1, 7, 2021, Available from: https://doi.org/10.1186/s13045-020-01014-w.

38. Bouard, D., Alazard-Dany, D., Cosset, F.-L., Viral vectors: From virology to transgene expression. *Br. J. Pharmacol.* [Internet], 157, 2, 153–165, 2009, Available from: https://pubmed.ncbi.nlm.nih.gov/18776913.
39. Ingusci, S., Verlengia, G., Soukupova, M., Zucchini, S., Simonato, M., Gene therapy tools for brain diseases. *Front. Pharmacol.* [Internet], 10, 724, 2019, Available from: https://pubmed.ncbi.nlm.nih.gov/31312139.
40. National Research Council (US) Committee on Mapping and Sequencing the Human Genome, *Mapping and sequencing the human genome*, National Academies Press (US), Washington (DC), 1988, 2, Introduction, Available from: https://www.ncbi.nlm.nih.gov/books/NBK2182.
41. Reuter, J.A., Spacek, D.V., Snyder, M.P., High-throughput sequencing technologies. *Mol. Cell* [Internet], 58, 4, 586–597, 2015, Available from: https://pubmed.ncbi.nlm.nih.gov/26000844.
42. Lander, E.S., Linton, L.M., Birren, B. *et al.*, Initial sequencing and analysis of the human genome. *Nat.* [Internet], 409, 6822, 860–921, 2001, Available from: https://doi.org/10.1038/35057062.
43. Saghaleyni, R., Sheikh Muhammad, A., Bangalore, P., Nielsen, J., Robinson, J.L., Machine learning-based investigation of the cancer protein secretory pathway. *PLoS Comput. Biol.* [Internet], 17, 4, e1008898, 2021, Available from: https://doi.org/10.1371/journal.pcbi.1008898.
44. Kourou, K., Exarchos, T.P., Exarchos, K.P., Karamouzis, M.V., Fotiadis, D.I., Machine learning applications in cancer prognosis and prediction. *Comput. Struct. Biotechnol. J.* [Internet], 13, 8–17, 2015, Available from: https://www.sciencedirect.com/science/article/pii/S2001037014000464.
45. Alhasan, A.S., Clinical applications of artificial intelligence, machine learning, and deep learning in the imaging of gliomas: A systematic review. *Cureus* [Internet], 13, 11, e19580–e19580, 2021, Available from: https://pubmed.ncbi.nlm.nih.gov/34926051.
46. Kourou, K., Exarchos, K.P., Papaloukas, C., Sakaloglou, P., Exarchos, T., Fotiadis, D.I., Applied machine learning in cancer research: A systematic review for patient diagnosis, classification and prognosis. *Comput. Struct. Biotechnol. J.* [Internet], 19, 5546–5555, 2021, Available from: https://pubmed.ncbi.nlm.nih.gov/34712399.
47. Lino, C.A., Harper, J.C., Carney, J.P., Timlin, J.A., Delivering CRISPR: A review of the challenges and approaches. *Drug Deliv.* [Internet], 25, 1, 1234–1257, 2018, Available from: https://pubmed.ncbi.nlm.nih.gov/29801422.
48. Gupta, R.M. and Musunuru, K., Expanding the genetic editing tool kit: ZFNs, TALENs, and CRISPR-Cas9. *J. Clin. Invest.* [Internet], 124, 10, 4154–4161, 2014, Available from: https://pubmed.ncbi.nlm.nih.gov/25271723.
49. Zhu, Y., Ong, C.S., Huttley, G.A., Machine learning techniques for classifying the mutagenic origins of point mutations. *Genet.* [Internet], 215, 1, 25–40, 2020, Available from: https://pubmed.ncbi.nlm.nih.gov/32193188.
50. Stottmann, R. and Beier, D., ENU mutagenesis in the mouse. *Curr. Protoc. Hum. Genet.*, 82, 15.4.1–10, 2014.

51. Olivier, M., Hollstein, M., Hainaut, P., TP53 mutations in human cancers: Origins, consequences, and clinical use. *Cold Spring Harb. Perspect. Biol.* [Internet], 2, 1, a001008–a001008, 2010, Available from: https://pubmed.ncbi.nlm.nih.gov/20182602.
52. Alagoz, M. and Kherad, N., Advance genome editing technologies in the treatment of human diseases: CRISPR therapy (review). *Int. J. Mol. Med.* [Internet], 46, 2, 521–534, 2020, Available from: https://pubmed.ncbi.nlm.nih.gov/32467995.
53. Uddin, M., Wang, Y., Woodbury-Smith, M., Artificial intelligence for precision medicine in neurodevelopmental disorders. *NPJ Digit. Med.*, 2, 1, 112, 2019.
54. Shen, M.W., Arbab, M., Hsu, J.Y. *et al.*, Predictable and precise template-free CRISPR editing of pathogenic variants. *Nat. [Internet]*, 563, 7733, 646–651, 2018, Available from: https://doi.org/10.1038/s41586-018-0686-x.
55. Sniecinski, I. and Seghatchian, J., Artificial intelligence: A joint narrative on potential use in pediatric stem and immune cell therapies and regenerative medicine. *Transfus. Apher. Sci. Off. J. World Apher. Assoc. Off. J. Eur. Soc. Haemapheresis.*, 57, 3, 422–424, 2018.
56. Mamoshina, P., Ojomoko, L., Yanovich, Y. *et al.*, Converging blockchain and next-generation artificial intelligence technologies to decentralize and accelerate biomedical research and healthcare. *Oncotarget*, 9, 5, 5665–5690, 2018.
57. Heathman, T.R.J., Rafiq, Q.A., Chan, A.K.C. *et al.*, Characterization of human mesenchymal stem cells from multiple donors and the implications for large scale bioprocess development. *Biochem. Eng. J.* [Internet], 108, 14–23, 2016, Available from: https://www.sciencedirect.com/science/article/pii/S1369703X15300073.
58. Pigeau, G.M., Csaszar, E., Dulgar-Tulloch, A., Commercial scale manufacturing of allogeneic cell therapy. *Front. Med.*, 5, 233, 2018.
59. Bulaklak, K. and Gersbach, C.A., The once and future gene therapy. *Nat. Commun.*, 11, 1, 5820, 2020.
60. Burger, S.R., Current regulatory issues in cell and tissue therapy. *Cytotherapy*, 5, 4, 289–298, 2003.
61. Moutsatsou, P., Ochs, J., Schmitt, R.H., Hewitt, C.J., Hanga, M.P., Automation in cell and gene therapy manufacturing: From past to future. *Biotechnol. Lett.*, 41, 11, 1245–1253, 2019.
62. Sharon, D. and Kamen, A., Advancements in the design and scalable production of viral gene transfer vectors. *Biotechnol. Bioeng.*, 115, 1, 25–40, 2018.
63. Bhushan, N., Hadpe, S., Rathore, A.S., Chemometrics applications in biotech processes: Assessing process comparability. *Biotechnol. Prog.*, 28, 1, 121–128, 2012.
64. Tulsyan, A., Garvin, C., Ündey, C., Advances in industrial biopharmaceutical batch process monitoring: Machine-learning methods for small data problems. *Biotechnol. Bioeng.*, 115, 8, 1915–1924, 2018.

65. Solle, D., Hitzmann, B., Herwig, C. *et al.*, Between the poles of data-driven and mechanistic modeling for process operation. *Chem. Ing. Tech.* [Internet], 89, 5, 542–561, 2017, Available from: https://doi.org/10.1002/cite.201600175.
66. Glassey, J., Multivariate data analysis for advancing the interpretation of bioprocess measurement and monitoring data. *Adv. Biochem. Eng. Biotechnol.*, 132, 167–191, 2013.
67. Li, B., Ryan, P.W., Ray, B.H., Leister, K.J., Sirimuthu, N.M.S., Ryder, A.G., Rapid characterization and quality control of complex cell culture media solutions using raman spectroscopy and chemometrics. *Biotechnol. Bioeng.*, 107, 2, 290–301, 2010.
68. Schaub, J., Clemens, C., Kaufmann, H., Schulz, T.W., Advancing biopharmaceutical process development by system-level data analysis and integration of omics data. *Adv. Biochem. Eng. Biotechnol.*, 127, 133–163, 2012.
69. Grzesik, P. and Warth, S.C., One-time optimization of advanced T cell culture media using a machine learning pipeline. *Front. Bioeng. Biotechnol.*, 9, 614324, 2021.
70. Jr D and Irion, S., Using machine learning for critical quality attribute discovery in cell therapy manufacture. *Cell Gene Ther. Insights*, 5, 85–96, 2019 Feb 14.
71. Rahmatallah, Y., Emmert-Streib, F., Glazko, G., Comparative evaluation of gene set analysis approaches for RNA-seq data. *BMC Bioinform.* [Internet], 15, 1, 397, 2014, Available from: https://doi.org/10.1186/s12859-014-0397-8.
72. Li, W.V. and Li, J.J., Modeling and analysis of RNA-seq data: A review from a statistical perspective. *Quant. Biol.* [Internet], 6, 3, 195–209, 2018, Available from: https://doi.org/10.1007/s40484-018-0144-7.
73. Yu, H., Samuels, D.C., Zhao, Y.-Y., Guo, Y., Architectures and accuracy of artificial neural network for disease classification from omics data. *BMC Genomics*, 20, 1, 167, 2019.
74. Davis, S., Button-Simons, K., Bensellak, T. *et al.*, Leveraging crowdsourcing to accelerate global health solutions. *Nat. Biotechnol.*, 37, 8, 848–850, 2019.
75. Filipp, F.V., Opportunities for artificial intelligence in advancing precision medicine. *Curr. Genet. Med. Rep.*, 7, 4, 208–213, 2019.
76. Shawe-Taylor, J. and Sun, S., A review of optimization methodologies in support vector machines. *Neurocomputing* [Internet], 74, 17, 3609–3618, 2011, Available from: https://www.sciencedirect.com/science/article/pii/S0925231211004371.
77. Wang, D. and Gu, J., Integrative clustering methods of multi-omics data for molecule-based cancer classifications. *Quant. Biol.* [Internet], 4, 1, 58–67, 2016, Available from: https://doi.org/10.1007/s40484-016-0063-4.
78. Tanaka, I., Furukawa, T., Morise, M., The current issues and future perspective of artificial intelligence for developing new treatment strategy in non-small cell lung cancer: Harmonization of molecular cancer biology and artificial intelligence. *Cancer Cell Int.*, 21, 1, 454, 2021.

79. Biswas, N. and Chakrabarti, S., Artificial intelligence (AI)-based systems biology approaches in multi-omics data analysis of cancer. *Front. Oncol.*, 10, 588221, 2020.
80. Wilson, S. and Filipp, F.V., A network of epigenomic and transcriptional cooperation encompassing an epigenomic master regulator in cancer. *NPJ Syst. Biol. Appl.*, 4, 24, 2018.
81. Engebretsen, S. and Bohlin, J., Statistical predictions with glmnet. *Clin. Epigenet.*, 11, 1, 123, 2019.
82. Ravera, S., Podestà, M., Sabatini, F. *et al.*, Discrete changes in glucose metabolism define aging. *Sci. Rep.*, 9, 1, 10347, 2019.
83. Kim, K., Doi, A., Wen, B. *et al.*, Epigenetic memory in induced pluripotent stem cells. *Nature*, 467, 7313, 285–290, 2010.
84. Volpato, V. and Webber, C., Addressing variability in iPSC-derived models of human disease: Guidelines to promote reproducibility. *Dis. Model. Mech.*, 13, 1, 2020.
85. Zhang, H., Shao, X., Peng, Y. *et al.*, A novel machine learning based approach for iPS progenitor cell identification. *PLoS Comput. Biol.*, 15, 12, e1007351, 2019.
86. Walczak, S. and Cerpa, N., *Artificial neural networks* [Internet], Third E, RABT Meyers, E of PS and T (Eds.), pp. 631–645, Academic Press, New York, 2003, Available from: https://www.sciencedirect.com/science/article/pii/B0122274105008371.
87. Kusumoto, D. and Yuasa, S., The application of convolutional neural network to stem cell biology. *Inflamm. Regen.*, 39, 14, 2019.
88. Fan, K., Zhang, S., Zhang, Y., Lu, J., Holcombe, M., Zhang, X., A machine learning assisted, label-free, non-invasive approach for somatic reprogramming in induced pluripotent stem cell colony formation detection and prediction. *Sci. Rep.*, 7, 1, 13496, 2017.
89. Mota, S.M., Rogers, R.E., Haskell, A.W. *et al.*, Automated mesenchymal stem cell segmentation and machine learning-based phenotype classification using morphometric and textural analysis. *J. Med. Imaging (Bellingham, Wash.)*, 8, 1, 14503, 2021.
90. Zhu, Y., Huang, R., Wu, Z., Song, S., Cheng, L., Zhu, R., Deep learning-based predictive identification of neural stem cell differentiation. *Nat. Commun.*, 12, 1, 2614, 2021.
91. Buggenthin, F., Buettner, F., Hoppe, P.S. *et al.*, Prospective identification of hematopoietic lineage choice by deep learning. *Nat. Methods*, 14, 4, 403–406, 2017.
92. Srinivasan, M., Thangaraj, S.R., Ramasubramanian, K., Thangaraj, P.P., Ramasubramanian, K.V., Exploring the current trends of artificial intelligence in stem cell therapy: A systematic review. *Cureus*, 13, 12, e20083, 2021.
93. Lee, A.S., Tang, C., Rao, M.S., Weissman, I.L., Wu, J.C., Tumorigenicity as a clinical hurdle for pluripotent stem cell therapies. *Nat. Med.*, 19, 8, 998–1004, 2013.

94. Taninaga, J., Nishiyama, Y., Fujibayashi, K. *et al.*, Prediction of future gastric cancer risk using a machine learning algorithm and comprehensive medical check-up data: A case-control study. *Sci. Rep.* [Internet], 9, 1, 12384, 2019, Available from: https://doi.org/10.1038/s41598-019-48769-y.
95. Zrimec, J., Börlin, C.S., Buric, F. *et al.*, Deep learning suggests that gene expression is encoded in all parts of a co-evolving interacting gene regulatory structure. *Nat. Commun.* [Internet], 11, 1, 6141, 2020, Available from: https://doi.org/10.1038/s41467-020-19921-4.
96. Mudge, J.M. and Harrow, J., The state of play in higher eukaryote gene annotation. *Nat. Rev. Genet.*, 17, 12, 758–772, 2016.
97. Kulmanov, M., Khan, M.A., Hoehndorf, R., Wren, J., DeepGO: Predicting protein functions from sequence and interactions using a deep ontology-aware classifier. *Bioinformatics*, 34, 4, 660–668, 2018.
98. Hashemifar, S., Neyshabur, B., Khan, A.A., Xu, J., Predicting protein-protein interactions through sequence-based deep learning. *Bioinformatics*, 34, 17, i802–i810, 2018.
99. de Jongh, R.P.H., van Dijk, A.D.J., Julsing, M.K., Schaap, P.J., de Ridder, D., Designing eukaryotic gene expression regulation using machine learning. *Trends Biotechnol.*, 38, 2, 191–201, 2020.
100. Tabl, A.A., Alkhateeb, A., ElMaraghy, W., Rueda, L., Ngom, A., A machine learning approach for identifying gene biomarkers guiding the treatment of breast cancer. *Front. Genet.*, 10, 256, 2019.
101. Nicholson, J.K., Wilson, I.D., Lindon, J.C., Pharmacometabonomics as an effector for personalized medicine. *Pharmacogenomics*, 12, 1, 103–111, 2011.
102. Doestzada, M., Vila, A.V., Zhernakova, A. *et al.*, Pharmacomicrobiomics: A novel route towards personalized medicine? *Protein Cell*, 9, 5, 432–445, 2018.
103. Vidyasagar, M., Identifying predictive features in drug response using machine learning: Opportunities and challenges. *Annu. Rev. Pharmacol. Toxicol.*, 55, 15–34, 2015.
104. Chary, M.A., Manini, A.F., Boyer, E.W., Burns, M., The role and promise of artificial intelligence in medical toxicology. *J. Med. Toxicol.* [Internet], 16, 4, 458–464, 2020, Available from: http://europepmc.org/abstract/MED/32215849.
105. Sullivan, K.M., Goldmuntz, E.A., Keyes-Elstein, L. *et al.*, Myeloablative autologous stem-cell transplantation for severe scleroderma. *N. Engl. J. Med.*, 378, 1, 35–47, 2018.
106. Franks, J.M., Martyanov, V., Wang, Y. *et al.*, Machine learning predicts stem cell transplant response in severe scleroderma. *Ann. Rheumatol. Dis.* [Internet], 79, 12, 1608 LP–1615, 2020, Available from: http://ard.bmj.com/content/79/12/1608.abstract.
107. Franks, J.M., Martyanov, V., Cai, G. *et al.*, A machine learning classifier for assigning individual patients with systemic sclerosis to intrinsic molecular subsets. *Arthritis Rheumatol. (Hoboken, N.J.)*, 71, 10, 1701–1710, 2019.

108. Shipp, M.A., Ross, K.N., Tamayo, P. *et al.*, Diffuse large B-cell lymphoma outcome prediction by gene-expression profiling and supervised machine learning. *Nat. Med.*, 8, 1, 68–74, 2002.
109. Mehrian, M., Lambrechts, T., Marechal, M., Luyten, F.P., Papantoniou, I., Geris, L., Predicting in vitro human mesenchymal stromal cell expansion based on individual donor characteristics using machine learning. *Cytotherapy*, 22, 2, 82–90, 2020.
110. Kandasamy, K., Chuah, J.K.C., Su, R. *et al.*, Prediction of drug-induced nephrotoxicity and injury mechanisms with human induced pluripotent stem cell-derived cells and machine learning methods. *Sci. Rep.* [Internet], 5, 1, 12337, 2015, Available from: https://doi.org/10.1038/srep12337.

17

Future Prospects and Challenges in the Implementation of AI and ML in Pharma Sector

Prashant Pokhriyal[1], Vivek P. Chavda[2] and Mili Pathak[1]*

[1]Process Science, Intas Pharmaceuticals Ltd. (Biopharma Division), Ahmedabad, Gujarat, India
[2]Department of Pharmaceutic and Pharmaceutical Technology, L. M. College of Pharmacy, Ahmedabad, India

Abstract
Drug manufacture is among the most significant businesses on the planet. For long, this business has been a key productive member of society, and it will remain to be for several years to come. It's difficult to fathom living without pharmaceuticals that treat ailments and enable people live longer, better lives. Drug industry must improve their manufacturing techniques in order to guarantee that operation is both efficient and robust. Artificial intelligence may assist by offering a third-party view on how the medication manufacturing process should be run and recommending improvements in equipment for optimal efficiency. It's vital to get through the jargon and cacophony as we approach closer to a future where AI/ML is more integrated into R&D. When forming judgments regarding data, it's also critical to remember that the scientific process isn't defunct. This will aid in distinguishing hope from hype and lead to more informed decisions on the best use of AI/ML in drug research. However, there are many challenges and hurdles to be handled for the successful AI/ML implementation in pharmaceutical industry.

***Keywords*:** Artificial intelligence (AI), bioinformatics, machine learning, pharma sector, modeling

**Corresponding author*: mpathak38@gmail.com

Vivek Chavda, Krishnan Anand and Vasso Apostolopoulos (eds.) Bioinformatics Tools for Pharmaceutical Drug Product Development, (401–416) © 2023 Scrivener Publishing LLC

17.1 Current Scenario

Although the medication manufacturing process is lengthy and complex, it is critical to understand the fundamentals of how this business functions. It is a procedure used in the pharmaceutical industry to synthesize medications on a large scale. The drug manufacturing technique is divided into several parts, each of which has an influence on the finished product's efficacy and uniformity. In accordance with the "Eroom's law", the returns in pharmaceutical sector are declining as a whole [1], despite the industries' desperate efforts. A counteractive measure is to implement Artificial Intelligence based tools, which can mimic human intelligence and decision making. The application of artificial intelligence (AI) tools in key areas is presumed to save an estimated USD 150 billion in healthcare expenses for United States alone [2]. The regulatory agencies are also pushing for the use of modeling based techniques for the drug manufacturers [3]. The application areas of AI spans from drug discovery and design, process development, manufacturing, compliance, clinical trial design and implementation, to pharmaceutical product management including marketing [4]. The estimates of total number of companies utilizing AI for drug discovery range from 230 [5] to 341 [6]. Around 40 % of them use AI to identify new drug candidates, 28 % to identify new drug targets and 17 % for drug design [7]. Some recent AI platforms like 3N-MCTS [8], DeepTox [9], PrOCTOR [10], SPiDER [11], RASAR [12], AiCURE [13], DeepDDI [14], PADME [15], DeepDTnet [16] etc. have sprung up in early stage drug discovery which reflects high involvement of research efforts put in this domain. Computational drug design, generally dependent on traditional *de novo* approaches to predict target protein structures or drug-protein interactions are gradually being replaced by more complex and efficient deep learning methods [17]. Bioinformatics, another *in silico* approach, hugely benefits from the AI approaches for data mining, protein designing, and glycobiology to name a few [18, 19]. New and complex data being poured into biological databases are creating new possibilities through AI for bioinformaticians. However depending on only one algorithm makes the data pipeline vulnerable to failure [20], necessitating implementation of multiple algorithms simultaneously [21]. This trend is also going to translate to more complex deep learning architectures in bioinformatics [22]. Much work has also been done on integrating AI to already established bioinformatics frameworks [23].

AI can be a great asset [18] for inchoate fields like application of Synthetic Biology in pharmaceuticals [24]. As part of hybrid models, AI can be combined with statistics [25], Genome Scale Modeling [26], image analysis [27], traditional chemical engineering principles like CFD [28], chromatography modeling [29], kinetic modeling [30], and monitoring and control [31]. These hybrid models can offset the limitations of poorly developed mechanistic models, and more research is expected to be done on them in the future.

Though empirical correlations are well-established for scaling-up/ scaling-down, oftentimes they may prove to be insufficient, leading to organizations incurring losses [32], and more advanced analytics are desirable [33]. A few examples demonstrate application of AI for this task [33, 34]. Commentaries on factories of the future envision an increased integration of AI to the pharmaceutical manufacturing [35–38] to improve different manufacturing operations through data mining [39], machine vision [40], predictive maintenance [41], automated quality control [42], digital Quality management System (QMS) [43], augmented reality [44, 45] etc.

End-to-end automation of processes combined with AI under human supervision will be a big boost to pharma productivity [35]. Regulatory agencies are continuously vying to industries for Process Analytical Technologies (PAT) [46], which greatly improves control over the processes in R&D and manufacturing. Within this framework, researchers' efforts have resulted in the implementation of AI in monitoring and control [47–49], a big change from a time when the analysis of data generated by the monitoring instruments was almost entirely done by statistics. This improved control generated by AI is a big boost for Continuous pharmaceutical manufacturing [50–52]. An automated, AI-powered, on-demand chemical synthesis platform, denominated as "Chemputer" is deemed as a next-gen revolutionary technology [53]. In the wake of the abovementioned applications and prospects, regulatory compliance is deemed to drastically enhance [54], especially in quality assurance [55] and quality control functions [56].

About half of the budget out of approx. USD 2 billion allocated for developing a new drug is spent on clinical trial phases [57], with the probability of success hovering below 20 % [58]. With such high stakes, AI algorithms can be infused into the schemes for patient cohort selection and recruitment [57], with several case studies [59–61]. The industry is also moving towards off-site decentralized clinical trials [62, 63], with AI being its integral part [64–66].

The advent of SARS-CoV has ignited a renewed interest in these technologies for vaccine development [67–81], and recently the number of publications for "*in silico vaccine*" has significantly increased in a short period [82]. Just like pharmaceuticals, AI is also helpful at every stage of the vaccine development process [83], but not sans the challenges. The data sets required for data-hungry AI algorithms in vaccine development are small and not of good quality [84], especially for new diseases. Recent approaches based on deep learning have significantly decreased the vaccine development times [67]. AI is also becoming a part of successful drug management and marketing campaigns, such as for market positioning [85], market forecasting and analysis [86, 87], product pricing [88], product lifecycle management [89] etc. Figure 17.1 summarizes challenges for the implementation of AI/ML in pharmaceutical Sector.

The data-intensive field of precision medicine and personalized health products can be advanced by the application of AI [90]. Some AI tools [91, 92] and use cases of precision medicine for neurodevelopment disorders [93], disease management [94] and cancer immunotherapy [95] can be found in the literature. However precision therapy requires more accurate data points for AI algorithms, otherwise inconsistencies and bias would be incorporated [90]. It is expected that AI will be employed more broadly for parsing complicated data and tracking prolonged treatment response [93].

One caveat here is that the disruption through data analytics is generally focused towards drug discovery [96] and applications of these techniques

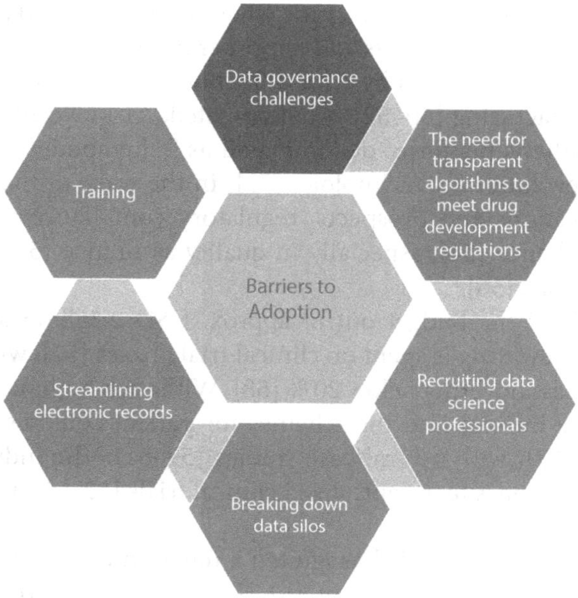

Figure 17.1 Summary of the challenges for the implementation of AI/ML in pharmaceutical sector.

in process development/bioprocessing are seen as complementary to existing frameworks [97] and are not able to move beyond Proof-of-Concept Stage [98]. This deliberation limits the full potential of AI in process development-intensive generics and biosimilars.

The need for humungous datasets for AI algorithms has changed the perception of data recording systems like historian and Electronic Laboratory Notebooks [99] from "desirable" to "necessary". Initiatives like FAIR [100], ATOM consortium [101] and MELLODDY can help to mitigate risks, provide competitive advantage and diversify data analytics portfolio [97], and many such open-source partnerships between government, industry and academics are the need of the hour. Even with the hype surrounding AI, many scientists are still unaware of its application [102]. Data preprocessing, one of the most time-consuming steps in the AI framework, is even more acute in the case of heterogeneous pharmaceutical data [103]. Though it may provide answers, preprocessing and managing the legacy data kept in data silos is going to take much more than sincere efforts by data scientists and database engineers. Some undertakings like eTOX [104] and MELLODDY have been successful in this regard.

Internet of Things (IoT), interconnected digital frameworks are increasingly becoming important of pharmaceutical industry [105, 106], but the data generated from this technology can have much more potential in manufacturing, supply chain, warehousing [107] etc. if coupled with AI.

AI can help in domains like pharmacovigilance, to muster and analyze datasets and conclude about side effects [108–110]. The adverse event case processing using can even be linked to screen candidates in discovery stage [111]. Continuous Process Verification (CPV), another post-regulatory approval step is also expected to embrace AI in the near future [112]. Some advanced technologies like deep learning [113], NLP (Natural Language Processing) [114], nanorobots [115], and combination drug delivery systems [116] are also gaining traction.

But with advancements comes more challenges, which is also true in the case of practical AI implementation, which are more acute in biopharmaceuticals [117]. Companies and investors are still hesitant in implementing AI in the organizations citing high costs, and though recent efforts have been made [118], quantifying Return over Investment of AI is still hazy. Other than capital, developing accurate and robust AI systems require time and human resources with subject matter expertise, the latter being scanter in the pharmaceutical industry. This, however, has not deterred industries to move forward as companies are increasingly willing to invest for AI in pharmaceuticals [119], and these investments are estimated to grow at a CAGR of 22 % [120]. "Machine learning can help plan chemical synthesis pathways and help identify which chemical parts within a molecule contribute to particular properties," adds Jensen [121]. "Also, this may ultimately lead us to explore new chemical spaces, increase chemical diversity, and give us a larger opportunity to identify suitable compounds that will have specific biological functions." AI/ML based technologies with omics helped a lot for the fast-track vaccine development of COVID-19 [72, 74, 75, 122–124].

17.2 Way Forward

Academic institutions should step up and design desired curriculum and training for students [125], and industries should focus on creating diversified skillsets in subject matter expertise and AI. One promising aspect is that big Pharma companies are increasingly collaborating with tech giants and acquiring AI start-ups to better leverage their data (For more details, readers can refer Paul *et al.* [4]). With the onset of AI, some ideas on the extreme end of spectrum proclaim mass job layoffs [4] and depreciation in demand of wet-lab skills [125]. However, the transition would certainly benefit humankind and only alter the job descriptions, but not the requirement of skilled workforce [126]. AI should be implemented in a step-by-step manner, prioritizing those departments first where the benefit to investment ratio is higher, and then gradually incorporating it to other 'good-to-have' realms, by scaling AI across the entire value chain [127]. However, along with technical know-how, complete AI adoption will also be dependent on the cultural shift in the organization. The FOMO (Fear Of Missing Out) behind AI adoption is far from just a hype [128], and it is a high time when pharmaceutical organizations start pulling up their socks for the next AI revolution.

Drug discovery and patients may benefit greatly from a mix of proper knowledge of both R&D and modern ML/AI approaches. AI/ML technology deployment and visualization may provide user-friendly frameworks for maximizing productivity and encouraging the usage of innovative approaches in R&D. Nevertheless, it is critical to comprehend the distinction between causality and correlation, as well as to recognize that the development of powerful prediction skills does not make the current scientific outdated. Plausible inference still needs good statistical judgement, which is especially important in drug development because of the direct influence on patient health and safety. This emphasizes the need of having a broad grasp of ML/AI approaches as well as enough domain-specific expertise in R&D for their optimum usage in drug development.

References

1. Scott, K., Pharma's broken business model - Part 1: An industry on the brink of terminal decline, pp. 1–11, Endpoints.com, 2018. https://endpts.com/pharmas-broken-business-model-an-industry-on-the-brink-of-terminal-decline/
2. Accenture, Artificial intelligence: Healthcare's new nervous system. *Accent. Rep.*, 1–8, 2017. https://www.accenture.com/au-en/insights/health/artificial-intelligence-healthcare
3. Chatterjee, S., Moore, C.M.V., Nasr, M.M., An overview of the role of mathematical models in implementation of quality by design paradigm for drug development and manufacture, in: *Comprehensive Quality by Design for Pharmaceutical Product Development and Manufacture*, pp. 9–24, John Wiley & Sons, Inc., Hoboken, NJ, USA, 2017.
4. Paul, D., Sanap, G., Shenoy, S., Kalyane, D., Kalia, K., Tekade, R.K., Artificial intelligence in drug discovery and development. *Drug Discovery Today* [Internet], 26, 1, 80–93, 2021, Available from: https://pubmed.ncbi.nlm.nih.gov/33099022.
5. Smith, S., 230 Startups using artificial intelligence in drug discovery, *BenchSci.*, 2017. https://blog.benchsci.com/startups-using-artificial-intelligence-in-drug-discovery
6. Buvailo, A., 341 Companies applying artificial intelligence in drug discovery and development, *BioPharmaTrend.* https://www.biopharmatrend.com/m/companies/ai/
7. Deloitte, Intelligent drug discovery powered, AI - A report from the Deloitte Centre for Health Solutions, 2019. https://www2.deloitte.com/us/en/insights/industry/life-sciences/artificial-intelligence-biopharma-intelligent-drug-discovery.html
8. Segler, M.H.S., Preuss, M., Waller, M.P., Planning chemical syntheses with deep neural networks and symbolic AI. *Nature*, 555, 7698, 604–610, 2018.
9. Mayr, A., Klambauer, G., Unterthiner, T., Hochreiter, S., DeepTox: Toxicity prediction using deep learning. *Front. Environ. Sci.*, 3, 1–29, Feb, 2016.
10. Gayvert, K.M., Madhukar, N.S., Elemento, O., A data-driven approach to predicting successes and failures of clinical trials. *Cell Chem. Biol.*, 23, 10, 1294–1301, 2016.
11. Rodrigues, T., Werner, M., Roth, J. *et al.*, Machine intelligence decrypts β-lapachone as an allosteric 5-lipoxygenase inhibitor. *Chem. Sci.*, 9, 34, 6899–6903, 2018.
12. Luechtefeld, T., Marsh, D., Rowlands, C., Hartung, T., Machine learning of toxicological big data enables read-across structure activity relationships (RASAR) outperforming animal test reproducibility. *Toxicol. Sci.*, 165, 1, 198–212, 2018.

13. Bain, E.E., Shafner, L., Walling, D.P. *et al.*, Use of a novel artificial intelligence platform on mobile devices to assess dosing compliance in a phase 2 clinical trial in subjects with schizophrenia. *JMIR mHealth uHealth*, 5, 2, e18, 2017.
14. Ryu, J.Y., Kim, H.U., Lee, S.Y., Deep learning improves prediction of drug–drug and drug–food interactions. *Proc. Natl. Acad. Sci.*, 115, 18, E4304–E4311, 2018.
15. Feng, Q., Dueva, E., Cherkasov, A., Ester, M., PADME: A deep learning-based framework for drug-target interaction prediction. *Arvix*, 1–29, 2018. https://arxiv.org/abs/1807.09741
16. Zeng, X., Zhu, S., Lu, W. *et al.*, Target identification among known drugs by deep learning from heterogeneous networks. *Chem. Sci.*, 11, 7, 1775–1797, 2020.
17. Hessler, G. and Baringhaus, K.-H., Artificial intelligence in drug design. *Molecules*, 23, 10, 2520, 2018.
18. Nicolas, J., Artificial intelligence and bioinformatics, in: *A Guided Tour of Artificial Intelligence Research*, P. Marquis, O. Papini, H. Prade (Eds.), pp. 209–264, Springer International Publishing, Cham, 2020.
19. Raj, V.S., Priyadarshini, A., Yadav, M.K., Pandey, R.P., Gupta, A., Vibhuti, A., Artificial intelligence in bioinformatics, in: *Biomedical Data Mining for Information Retrieval*, pp. 21–51, John Wiley & Sons, Ltd, 2021. https://onlinelibrary.wiley.com/doi/abs/10.1002/9781119711278.ch2
20. Naresh, E., Vijaya Kumar, B.P., Ayesha, Shankar, S.P., Impact of machine learning in bioinformatics research, in: *Statistical Modelling and Machine Learning Principles for Bioinformatics Techniques, Tools, and Applications*, K.G. Srinivasa, G.M. Siddesh, S.R. Manisekhar (Eds.), pp. 41–62, Springer Singapore, Singapore, 2020.
21. Wong, K.-C., Li, Y., Zhang, Z., Unsupervised learning in genome informatics, in: *Unsupervised Learning Algorithms*, pp. 405–448, Springer International Publishing, Cham, 2016.
22. Min, S., Lee, B., Yoon, S., Deep learning in bioinformatics. *Brief. Bioinform.*, 18, 5, bbw068, 2016.
23. Auslander, N., Gussow, A.B., Koonin, E.V., Incorporating machine learning into established bioinformatics frameworks. *Int. J. Mol. Sci.*, 22, 6, 2903, 2021.
24. Trosset, J.-Y. and Carbonell, P., Synthetic biology for pharmaceutical drug discovery. *Drug Des. Devel. Ther.*, 9, 6285, 2015.
25. Narayanan, H., Sokolov, M., Butté, A., Morbidelli, M., Decision tree-PLS (DT-PLS) algorithm for the development of process: Specific local prediction models. *Biotechnol. Prog.*, 35, 4, 2019.
26. Zampieri, G., Vijayakumar, S., Yaneske, E., Angione, C., Machine and deep learning meet genome-scale metabolic modeling. *PLoS Comput. Biol.*, 15, 7, e1007084, 2019.

27. David, L., Arús-Pous, J., Karlsson, J. *et al.*, Applications of deep-learning in exploiting large-scale and heterogeneous compound data in industrial pharmaceutical research. *Front. Pharmacol.*, 10, November 2019, 1–16, 2019.
28. Mosavi, A., Shamshirband, S., Salwana, E., Chau, Kw, Tah, J.H.M., Prediction of multi-inputs bubble column reactor using a novel hybrid model of computational fluid dynamics and machine learning. *Eng. Appl. Comput. Fluid Mech.*, 13, 1, 482–492, 2019.
29. Wang, G., Briskot, T., Hahn, T., Baumann, P., Hubbuch, J., Estimation of adsorption isotherm and mass transfer parameters in protein chromatography using artificial neural networks. *J. Chromatogr. A*, 1487, 211–217, 2017.
30. O'Brien, C.M., Zhang, Q., Daoutidis, P., Hu, W.S., A hybrid mechanistic-empirical model for in silico mammalian cell bioprocess simulation. *Metab. Eng.*, 66, March, 31–40, 2021.
31. Munir, N., Nugent, M., Whitaker, D., McAfee, M., Machine learning for process monitoring and control of hot-melt extrusion: Current state of the art and future directions. *Pharmaceutics*, 13, 9, 1432, 2021.
32. Carpio, M., Current challenges with cell culture scale-up for biologics production. *BioPharm Int.*, 33, 10, 23–27, 2020.
33. Wolszon, Z., Improving predictability of cell culture processes during biologics manufacturing scale-up through hybrid modeling, 2020.
34. Bayer, B., Striedner, G., Duerkop, M., Hybrid modeling and intensified DoE: An approach to accelerate upstream process characterization. *Biotechnol. J.*, 15, 9, 2000121, 2020.
35. Arden, N.S., Fisher, A.C., Tyner, K., Yu, L.X., Lee, S.L., Kopcha, M., Industry 4.0 for pharmaceutical manufacturing: Preparing for the smart factories of the future. *Int. J. Pharm.*, 602, 120554, 2021.
36. Rantanen, J. and Khinast, J., The future of pharmaceutical manufacturing sciences. *J. Pharm. Sci.*, 104, 11, 3612–3638, 2015.
37. Owczarek, D., The future of pharmaceutical manufacturing process: Artificial intelligence, nexocode, 2021. https://nexocode.com/blog/posts/ai-in-pharmaceutical-manufacturing/
38. Markarian, J., Industry 4.0 in biopharmaceutical manufacturing. *BioPharm Int.*, 38, 7, 36–38, 2018.
39. Charaniya, S., Hu, W.-S., Karypis, G., Mining bioprocess data: Opportunities and challenges. *Trends Biotechnol.*, 26, 12, 690–699, 2008.
40. Vijay, Y. and Kennedy, C., Vision inspection using machine learning/artificial intelligence | Pharmaceutical engineering, ISPE, 2020. https://ispe.org/pharmaceutical-engineering/november-december-2020/vision-inspection-using-machine
41. Otto, S., The case for predictive maintenance, *Pharma Manuf.*, 2019. https://www.pharmamanufacturing.com/articles/2019/the-case-for-predictive-maintenance/
42. Han, Y., Makarova, E., Ringel, M., Telpis, V., Digitization, automation, and online testing: The future of pharma quality control, pp. 1–12, McKinsey Co.,

3 January 2019. https://www.mckinsey.com/industries/life-sciences/our-insights/digitization-automation-and-online-testing-the-future-of-pharma-quality-control

43. Chapman, J., How AI tools will transform quality management in the life sciences, Pharamaceutical Online, 1, 2018. https://www.pharmaceuticalonline.com/doc/how-ai-tools-will-transform-quality-management-in-the-life-sciences-0001
44. Stracquatanio, A., Harnessing augmented reality in pharmaceutical manufacturing, Pharmaceutical online, 2018. https://www.pharmaceuticalonline.com/doc/harnessing-augmented-reality-in-pharmaceutical-manufacturing-0001
45. Kavanaugh, D., Lenich, R., Iles-smith, P., Sheehy, P., Biotechnology roadmap - Automated facility. *Bioforum*, 1–34, 2017. https://www.biophorum.com/wp-content/uploads/bp_downloads/Automated-Facility.pdf
46. USFDA, GMP's for the 21st century, Department of Health and Human Services, 2007. https://www.fda.gov/about-fda/center-drug-evaluation-and-research-cder/pharmaceutical-quality-21st-century-risk-based-approach-progress-report
47. Bocklitz, T., Schmitt, M., Popp, J., Optical molecular spectroscopy in combination with artificial intelligence for process analytical technology. *Spectrosc. (Santa Monica)*, 35, 6, 28–32, 2020.
48. Takahashi, M.B., Leme, J., Caricati, C.P., Tonso, A., Fernández Núñez, E.G., Rocha, J.C., Artificial neural network associated to UV/Vis spectroscopy for monitoring bioreactions in biopharmaceutical processes. *Bioprocess Biosyst. Eng.*, 38, 6, 1045–1054, 2015.
49. Tulsyan, A., Garvin, C., Undey, C., Machine-learning for biopharmaceutical batch process monitoring with limited data. *IFAC-PapersOnLine*, 51, 18, 126–131, 2018.
50. Roggo, Y., Jelsch, M., Heger, P., Ensslin, S., Krumme, M., Deep learning for continuous manufacturing of pharmaceutical solid dosage form. *Eur. J. Pharm. Biopharm.*, 153, 95–105, 2020.
51. Domokos, A., Nagy, B., Szilágyi, B., Marosi, G., Nagy, Z.K., Integrated continuous pharmaceutical technologies—A review. *Org. Process Res. Dev.*, 25, 4, 721–739, 2021.
52. Rajamanickam, V., Spadiut, O., Herwig, C., Data science, modeling, and advanced PAT tools enable continuous culture. *Bioprocess Int.*, 16, 4, 20–25, 2018.
53. Gromski, P.S., Granda, J.M., Cronin, L., Universal chemical synthesis and discovery with 'The Chemputer.' *Trends Chem.*, 2, 1, 4–12, 2020.
54. Zonnenberg, J.P., Improving digital quality in the pharmaceutical industry, *Pharma Manuf.*, 2018. https://www.pharmamanufacturing.com/articles/2018/improving-digital-quality-in-the-pharmaceutical-industry/
55. Foster, T., Makarova, E., Telpis, V., Making quality assurance smart, McKinsey Co., January 2021. https://www.mckinsey.com/industries/life-sciences/our-insights/making-quality-assurance-smart

56. Haigney, S., A new view on quality control? *BioPharm Int.*, 34, 11, 10–14, 2021.
57. Harrer, S., Shah, P., Antony, B., Hu, J., Artificial intelligence for clinical trial design. *Trends Pharmacol. Sci.* [Internet], 40, 8, 577–591, 2019, Available from: https://www.sciencedirect.com/science/article/pii/S0165614719301300.
58. Wong, C.H., Siah, K.W., Lo, A.W., Estimation of clinical trial success rates and related parameters. *Biostatistics* [Internet], 20, 2, 273–286, 2019, Available from: https://doi.org/10.1093/biostatistics/kxx069.
59. Helgeson, J., Rammage, M., Urman, A. *et al.*, Clinical performance pilot using cognitive computing for clinical trial matching at Mayo Clinic. *J. Clin. Oncol.*, 36, 15_suppl, e18598–e18598, 2018.
60. Haddad, T., Helgeson, J.M., Pomerleau, K.E. *et al.*, Accuracy of an artificial intelligence system for cancer clinical trial eligibility screening: Retrospective pilot study. *JMIR Med. Inform.*, 9, 3, 1–7, 2021.
61. Chaudhari, N., Ravi, R., Gogtay, N., Thatte, U., Recruitment and retention of the participants in clinical trials: Challenges and solutions. *Perspect. Clin. Res.*, 11, 2, 64, 2020.
62. Van Norman, G.A., Decentralized clinical trials: The future of medical product development? *JACC Basic Transl. Sci.*, 6, 4, 384–387, 2021.
63. Agrawal, G., Moss, R., Raschke, R., Wurzer, S., Xue, J., No place like home? Stepping up the decentralization of clinical trials, McKinsey Co., June 2021. https://www.mckinsey.com/industries/life-sciences/our-insights/no-place-like-home-stepping-up-the-decentralization-of-clinical-trials
64. Moss, N., Decentralized trials fuel AI revolution in clinical research, Contract PHARMA, 2020. https://www.contractpharma.com/issues/2020-11-01/view_features/decentralized-trials-fuel-ai-revolution-in-clinical-research/
65. Taylor, K. and Properzi, F., Intelligent clinical trials, p. 34, Deloitte Insights, 2020. https://www2.deloitte.com/us/en/insights/industry/life-sciences/artificial-intelligence-in-clinical-trials.html
66. The future of clinical trials: The promise of AI and the role of big tech, CBInsights, 2021. https://www.cbinsights.com/research/clinical-trials-ai-tech-disruption/
67. Yang, Z., Bogdan, P., Nazarian, S., An in silico deep learning approach to multi-epitope vaccine design: A SARS-CoV-2 case study. *Sci. Rep.*, 11, 1, 1–21, 2021.
68. Lv, H., Shi, L., Berkenpas, J.W. *et al.*, Application of artificial intelligence and machine learning for COVID-19 drug discovery and vaccine design. *Brief. Bioinform.*, 22, 6, 19, 2021.
69. Chavda, V.P. and Apostolopoulos, V., Omicron variant (B.1.1.529) of SARS-CoV-2: Threat for the elderly? *Maturitas* [Internet], 158, 78–81, 2022, Available from: https://doi.org/10.1016/j.maturitas.2022.01.011.
70. Chavda, V.P., Vora, L.K., Vihol, D.R., COVAX-19® vaccine: Completely blocks virus transmission to non-immune individuals. *Clin. Complement.*

Med. Pharmacol. [Internet], 1, 1, 100004, 2021, Available from: https://www.sciencedirect.com/science/article/pii/S2772371221000048.
71. Basu, D., Chavda, V.P., Mehta, A.A., Therapeutics for COVID-19 and post COVID-19 complications: An update. *Curr. Res. Pharmacol. Drug Discovery* [Internet], 3, 1, 1, 100086, 2022, Available from: https://www.sciencedirect.com/science/article/pii/S2590257122000062.
72. Chavda, V.P., Kapadia, C., Soni, S. *et al.*, A global picture: Therapeutic perspectives for COVID-19. *Immunotherapy* [Internet], 14, 351–371, 2022. 10.2217/imt-2021–0168, Available from: https://doi.org/10.2217/imt-2021-0168.
73. Chavda, V.P. and Apostolopoulos, V., Global impact of delta plus variant and vaccination. *Expert Rev. Vaccines* [Internet], 21, 597–600, 2022. null-null. Available from: https://doi.org/10.1080/14760584.2022.2044800.
74. Chavda, V.P., Hossain, M.K., Beladiya, J., Apostolopoulos, V., Nucleic acid vaccines for COVID-19: A paradigm shift in the vaccine development arena. *Biologics*, 1, 3, 337–356, 2021.
75. Chavda, V.P., Bezbaruah, R., Athalye, M. *et al.*, Replicating viral vector-based vaccines for COVID-19: Potential avenue in vaccination arena. *Viruses*, 14, 4, 759–779, 2022.
76. Chavda, V.P., Feehan, J., Apostolopoulos, V., A veterinary vaccine for SARS-CoV-2: The first COVID-19 vaccine for animals. *Vaccines*, 9, 6, 631–633, 2021.
77. Chavda, V.P., Patel, A.B., Vaghasiya, D.D., SARS-CoV-2 variants and vulnerability at the global level. *J. Med. Virol.* [Internet], 94, 2986–3005, 2022, Available from: https://doi.org/10.1002/jmv.27717.
78. Chavda, V.P., Pandya, R., Apostolopoulos, V., DNA vaccines for SARS-CoV-2: Toward third-generation vaccination era. *Expert Rev. Vaccines*, 20, 12, 1549–1560, 2021.
79. Chavda, V.P. and Apostolopoulos, V., Is booster dose strategy sufficient for omicron variant of SARS-CoV-2? *Vaccines*, 10, 3, 367–372, 2022.
80. Chavda, V.P., Patel, A.B., Vihol, D. *et al.*, Herbal remedies, nutraceuticals, and dietary supplements for COVID-19 management: An update. *Clin. Complement. Med. Pharmacol.* [Internet], 2, 1, 100021, 2022, Available from: https://www.sciencedirect.com/science/article/pii/S2772371222000031.
81. Chavda, V.P., Vora, L.K., Pandya, A.K., Patravale, V.B., Intranasal vaccines for SARS-CoV-2: From challenges to potential in COVID-19 management. *Drug Discovery Today* [Internet], 26, 11, 2619–2636, 2021, Available from: https://www.sciencedirect.com/science/article/pii/S1359644621003317.
82. Nevmerzhitskaya, A., Gromova, M., Pfleiderer, M., Designing vaccines: The role of artificial intelligence and digital health, part 1. *Bioprocess Int.*, 19, 24–33, 2021.
83. Mohanty, E. and Mohanty, A., Role of artificial intelligence in peptide vaccine design against RNA viruses. *Inform. Med. Unlocked*, 26, 100768, 2021.
84. Naudé, W., Artificial intelligence vs COVID-19: Limitations, constraints and pitfalls. *AI Soc.*, 35, 3, 761–765, 2020.

85. Chiu, C.-Y., Chen, Y.-F., Kuo, I.-T., Ku, H.C., An intelligent market segmentation system using k-means and particle swarm optimization. *Expert Syst. Appl.*, 36, 3, Part 1, 4558–4565, 2009.
86. Singh, J., Flaherty, K., Sohi, R.S. *et al.*, Sales profession and professionals in the age of digitization and artificial intelligence technologies: Concepts, priorities, and questions. *J. Pers. Sell. Sales Manage.*, 39, 1, 2–22, 2019.
87. Milgrom, P.R. and Tadelis, S., How artificial intelligence and machine learning can impact market design, NBER, 2018. https://www.nber.org/papers/w24282
88. de Jesus, A., AI for pricing – Comparing 5 current applications, Emerj, 2019. https://emerj.com/ai-sector-overviews/ai-for-pricing-comparing-5-current-applications/
89. E-VAI - the artificial intelligence platform from Eularis changes the rules of the marketing in pharma, CISION PR Newswire, 2015. https://www.prnewswire.com/news-releases/e-vai--the-artificial-intelligence-platform-from-eularis-changes-the-rules-of-the-marketing-in-pharma-300142785.html
90. Schork, N.J., Artificial intelligence and personalized medicine, in: *Precision Medicine in Cancer Therapy*, D.D. Von Hoff and H. Han (Eds.), pp. 265–283, Springer International Publishing, Cham, 2019.
91. Daouda, T., Perreault, C., Lemieux, S., pyGeno: A Python package for precision medicine and proteogenomics. *F1000Research*, 5, 0, 381, 2016.
92. Blasiak, A., Khong, J., Kee, T., CURATE.AI: Optimizing personalized medicine with artificial intelligence. *SLAS Technol. Transl. Life Sci. Innov.*, 25, 2, 95–105, 2020.
93. Uddin, M., Wang, Y., Woodbury-Smith, M., Artificial intelligence for precision medicine in neurodevelopmental disorders. *NPJ Digit. Med.*, 2, 1, 2019.
94. Subramanian, M., Wojtusciszyn, A., Favre, L. *et al.*, Precision medicine in the era of artificial intelligence: Implications in chronic disease management. *J. Transl. Med.*, 18, 1, 1–12, 2020.
95. Sherafat, E., Force, J., Măndoiu, I.I., Semi-supervised learning for somatic variant calling and peptide identification in personalized cancer immunotherapy. *BMC Bioinform.*, 21, 18, 1–18, 2020.
96. Lamberti, M.J., Wilkinson, M., Donzanti, B.A. *et al.*, A study on the application and use of artificial intelligence to support drug development. *Clin. Ther.*, 41, 8, 1414–1426, 2019.
97. von Stosch, M., Portela, R.M., Varsakelis, C., A roadmap to AI-driven *in silico* process development: Bioprocessing 4.0 in practice. *Curr. Opin. Chem. Eng.*, 33, 100692, 2021.
98. McKinsey, Digital manufacturing – Escaping pilot purgatory, p. 24, Digit. McKinsey, 2018. https://www.mckinsey.com/business-functions/operations/our-insights/how-digital-manufacturing-can-escape-pilot-purgatory
99. Machina, H.K. and Wild, D.J., Electronic laboratory notebooks progress and challenges in implementation. *J. Lab. Autom.*, 18, 4, 264–268, 2013.

100. Wise, J., de Barron, A.G., Splendiani, A. *et al.*, Implementation and relevance of FAIR data principles in biopharmaceutical R&D. *Drug Discovery Today*, 24, 4, 933–938, 2019.
101. Hinkson, I.V., Madej, B., Stahlberg, E.A., Accelerating therapeutics for opportunities in medicine: A paradigm shift in drug discovery. *Front. Pharmacol.*, 11, June, 1–7, 2020.
102. Smith, S., 6 things we learned about artificial intelligence in drug discovery from 330 scientists, BenchSci, 2018. https://blog.benchsci.com/6-things-we-learned-about-artificial-intelligence-in-drug-discovery-from-330-scientists
103. Casola, G., Siegmund, C., Mattern, M., Sugiyama, H., Data mining-based algorithm for pre-processing biopharmaceutical manufacturing records, in: *Computer Aided Chemical Engineering*, pp. 2263–2268, Elsevier Masson SAS, 2018. https://scienceon.kisti.re.kr/srch/selectPORSrchArticle.do?cn=NART95820946
104. Sanz, F., Pognan, F., Steger-Hartmann, T. *et al.*, Legacy data sharing to improve drug safety assessment: The eTOX project. *Nat. Rev. Drug Discovery*, 16, 12, 811–812, 2017.
105. Singh, M., Sachan, S., Singh, A., Singh, K.K., Internet of Things in pharma industry: Possibilities and challenges, in: *Emergence of Pharmaceutical Industry Growth with Industrial IoT Approach*, pp. 195–216, Elsevier, 2020. https://www.sciencedirect.com/science/article/pii/B9780128195932000078?via%3Dihub
106. Sharma, A., Kaur, J., Singh, I., Internet of Things (IoT) in pharmaceutical manufacturing, warehousing, and supply chain management. *SN Comput. Sci.*, 1, 4, 232, 2020.
107. Ding, Y. and Feng, D., Intelligent warehousing based on the Internet of Things technology, in: *Proceedings of the 2nd International Conference on Advances in Artificial Intelligence*, pp. 51–55, ACM, New York, NY, USA, 2018.
108. Hauben, M. and Hartford, C.G., Artificial intelligence in pharmacovigilance: Scoping points to consider. *Clin. Ther.*, 43, 2, 372–379, 2021.
109. Murali, K., Kaur, S., Prakash, A., Medhi, B., Artificial intelligence in pharmacovigilance: Practical utility. *Indian J. Pharmacol.*, 51, 6, 373, 2019.
110. Huysentruyt, K., Kjoersvik, O., Dobracki, P. *et al.*, Validating intelligent automation systems in pharmacovigilance: Insights from good manufacturing practices. *Drug Saf.*, 44, 3, 261–272, 2021.
111. Schmider, J., Kumar, K., LaForest, C., Swankoski, B., Naim, K., Caubel, P.M., Innovation in pharmacovigilance: Use of artificial intelligence in adverse event case processing. *Clin. Pharmacol. Ther.*, 105, 4, 954–961, 2019.
112. Manzano, T., PDA study explores role of A.I. @ in CPV. PDA, 2020. https://www.pda.org/pda-letter-portal/home/full-article/pda-study-explores-role-of-a.i.-in-cpv
113. Chen, H., Engkvist, O., Wang, Y., Olivecrona, M., Blaschke, T., The rise of deep learning in drug discovery. *Drug Discovery Today [Internet]*, 23, 6,

1241–1250, 2018, Available from: https://www.sciencedirect.com/science/article/pii/S1359644617303598.
114. Sheikhalishahi, S., Miotto, R., Dudley, J.T., Lavelli, A., Rinaldi, F., Osmani, V., Natural language processing of clinical notes on chronic diseases: Systematic review. *JMIR Med. Inform.*, 7, 2, e12239, 2019.
115. Fu, J. and Yan, H., Controlled drug release by a nanorobot. *Nat. Biotechnol.*, 30, 5, 407–408, 2012.
116. Tsigelny, I.F., Artificial intelligence in drug combination therapy. *Brief. Bioinform.*, 20, 4, 1434–1448, 2019.
117. Steinwandter, V., Borchert, D., Herwig, C., Data science tools and applications on the way to Pharma 4.0. *Drug Discovery Today*, 24, 9, 1795–1805, 2019.
118. Varsakelis, D. and von Stosch, P., Show me the money! Process modeling in pharma from the investor's point of view. *Processes*, 7, 9, 596, 2019.
119. Batra, G., Queirolo, A., Santhanam, N., Artificial intelligence: The time to act is now, December) 12, 2017. https://www.mckinsey.com/industries/advanced-electronics/our-insights/artificial-intelligence-the-time-to-act-is-now
120. Growthinsight—RoleofAIinthepharmaceuticalindustry,Global,2018–2022. https://www.researchandmarkets.com/reports/4846380/growth-insight-role-of-ai-in-the-pharmaceutical
121. Koperniak, S., Applying machine learning to challenges in the pharmaceutical industry [Internet], 2022, Available from: https://news.mit.edu/2018/applying-machine-learning-to-challenges-in-pharmaceutical-industry-0517. https://news.mit.edu/2018/applying-machine-learning-to-challenges-in-pharmaceutical-industry-0517
122. Vivek, C., Patel, C., Bhadani, J., Metabolomics: At a glance. *Res. Rev. J. Drug Formulation Dev. Prod.*, 4, 1, 23–30, 2017.
123. Chavda, V., Sheta, S., Changani, D., Chavda, D., New bioinformatics platform-based approach for drug design [Internet]. *Comput. Bioinf.*, 101–120, 2021, Available from: https://doi.org/10.1002/9781119654803.ch6.
124. Chavda, V.P., Nanotherapeutics and nanobiotechnology, in: *Applications of Targeted Nano Drugs and Delivery Systems*, pp. 1–13, Elsevier, 2019. https://www.elsevier.com/books/applications-of-targeted-nano-drugs-and-delivery-systems/mohapatra/978-0-12-814029-1
125. Fleming, N., How artificial intelligence is changing drug discovery. *Nature.*, 557, 7707, S55–S57, 2018.
126. Ronanki, R. and Davenport, T., Artificial intelligence for the real world. *Harv. Bus. Rev.*, February, 1–10, 2018. https://hbsp.harvard.edu/product/R1801H-PDF-ENG
127. Kudumala, A., Ressler, D., Miranda, W., Scaling up AI across the life sciences value chain, Deloitte Insights, 2020. https://www2.deloitte.com/us/en/insights/industry/life-sciences/ai-and-pharma.html

128. Hargreaves, B., Pharma companies slow to adopt AI will be 'left behind.' Outsourcing Pharma, 2019. https://www.outsourcing-pharma.com/Article/2019/12/11/IQVIA-on-the-adoption-of-AI-and-machine-learning

Index

Printed in the USA/Agawam, MA
September 16, 2026

910661.139